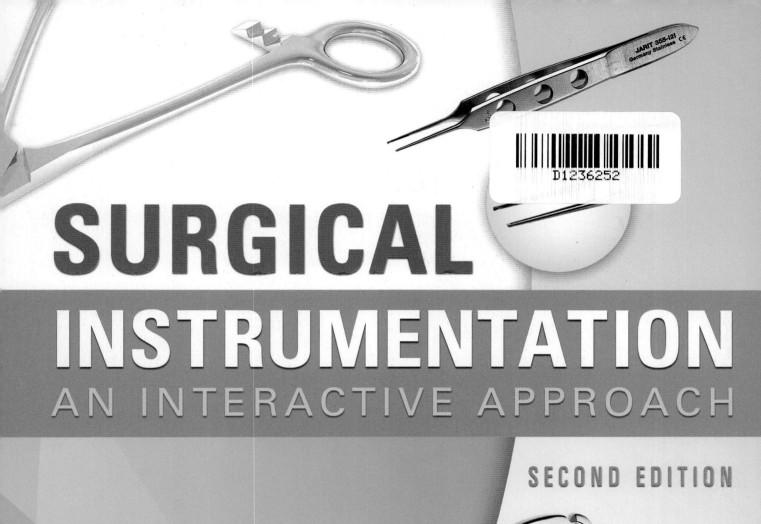

SURGICAL
INSTRUMENTATION
AN INTERACTIVE APPROACH

SECOND EDITION

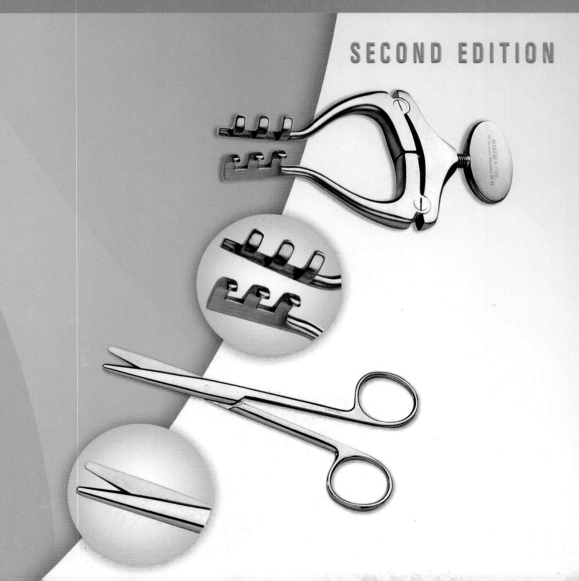

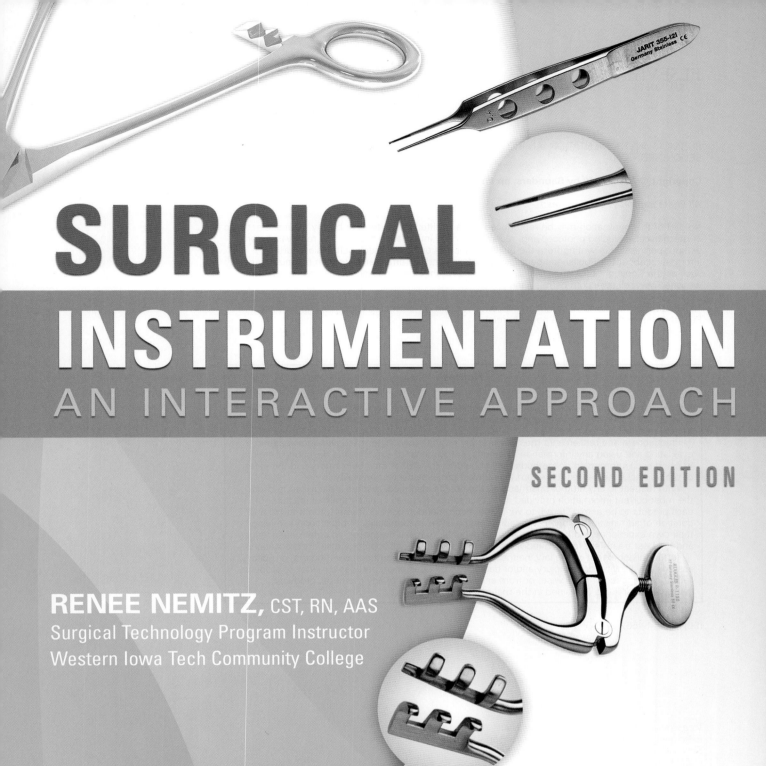

SURGICAL INSTRUMENTATION

AN INTERACTIVE APPROACH

SECOND EDITION

RENEE NEMITZ, CST, RN, AAS
Surgical Technology Program Instructor
Western Iowa Tech Community College

ELSEVIER

3251 Riverport Lane
St. Louis, Missouri 63043

SURGICAL INSTRUMENTATION: AN INTERACTIVE APPROACH,
SECOND EDITION

ISBN: 978-1-4557-0719-5

Notices

Knowledge and best practice in this field are constantly changing. As new research and experience broaden our understanding, changes in research methods, professional practices, or medical treatment may become necessary.

Practitioners and researchers must always rely on their own experience and knowledge in evaluating and using any information, methods, compounds, or experiments described herein. In using such information or methods they should be mindful of their own safety and the safety of others, including parties for whom they have a professional responsibility.

With respect to any drug or pharmaceutical products identified, readers are advised to check the most current information provided (i) on procedures featured or (ii) by the manufacturer of each product to be administered, to verify the recommended dose or formula, the method and duration of administration, and contraindications. It is the responsibility of practitioners, relying on their own experience and knowledge of their patients, to make diagnoses, to determine dosages and the best treatment for each individual patient, and to take all appropriate safety precautions.

To the fullest extent of the law, neither the Publisher nor the authors, contributors, or editors, assume any liability for any injury and/or damage to persons or property as a matter of products liability, negligence or otherwise, or from any use or operation of any methods, products, instructions, or ideas contained in the material herein.

ISBN: 978-1-4557-0719-5

Vice President and Publisher: Andrew Allen
Executive Content Strategist: Jennifer Janson
Senior Content Development Specialist: Kelly Brinkman
Publishing Services Manager: Julie Eddy
Senior Project Manager: Marquita Parker
Designer: Jessica Williams
All Photography by Frank Pronesti

Printed in China

Last digit is the print number: 9 8 7 6 5 4 3 2 1

Reviewers

DANA E. BANCER, CST, AAS
Associate Professor and Program Manager
Surgical Technology
Daytona State College
Daytona Beach, Florida

JULIA HINKLE, RN, MHS, CNOR
Professor and Program Chair
Surgical Technology
Ivy Tech Community College
Evansville, Indiana

GINNY SCHIMANSKY, CST
Clinical Instructor
Surgical Technology
College of Health, Human and Public Services
Daytona State College
Daytona Beach, Florida

JACOB MUTH, CST
Instructor
Surgical Technology
Great Lakes Institute of Technology
Erie, Pennsylvania

Dedication

To all my students—past, present, and future.
You are the reason for the inception, development, and
completion of this project.

Acknowledgments

I discovered throughout this project how blessed I am to have such incredible people in my life. I would like to acknowledge and sincerely thank the following people for their help, contributions, effort, and time.

First, to my husband, Rollin. Thank you for believing in me. Without your support, this project would not be a reality. To my young daughters, Madison, Miranda, and Melia, who truly believe this is the longest book ever, for all the sacrifices you each made to let Mom work. To my parents, Marilyn and Dick Kreisel, for raising me to believe that I could accomplish anything and for all the time you spent with the girls during this project.

To the fantastic staff at Elsevier: Jennifer Janson and Kelly Brinkman. Thanks for your support, patience, and guidance. Without you, this project would not be a reality. I'm particularly grateful to Michael Ledbetter for sharing my ideas and believing in this project. Thanks for all your encouragement and fortitude.

Special thanks to Marsha McArthur, Product Manager of surgical instruments at Integra Life-Sciences Corporation (JARIT, Padgett, Ruggles, and R&B), who allowed us to photograph countless images for this book. Without her trust and access to the instruments, this book would not have been possible!

Also thanks to the following companies for working with us to photograph their instruments for the project: Stryker Corporation, DePuy, Miltex, Autosuture, and ACMI.

I would also like to thank Frank Pronesti and Gary Deamer at Heirloom Studio in Yardley, Pennsylvania, for providing their beautiful, high-resolution photography for all the instruments in this book. And thank you to Elizabeth Pronesti, for her consulting during the many photo shoots we had during the first edition of this text.

To my friend, Chris Keegan, CST, MS, FAST. I thank you for all you have done throughout this project. Your time, encouragement, and wisdom are immeasurable. I would not have made it through this without you. To Clifford Smith, MSN, BSEd, ONC, CRNFA, for all the time you spent helping with revisions and your contributions to the Orthopedic chapter in the first edition of the book. I am so grateful to you. Karen Lipinski, CSTFA, thank you for your contributions to the Cardiovascular Thoracic chapter in the first edition.

Thanks to Master Key Consulting in St. Louis, Missouri, for your hard work developing the interactive portion of this project. A special thanks to Peggy Maley, RN, BSN, SNOR, RNFA, and the entire Central Processing Department at Penn Prysbyterian Medical Center in Philadelphia, Pennsylvania, who graciously assisted us with a 2-day photo shoot for this new edition. Our thanks go out to the following facilities and surgical staff for allowing us to conduct on-site photo shoots for the first edition of this text: St. Luke's Hospital operating room, St. Louis, Missouri; Jane Spiller, RN, BS, Orthopedic team leader; Cynthia M. Clisham, RN, BSN, Associate Head Nurse-Clinical Educator; Virginia Babcock, RN, Head Nurse; Marsha Helms RN, Associate Head Nurse; Brenda Kelly, RN, BA, Vice President; Jerry Smith, Executive Assistant. Thanks also to Ruth E. Morse RN, MSN, CEN, CNA, BC, Director of Nursing Resources at Christiana Hospital, Wilmington, Delaware.

The willingness of all to work with our team was invaluable in developing this educational resource.

Preface

Instrumentation is one of the most important aspects of a surgical procedure. Surgical instruments can be considered an extension of the surgeon's hands. When the surgical team knows the proper name, handling, and use of each instrument, it enhances the quality of the surgical procedure. As a learner this can be extremely overwhelming due to the multitude of instruments and their similarities. Learning instruments is much more than just recalling the name. The idea for this text came about after years of watching my students struggle with this. They could often recall the names, categories, and specialty area, but could rarely explain what it was or how it was used. I saw a pressing need for a product that had not only clear, detailed photos, but also addressed common uses, gave insights about instruments, and allowed for interaction. Whether you are a student, surgical technologist, first assistant, registered nurse, or physician's assistant who is working in surgery, in central service, or product sales, this instrumentation book with interactive exercises will help you, the learner, gain vital core knowledge about instrumentation.

The text is organized into 14 chapters, starting with the basic instruments. Chapter 1 is an overview of instrumentation, followed by Chapter 2, designed to introduce the learner to the fundamental instruments. These are the basic essential instruments that can be seen in any instrument set, regardless of specialty area. The text then moves through commonly used instruments in the 12 different surgical specialty areas. Keep in mind that instruments may vary according to facility, surgeon, and procedure. To conserve space, some instruments may be addressed in one specialty area and are used by other specialties, but these will not be repeated. Within each chapter, the instruments are grouped according to their category - accessory, clamping and occluding, cutting and dissecting, grasping and holding, probing and dilating, retracting and exposing, suctioning and aspirating, suturing and stapling, or viewing.

Each page contains one to two instrument monographs with a consistent presentation of each, including:

- **Large, clear, full photo with detail.**
- **Name:** states proper instrument name.
- **Other name:** states alternate name or names that the instrument may be called.
- **Description:** briefly describes instrument characteristics.
- **Use(s):** lists common uses and/or areas of use.
- **Instrument insight:** explains key information about the instrument.
- **Caution:** expounds on some of the dangers that can happen when handling instruments.

Enhanced Evolve resources include the invaluable interactive component of this product. Access to the Evolve site requires a pin code (found in the inside front cover). Once registered, the interactive activities will give you the ability to interact with the instruments, taking your knowledge to the next level. No other product on the market offers this type of interaction. Included are:

- **Digital image library:** includes all of the photos from the book with the ability to zoom in and out, and rotating views of more than 100 instruments.
- **Audio pronunciation:** allows the learner to click on the audio icon and hear the proper name for each instrument.
- **Drop-and-drag exercise:** allows the learner to place instruments onto a Mayo tray from select procedures.
- **Timed audio identification exercises:** challenges the learner to identify the instrument in 5 seconds or less. The instrument is asked for, and the learner has to choose the correct instrument from a set of images.
- **Flash card exercises:** the learner clicks the card image, and it "flips" to reveal its name, category, and discipline.
- **Small fragment fixation set:** allows the learner to explore a small fragment set. This exercise lets the user open the set and investigate each tray. The learner can view animation of the tray being opened; roll over any item in the

instrument, screw, or plate trays; and click on it to view a close-up image and the name.

- **Large fragment fixation set:** allows the learner to explore a large fragment set. This exercise lets the user open each pan and investigate it; roll over any item in the instrument, screw, or plate pan; and click on it to view a close-up image and the name.
- **Other exercises:** allows the learner to fire a skin stapler; assemble the McIvor mouth gag and the bone cement system; and load a screwdriver, scalpel and clip, Stryker System 6 power, and TSP power (saws, drills, and reamers) and more.

To assist educators with course materials, all images are downloadable for use in lectures, handouts, and exams. With the high-quality photographs and interactive exercises, your institution will not have to budget thousands of dollars for instrument sets used for demonstration only.

Contents

1 Introduction to Surgical Instruments, *1*

2 Basic Instruments, *6*

3 General Instruments, *35*

4 Laparoscopic Instruments, *48*

5 Robotic Instruments, *74*

6 Obstetrics and Gynecologic Instruments, *81*

7 Genitourinary Instruments, *101*

8 Ophthalmic Instruments, *119*

9 Otorhinolaryngology Instruments, *139*

10 Oral Instruments, *185*

11 Plastic and Reconstructive Instruments, *197*

12 Orthopedic Instruments, *210*

13 Neurosurgical Instruments, *257*

14 Cardiovascular Thoracic Instruments, *291*

1

Introduction to Surgical Instruments

HISTORY

A surgical instrument is a specially designed device or apparatus used to carry out a specified task during a surgical procedure. Surgical instruments date back to prehistoric times when our early ancestors sharpened stones, flints, and animal teeth to perform surgery. Throughout history, surgical instruments have been created from a variety of materials, such as ivory, wood, bronze, iron, and silver. The discovery of anesthesia and asepsis in the eighteenth century and the development of stainless steel in the nineteenth century started the modern evolution of surgical instrumentation. The twentieth century brought many changes with the development of electrocautery, ultrasonic, and endoscopic devices. New materials, such as titanium, Vitallium, vanadium, carbides, and polymers, are being used in the manufacturing process of instruments. The twenty-first century has already seen advances in remote telesurgery, robotics, and image-guided systems, which have changed the way surgery is performed and how instruments are developed. The next generation of surgical systems and new materials will revolutionize the way surgical instruments are designed and created.

The vast majority of surgical instruments, however, are still manufactured from stainless steel. Stainless steel is a combination of carbon, chromium, iron, and other metals (alloys). This combination makes the instruments strong and resistant to wear and corrosion. During fabrication, one of three types of finishes is used on stainless steel instruments. The mirror finish is highly polished and reflects light. This causes a glare, but the instrument is highly resistant to corrosion. Satin or matte is a dull finish that reduces glare and is the preferred finish. Ebony is a black chromium finish that completely eliminates reflection and glare; instruments with this finish are used during laser procedures to prevent light beam deflection.

Gold plating on an instrument signifies that tungsten carbide was incorporated in the manufacturing process. Tungsten carbide is an extremely hard metal that is used to laminate scissor blades to increase and maintain sharpness and is inserted into the jaws of needle holders to increase strength and gripping abilities.

CARE AND HANDLING OF INSTRUMENTS

Surgical instruments are a large financial expense for medical facilities. Properly preparing, using, and processing instruments promotes patient safety, prolongs the life of the instrument, and decreases repair and replacement costs. All surgical instruments are designed for a specific use. Using them for any other purpose will damage or dull the instrument (e.g., using tissue scissors to cut drapes or dressings or using a hemostat to open a medication vial). Misuse of an instrument can also endanger patients. Simple steps can keep instruments in proper working order. Instruments should be handled individually or in small groups to prevent damage that might occur if they become entangled or are piled on top of one another. They should not be jostled around in the tray when setting up or looking for a certain item. Before, during, and after surgery, instruments should be placed onto the designated area. They should not be tossed or dropped. Heavy items and instruments should never be placed on top of another instrument. These types of mishandlings cause misalignment and dull blades and can damage instrument tips. To ensure patient safety, instruments should be inspected and tested before each surgical procedure. Instruments should be clean and free of debris, properly aligned, damage free, and in good working order.

During surgery, instruments should be wiped or rinsed with sterile water as they become soiled with blood and tissue. This ensures removal from the box lock, serrations, the jaws, and any crevice. Blood and tissue that is allowed to dry and harden can cause an instrument to become stiff and not work properly. This can also make the cleaning process difficult and interfere with the sterilization process. Nondisposable suction tips should be periodically irrigated with a syringe and sterile water to remove trapped blood and debris. Saline should not be used to wipe, rinse, or soak instruments. Exposure to saline will cause corrosion and pitting.

After the surgical procedure, all disposable sharps and blades should be removed and discarded in a sharps container. Instruments should be opened, disassembled, and submerged in water or enzymatic solution. The instruments should be placed in the solution so that they do not become entangled or damaged. Heavy instruments should be placed first, and lighter, more delicate ones should be placed on top. Sharp edges or tips should be placed so that they do not endanger the personnel who will be cleaning them. Delicate instruments, rigid endoscopes, cameras, and fiberoptic light cords should be separated to prevent damage. All cords should be loosely coiled. Power saws and drills should never be immersed in solutions.

Microsurgical Instruments

Microsurgical instruments are delicate. Proper care and handling are essential to prevent damage. Generally, special storage containers are used to protect the instruments. These racks keep the instruments separate and help in identification by providing a place to label them. One should not drop these instruments, allow them to become entangled with each other, or place heavy items on top of them. All microsurgical instruments should be inspected for damage before use. Care should be exercised when handling these instruments. Many have sharp tips that can easily compromise the integrity of gloves and/or skin. When passing instruments, a surgeon should be able to remain focused and not have to move away from the microscope. Ringed forceps (cups, scissors, and nippers) are passed by holding the instrument just above the rings on the shaft and positioning against the palm of the surgeon's hand so he or she can easily place fingers into the loops. The instrument should be held in this position until the surgeon is allowed to adjust his or her fingers. Additional instruments (picks, knives, elevators, and suction tips) should be passed with the tips slightly downward and positioned into the surgeon's hand onto the web between the thumb and index finger (pencil style). Microsurgical instruments should be immediately retrieved from the surgeon to prevent unintentional dropping from the field. After each use, blood and debris should be removed from all instruments. Instrument tips wiped clean with a moistened instrument wipe or a sponge and suction tips should be irrigated often with water.

Powered Instruments

Powered surgical instruments have historically corresponded with surgical needs, predominantly in procedures involving bone. This progression has been important because the complexity of these have required the use of different types of implants. The use of power instruments decreased the use of manual instruments thereby reducing surgery time and improving overall outcomes. Powered surgical instruments are used to perform orthopedic; neurosurgery; ear, nose, and throat (ENT); and oral procedures as well as procedures on other bodily systems. These devices perform cutting, driving, drilling, and reaming and are driven by batteries, compressed gas, and electrical power. Each instrument consists of one or more handpieces and related accessories as well as disposable and limited reuse items, such as burrs, saw blades, drill bits, and reamers. Power instruments should not be submerged in fluid or placed on top of other instruments. Power sources to these instruments should be disconnected or removed before the cleaning process begins.

PARTS OF AN INSTRUMENT

The overall design of an instrument is dependent on what function it will perform. All instruments have a basic standard design and will be modified according to function and type.

Components of this basic design include handles, ratchets, shanks, joints, jaws or blades, and tips (Figure 1-1).

Finger rings are on the proximal end and is the handle area of the instrument. Above the rings are shanks that define the length of the instrument, which is determined by the depth of the wound. Above the rings, attached to the shank may be ratchets that allow for the jaws to be closed and locked on tissues. Between the shanks and the jaw is the joint, which is where the two halves of the instrument are joined to permit for opening and closing. These joints are either a box lock or a screw joint. Beyond the joint are the jaws, which are the working portion of the instrument. The inner jaws, tips, and the shape determine how and on what tissues the instrument is used. Ringed instruments are placed in the palm of a surgeon's hand with the working end up.

Tissue forceps have a spring action joint at the distal end that holds the instrument open until compressed. The handle grip is where the surgeon's fingers are placed. The shanks determine the length of the forceps. The jaws and the tips are the working end of the forceps; these are determined by the type of tissue that is being grasped (Figure 1-2). Tissue forceps are held between the thumb and index finger with the distal joint end resting on the top of the hand like a pencil.

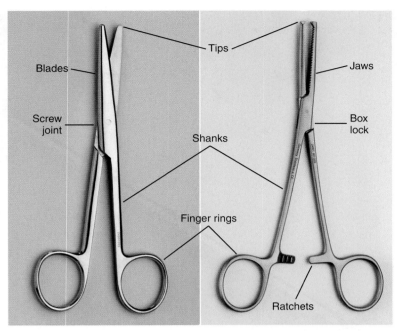

Figure 1-1 Mayo Scissors and kocher forceps illustrating the parts of a ringed instrument.

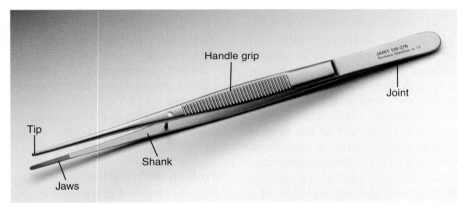

Figure 1-2 Plain tissue forceps illustrating the parts of a tissue forceps.

Retractors are used to hold a surgical wound open to expose the site that is being worked on. A handheld retractor will be designed with a handle, a shank, a blade or blades, and tips. The handle is where the retractor is grasped; this may be on one end or in the middle. The shank is responsible for the length and runs from the handle to the blade. The blade determines the depth to which the retractor is placed into the wound. The tip is at the end of the blade and differs according to where and how the retractor is utilized. The retractor that is pictured in Figure 1-3 is a double-ended retractor that has a blade on either end. The handle is positioned in the center. The position of the handle determines how the retractor is handed to a surgeon.

INSTRUMENT CATEGORIZATION

Whether an instrument is curved or straight, long or short, wide or narrow, sharp or dull, it is designed for a particular task. An instrument is categorized according to its function. The nine categories include accessory, clamping and occluding, cutting and dissecting, grasping and holding, probing and dilating, retracting and exposing, suctioning and aspirating, suturing and stapling, and viewing.

Accessory

An accessory is an instrument that does not fall into any of the other categories but has a specific function and is an integral part of the surgical procedure. An example of an accessory item is a mallet, electrosurgical pencil, lens warmer, screwdriver, or harmonic scalpel.

Clamping and Occluding

Clamping and occluding instruments are used to compress vessels and other tubular structures to impede or obstruct the flow of blood and other

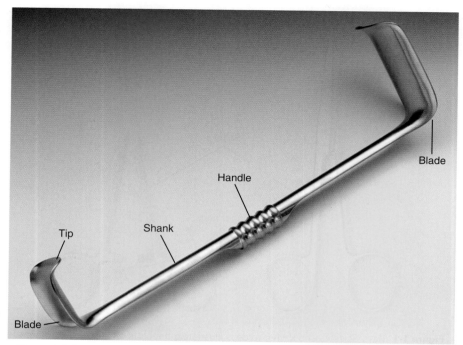

Figure 1-3 Richardson-Eastman double ended retractor illustrating the parts of a retractor.

fluids. These clamps are atraumatic ratcheted instruments that are straight, curved, or angled and have a variety of inner jaw patterns. These clamps may totally occlude or partially occlude the tissues between the jaws. A total occlusion clamp has the ability to completely compress or close the jaws at the initial engagement of the ratchet device. The partial occlusion clamp is capable of varying levels of compression. The jaws gradually come together as each increment of the ratcheting is employed. The most common example of a clamping and occluding instrument is the Crile hemostatic forceps or hemostat. Other examples are the Kelly forceps, Glover bulldog, Satinsky clamp, Doyen intestinal clamp, or Mixter forceps.

Cutting and Dissecting

Cutting and dissecting instruments are used to incise, dissect, and excise tissues. Cutting instruments have single or double razor-sharp edges or blades, such as a scalpel, scissors, or osteotomes. Dissecting instruments may have a cutting edge and come in a variety of designs. Examples include curettes, cone tip dissectors, and biopsy forceps.

Grasping and Holding

Grasping and holding instruments are designed to grip and manipulate body tissues. They are often used to stabilize tissue that is to be excised, dissected, repaired, or sutured. Tissue forceps are the nonratcheted style and are often referred to as pickups or thumbs. The tips may be smooth or serrated and may have interlocking teeth. They vary in size and shape according to use. Common examples of tissue forceps are Debakey, Adson, Cushing, Russian, and Ferris-Smith. The ratcheted type of grasping forceps can be curved or straight; the jaws may be smooth or serrated and have interlocking teeth or sharp prongs. Some examples are the Kocker forceps, Allis forceps, bone-holding forceps, and tenaculum.

Probing and Dilating

Probing instruments are used to explore a structure, opening, or tract. These instruments are often blunt, malleable, and wire-like instruments. Dilating instruments are used to gradually enlarge an orifice or tubular structure, to open a stricture, or to introduce another instrument. They come in sets numbered from the smallest to the largest. A few examples of dilators are Hanks, Van Buren, Bakes, and Mahoney.

Retracting and Exposing

Retracting and exposing instruments are designed to hold back or pull aside wound edges, organs, vessels, nerves, and other tissues to gain access to the operative site. They are generally referred to as retractors and are either manual (handheld) or self-retaining (stay open on their own). Retractors have one or more blades. These blades are used for holding back tissues without causing trauma and should not be confused with a cutting blade. Retractor blades are usually curved or angled and may be blunt or have sharp or dull prongs. The blades will vary in size according to the depth of the wound and the area of placement. Handheld retractors consist of a blade attached to some type of handle, which is pulled back or held in place by the user. Manual retractors are often used in pairs, one on each side of the wound. Some are double-ended, with a blade on each end with a slight variation in size or shape. Examples of handheld retractors are Parker, Joseph skin hook, Senn, Ragnell and Richardson. Self-retaining retractors are holding devices with two or more blades that spread the wound apart or hold tissues back. A self-retaining retractor has a ratchet, crank, spring, or locking device that holds it open. Some will have permanent attached blades, while others will have interchangeable blades that come in a variety of shapes, lengths, and widths, depending on the operative location. Screws, hooks, wing nuts, or clamping devices secure the blades in place. Some retractors attach directly to the operating room table for stability. Examples of self-retaining retractors are the Balfour, Omni tract, Bookwalter, Burford, Finochietto, Weitlaner, and Gelpi.

Suctioning and Aspirating

Suctioning and aspirating devices are used to remove blood, fluid, and debris from operative sites. These suction tips may be disposable or nondisposable and come in a variety of shapes and sizes according to use. Some examples of these hollow tips include the Yankauer, Frazier, Poole, and Barron.

Suturing and Stapling

Suturing instruments are used to ligate, repair, and approximate tissues during a surgical procedure. This mainly includes needle holders, which are used to hold curved suture needles, but also includes other items such as a knot pusher, endo stitch, and endo loops. Stapling devices are used to ligate, anastomose, or approximate tissues. Stainless steel, titanium, and Insorb absorbable material are used for stapling. Staples are designed to be noncrushing when inserted into the tissues to promote healing. A nondisposable stapler uses disposable stapling cartridges that have to be assembled during setup. Disposable staplers are assembled, packaged, and sterilized by the manufacturer. They are designed to be reloaded with a new cartridge for multiple uses on the same patient. Some examples of stapling devices are skin staplers, ligating clips, linear cutters, and intraluminal staplers.

Viewing

Viewing instruments allow visualization of a structure or cavity. Various examples include the nasal speculum, ridged and flexible endoscopes, and endoscopic camera.

Sets

Instruments are generally placed into sets according to the type of procedures that are performed at the facility. Typically, instruments from each category will be selected for the assembly of a set. These sets are then assembled, labeled, sterilized, and stored for later use. Instrument sets are often labeled according to the procedure, degree of the procedure (i.e., major or minor) or the specialty area. For instance, a hysterectomy set would be used to perform a hysterectomy, and an orthopedic basic set can be used for a number of orthopedic procedures.

2

ACCESSORY INSTRUMENTS

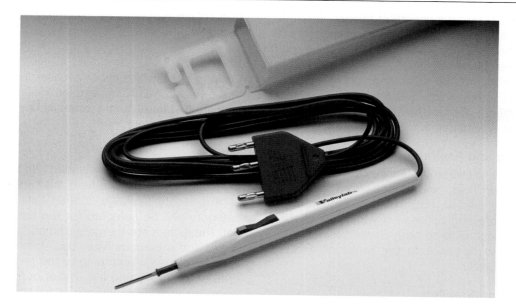

Instrument: ELECTROSURGICAL PENCIL

Other Names: Bovie, cautery, monopolar, diathermy

Use(s): Monopolar cautery uses electrical current to coagulate and cut blood vessels and tissues to provide homeostasis; also used for dissection.

Description: This is a disposable instrument that usually comes packaged with a blade tip and a holster. The current is activated by a switch or button on the pencil or with a foot pedal. There are several different types of interchangeable electrode tips that fit into the hand piece. Some of the common types of tips are blade, ball, needle, and extended blade tips.

Instrument Insight: All monopolar electrodes require a dispersive pad because the electricity enters the patient's body. Monopolar current travels from the generator, to the active electrode, and through the patient's body; the current is then captured by the dispersive pad, which channels it back to the generator, completing the closed circuit. A scratch pad is used to remove charred blood and tissue from the electrode tip. The tip may also be Teflon coated for ease in cleaning.

⚠ CAUTION: The tip of the pencil becomes hot after extended use. When not in use the pencil should be placed in the holster to prevent burning the drapes or the patient.

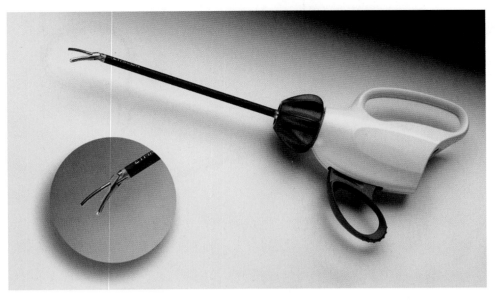

Instrument: HARMONIC SCALPEL
Other Names: Ultrasonic scalpel
Use(s): The harmonic scalpel is a grasping instrument that delivers ultrasonic energy between the jaws to coagulate and divide tissue by low-temperature cavitation.
Description: This device has a manufacturer-packaged disposable hand piece. A nondisposable cord and wrench are also needed. These two components need to be packaged and sterilized by the facility.
Instrument Insight: Blood and tissue can build up on the jaws and may need to be removed periodically with a moistened sponge.

CLAMPING AND OCCLUDING INSTRUMENTS

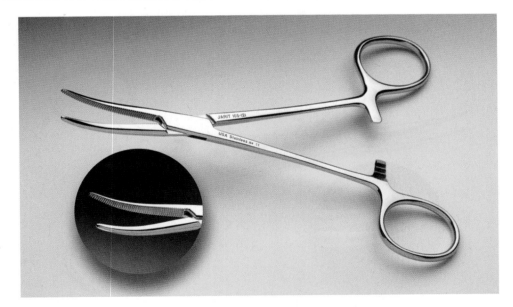

Instrument: CRILE FORCEPS
Other Names: Hemostat, snap, clamp, Kelly, stat
Use(s): Used for occluding bleeders before cauterization or ligation.
Description: A curved or straight clamp with horizontal serrations that run the complete length of the jaws.
Instrument Insight: The curved Crile is the most widely used clamp in all specialty areas.

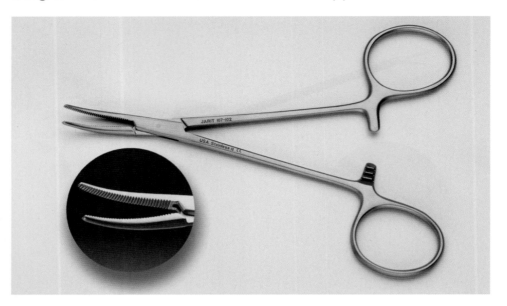

Instrument: HALSTEAD FORCEPS
Other Names: Mosquito, Hartman
Use(s): Used for occluding bleeders in small or superficial wounds before cauterization or ligation. Used often for delicate or small, confined procedures. Some examples are plastics, pediatric, thyroid, and hand procedures.

Description: A small, curved or straight clamp with fine tips and horizontal serrations that run the length of the jaws.
Instrument Insight: These forceps are much smaller than a Crile or a Kelly.

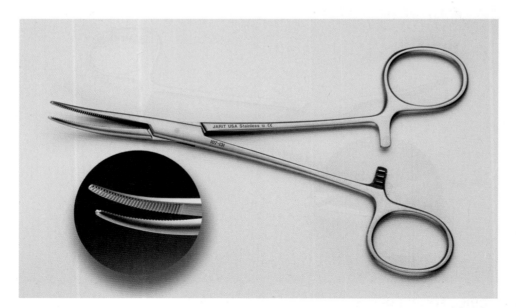

Instrument: KELLY FORCEPS
Other Names: Hemostat, Crile, clamp
Use(s): Used for occluding bleeders before cauterization or ligation.

Description: A curved or straight clamp with horizontal serrations that run about half the length of the jaws.

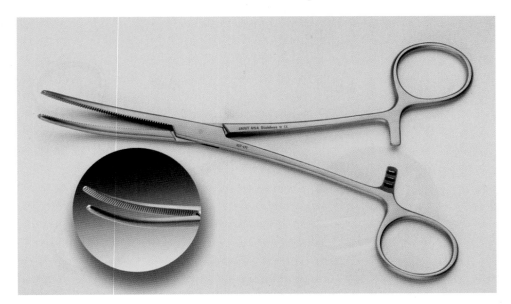

Instrument: ROCHESTER-PÉAN FORCEPS
Other Names: Péan, Mayo
Use(s): Used for occluding larger blood vessels and tissue before ligation, usually in a deeper wound or on heavier tissue.

Description: Curved or straight clamp that has heavier, broader jaws with horizontal serrations that run the length of the jaws.

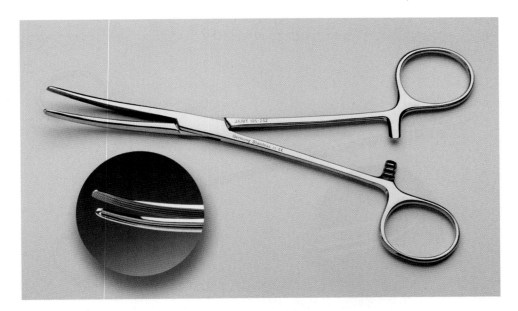

Instrument: CARMALT FORCEPS
Other Names: Carmalt, big curved
Use(s): Used for occluding larger blood vessels and tissue before ligation, usually in a deeper wound or on heavier tissue.

Description: Curved or straight clamp with a crosshatch pattern at the tips that continue with vertical serrations that run the length of the jaws.

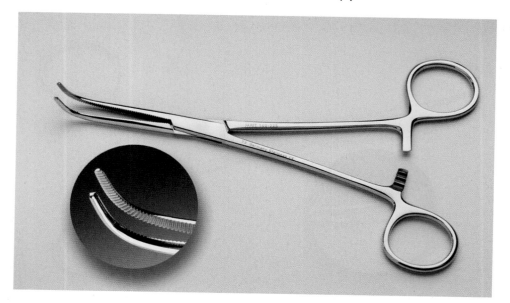

Instrument: MIXTER FORCEPS
Other Names: Right angle, Gemini, Lahey, obtuse clamp, ureter clamp
Use(s): Is used to clamp, dissect, and occlude tissue. Is often used to place a tie or vessel loop under and around a tubular structure such as a vessel or a duct, enabling the surgeon to grasp the ligature or loop and pull it up and around the structure to either ligate or retract.
Description: A 75° angle clamp with horizontal serrations that run the length of the jaws.

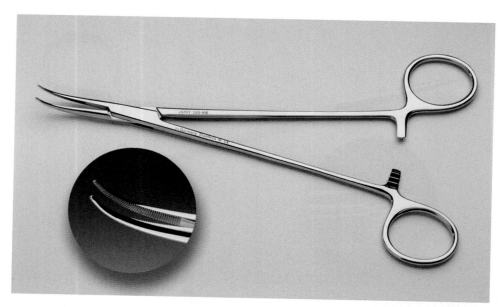

Instrument: ADSON FORCEPS
Other Names: Tonsil Schnidt, fancy clamp
Use(s): Clamps small vessels in a deep wound or holds tonsil sponges.
Description: A fine curved or straight clamp with horizontal serrations running halfway down the jaws. The shanks are longer than those of a Crile or a Kelly.

CUTTING AND DISSECTING INSTRUMENTS

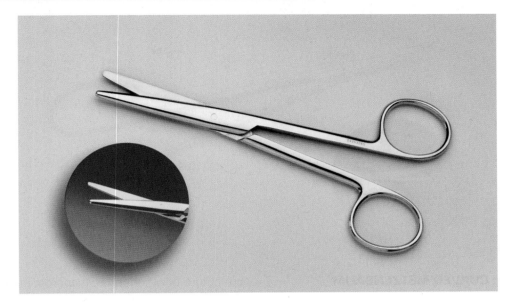

Instrument: STRAIGHT MAYO SCISSORS
Other Names: Suture scissors
Use(s): Used for cutting suture.
Description: Heavy scissors with straight blades.
Instrument Insight: Use the very tips of the scissors when cutting suture. Slightly rotate the scissors to visualize the knot or the appropriate length of the suture tail that will remain.

⚠ **CAUTION:** It is important to always check the screw to ensure it is fully tightened to prevent it from dropping into the wound.

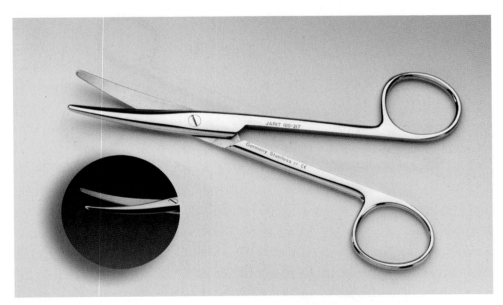

Instrument: CURVED MAYO SCISSORS
Other Names: Heavy tissue scissors
Use(s): Dissect or undermine heavy fibrous tissues.
Description: Heavy scissors with curved blades and blunt or sharp tips.
Instrument Insight: Tissue scissors are intended to cut tissue only and should never be used to cut other items. Inappropriate use of the scissors will cause the blades to become dull and not function properly.

⚠ **CAUTION:** It is important to always check the screw to ensure it is fully tightened to prevent it from dropping into the wound.

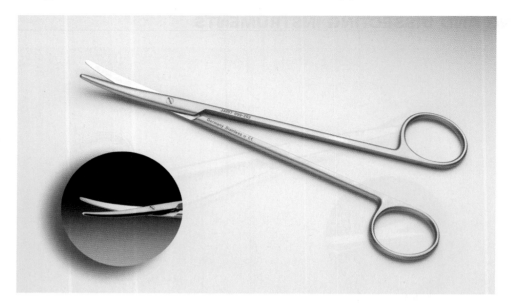

Instrument: CURVED METZENBAUM SCISSORS
Other Names: Metz, tissue scissors
Use(s): Dissect and undermine delicate tissues.
Description: Longer, thinner scissors with curved or straight blades that can have blunt or sharp tips.
Instrument Insight: Tissue scissors are intended to cut tissue only and should never be used to cut suture or other items. Inappropriate use of the scissors will cause the blades to become dull and not function properly.

⚠ **CAUTION:** It is important to always check the screw to ensure it is fully tightened to prevent it from dropping into the wound.

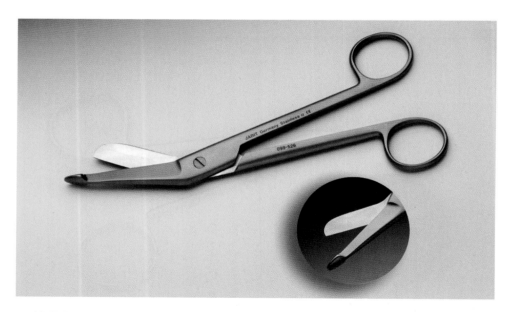

Instrument: LISTER BANDAGE SCISSORS
Other Names: Bandage scissors
Use(s): Cut dressings, drapes, and other items; also used in cesarean sections to open the uterus without harm to the baby.
Description: An angled blunt scissors in which the lower blade has a smooth, flattened tip.
Instrument Insight: The flattened tip is designed to give these scissors the ability to get under dressings or drapes and cut the material without harming the patient.

⚠ **CAUTION:** It is important to always check the screw to ensure it is fully tightened to prevent it from dropping into the wound.

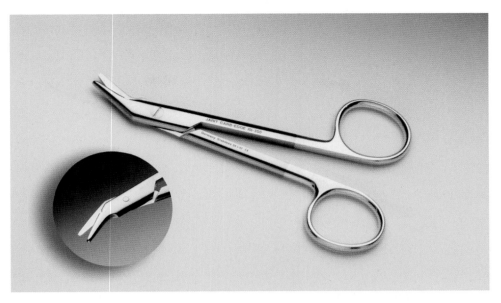

Instrument: WIRE SCISSORS
Other Names: Wire cutters
Use(s): Cut small-gauge wire and suture.
Description: Angled scissors with fine serrations on the blades and a circular notch in the inner jaws.
Instrument Insight: The serrations are intended to facilitate grasping the item being cut. When the wire is placed inside the notch, it gives the scissors the ability to exert additional pressure to cut heavier gauged wire.

⚠ **CAUTION:** It is important to always check the screw to ensure it is fully tightened to prevent it from dropping into the wound.

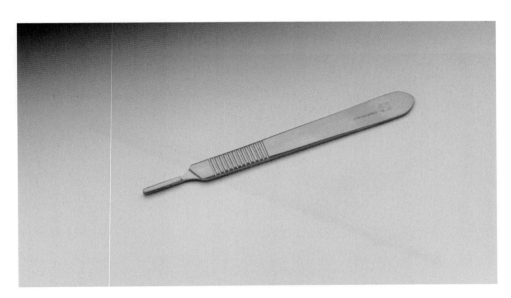

Instrument: #3 KNIFE HANDLE
Other Names: #3 handle, scalpel handle
Use(s): Knife handles are used to hold various blades to create a scalpel. Scalpels are used to make skin incisions or whenever a fine precision cut is necessary.
Description: A #3 handle holds blades 10, 11, 12, and 15.
Instrument Insight: Because the skin is not sterile, once the skin incision is made the scalpel should be removed from the mayo stand, isolated, and reused only to incise the skin.

⚠ **CAUTION:** Never retrieve the scalpel from the surgeon's hand after use; allow the surgeon to place it in the "neutral zone."

⚠ **CAUTION:** Never use fingers to load or unload a knife blade from the handle. Always use a needle holder.

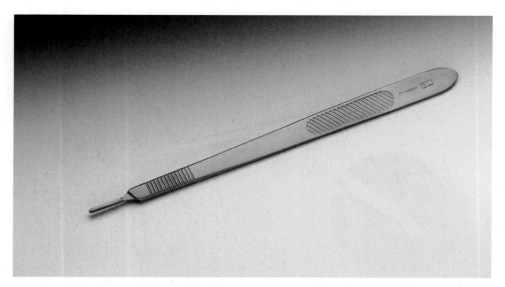

Instrument: #3 LONG KNIFE HANDLE
Other Names: Long knife, long handle
Use(s): Used for precision cutting deep within a wound.
Description: A #3 long knife handle holds blades 10, 11, 12, and 15.

⚠ **CAUTION:** Never retrieve the scalpel from the surgeon's hand after it is used; allow the surgeon to place it in the "neutral zone."

⚠ **CAUTION:** Never use fingers to load or unload a knife blade from the handle. Always use a needle holder.

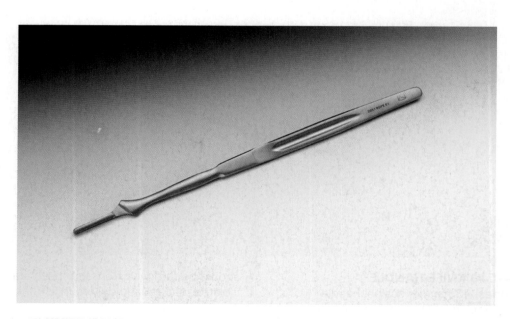

Instrument: #7 KNIFE HANDLE
Use(s): Used when precision cutting is needed in a confined space or a deep wound.
Description: A #7 knife handle holds blades 10, 11, 12, and 15.

⚠ **CAUTION:** Never retrieve the scalpel from the surgeon after it is used; allow the surgeon to place it in the "neutral zone."

⚠ **CAUTION:** Never use fingers to load or unload a knife blade from the handle. Always use a needle holder.

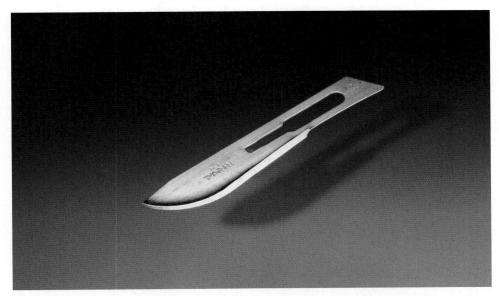

Instrument: #10 BLADE
Use(s): Used for making skin incisions.
Description: An extensive body blade with a curved cutting edge to the tip.
Instrument Insight: To load a scalpel blade onto a scalpel handle, grasp the blade with a straight hemostat or just above the opening on the noncutting side. Line up the grooves on the handle with the opening on the blade. Make sure that the angle of the blade matches the angle of the handle. Advance the blade onto the handle until it clicks in place. A scalpel blade is a single-patient use item that comes prepackaged and sterilized from the manufacturer.

⚠ **CAUTION:** Never use fingers to load or unload a knife blade from the handle. Always use a needle holder.

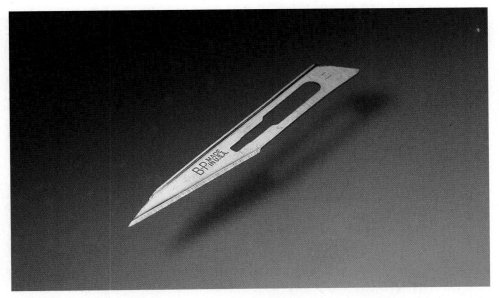

Instrument: #11 BLADE
Use(s): Used for puncturing the skin or to initiate the opening of an artery.
Description: An angled cutting edge that ascends to a sharp point.
Instrument Insight: The #11 blade is commonly loaded onto the #7 handle. A scalpel blade is a single-patient use item that comes prepackaged and sterilized from the manufacturer.

⚠ **CAUTION:** Never use fingers to load or unload a knife blade from the handle. Always use a needle holder.

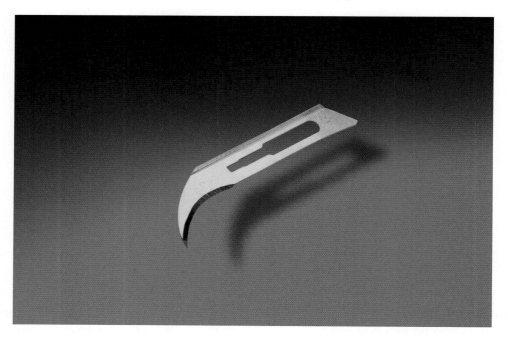

Instrument: #12 BLADE
Other name: Sickle knife
Use(s): A #12 blade is sometimes used during tonsillectomies, parotid surgeries, septoplasties, and during cleft palate procedures. It can also be utilized for removal of calculi in the ureter and the kidney (ureterolithotomies and pyelolithotomies).
Description: A small, crescent shaped blade sharpened along the inside edge of the curve.

Instrument Insight: The #12 blade is commonly loaded onto the #7 handle but may also be used on a #3 regular or long. A scalpel blade is a single-patient use item that comes prepackaged and sterilized from the manufacturer.

⚠ **CAUTION:** Never use fingers to load or unload a knife blade from the handle. Always use a needle holder.

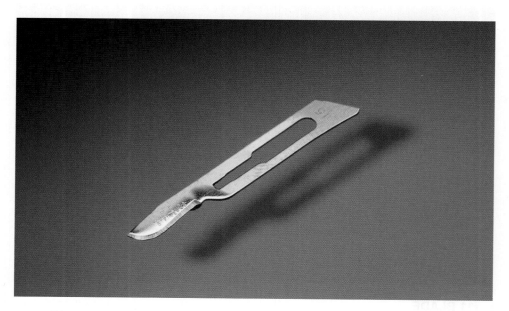

Instrument: #15 BLADE
Use(s): Used for creating small precise incisions.
Description: A narrow blade that has a small, rounded cutting edge.
Instrument Insight: Commonly used for pediatric or plastic/reconstructive surgery. A scalpel blade is a single-patient use item that comes prepackaged and sterilized from the manufacturer.

⚠ **CAUTION:** Never use fingers to load or unload a knife blade from the handle. Always use a needle holder.

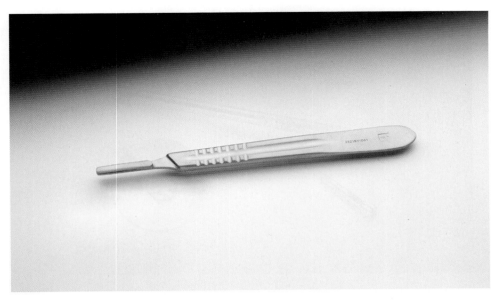

Instrument: #4 KNIFE HANDLE
Use(s): Used with the #20 blade to create a larger and/or deeper incision in heavy tissue areas.
Description: Has a larger tip to accommodate the larger blades.
Instrument Insight: The #4 handle will hold blades 20, 21, 22, 23, 24, and 25. Never use fingers to load or unload a knife blade from the handle. Always use a needle holder.

⚠ **CAUTION:** Never use fingers to load or unload a knife blade from the handle. Always use a needle holder.

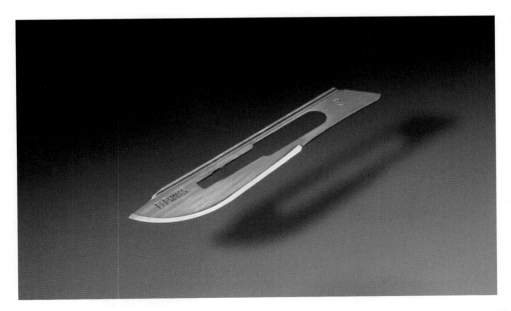

Instrument: #20 BLADE
Use(s): Used with the #4 handle to create a larger and/or deeper incision and on heavy tissues and bone.
Description: A broader body blade with a curved cutting edge to the tip.
Instrument Insight: Blades should never be loaded with your fingers.

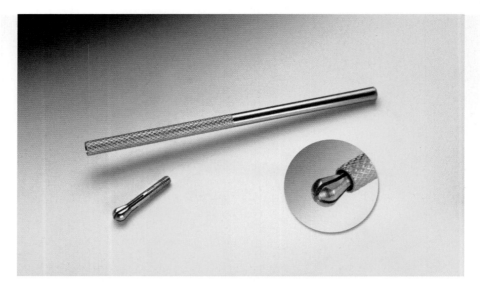

Instrument: BEAVER HANDLE

Other Names: Round handle

Use(s): Used when precision cutting is needed in a confined space or incising a small structure. The beaver knife is commonly used in ENT, ophthalmic, neurology, podiatry, and small orthopedic procedures.

Description: Round handle with a ball tip that screws into the handle to tighten the blade in place.

The rounded tip has a slot that accepts the blade. As the tip is screwed into the handle, it tightens to hold the blade. Many blades designed for specific purposes and procedures are available.

Instrument Insight: There are many types and shapes of blades that will fit on the Beaver handle depending on surgeon's preference and procedure being performed.

GRASPING AND HOLDING INSTRUMENTS

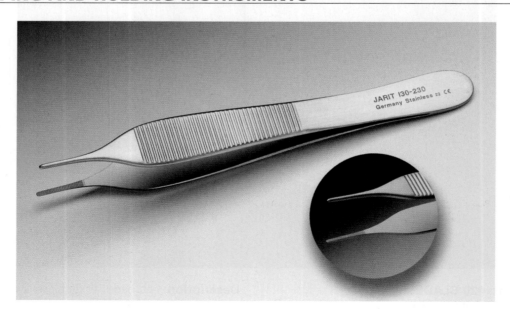

Instrument: PLAIN ADSON TISSUE FORCEPS

Other Names: Adson dressing forceps

Use(s): Used for grasping delicate tissue.

Description: Fine tips with horizontal serrations.

Instrument Insight: All of the Adson tissue forceps are the same size and shape. They are differentiated by the inner tips.

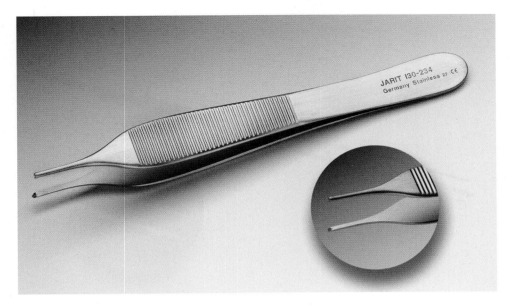

Instrument: TOOTHED ADSON TISSUE FORCEPS
Other Names: Adson with teeth, rat tooth
Use(s): Aligns the edges of the wound during stapling of the skin; grasps superficial tissues so that Steri-Strips can be placed.
Description: The fine tips have two small teeth on one side and one small tooth on the other side that fit together when closed.

Instrument Insight: All of the Adson tissue forceps are the same size and shape. They are differentiated by the inner tips.

⚠ **CAUTION:** Exercise care when handling forceps with teeth. The sharp teeth can easily compromise the integrity of your gloves and those of the surgeon.

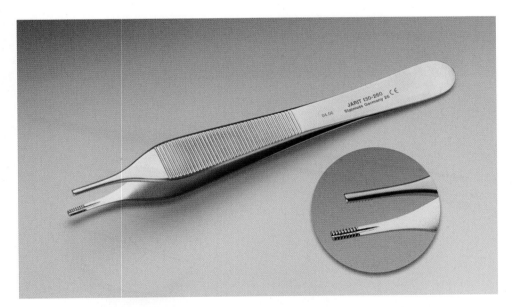

Instrument: BROWN-ADSON TISSUE FORCEPS
Other Names: Brown
Use(s): Used for grasping superficial delicate tissues. Often used in plastic or hand surgery.
Description: On each side of the tip there are two rows of multiple teeth that interlock when closed.
Instrument Insight: All Adson tissue forceps are the same size and shape. They are differentiated by the inner tips. It is important to ensure that the teeth are properly aligned and in working order before use.

⚠ **CAUTION:** Exercise care when handling forceps with teeth. The sharp teeth can easily compromise the integrity of your gloves, skin and those of the surgeon.

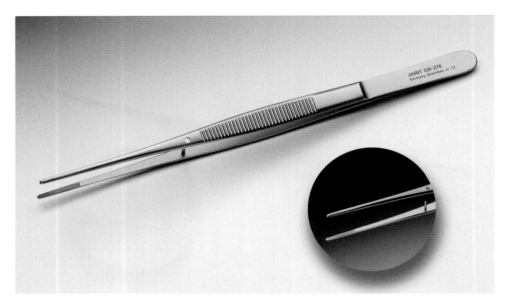

Instrument: PLAIN TISSUE FORCEPS
Other Names: Semken dressing forceps, smooth forceps, tissue forceps without teeth
Use(s): Used for grasping tissue and dressing application.

Description: Atraumatic tissue forceps with horizontal serrated tips that vary from fine to heavy.

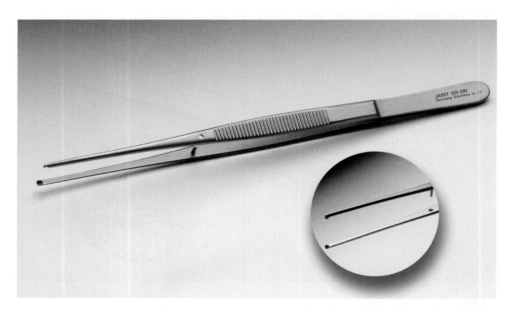

Instrument: TOOTHED TISSUE FORCEPS
Other Names: Semken tissue forceps, rat tooth, tissue forceps with teeth
Use(s): Used for grasping moderate to heavy tissue and used during wound closure.
Description: The tips have two teeth on one side and one tooth on the other side that fits between the opposite when closed.

Instrument Insight: It is important to ensure the teeth are properly aligned and in working order before use.

⚠ **CAUTION:** Exercise care when handling forceps with teeth. The sharp teeth can easily compromise the integrity of your gloves, skin and those of the surgeon.

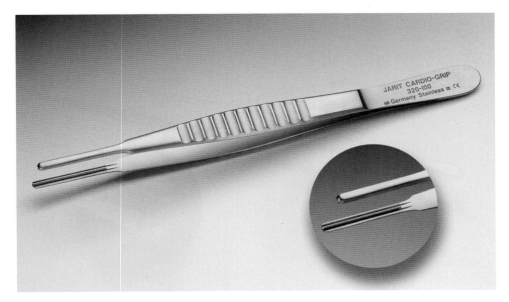

Instrument: DEBAKEY TISSUE FORCEPS
Other Names: DeBakey's, DeBakes
Use(s): Grasps numerous types of tissue; commonly used in cardiac, vascular surgery, and gastrointestinal procedures.
Description: An atraumatic tissue forceps with an elongated, narrowed blunt tip. A set of parallel fine serrations runs the length of one jaw with a center row of serrations on the opposite side that interlocks to grip when closed.
Instrument Insight: These are considered a vascular tissue forceps, but they are commonly used in all specialty areas because of the ability to securely grip without causing damage to the tissues.

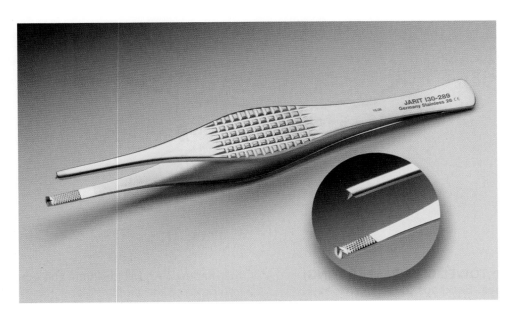

Instrument: FERRIS-SMITH TISSUE FORCEPS
Other Names: Big ugly's
Use(s): Grasps heavy tissue, muscle, and bone; often used in orthopedics, spinal, and obstetrics surgery.
Description: This is always the same size and shape. The tips have two to one interlocking large teeth followed by a crisscrossed pattern serration.
Instrument Insight: it is important to ensure that the teeth are properly aligned and in working order before use.

⚠ **CAUTION:** Exercise care when handling forceps with teeth. The sharp teeth can easily compromise the integrity of your gloves, skin and those of the surgeon.

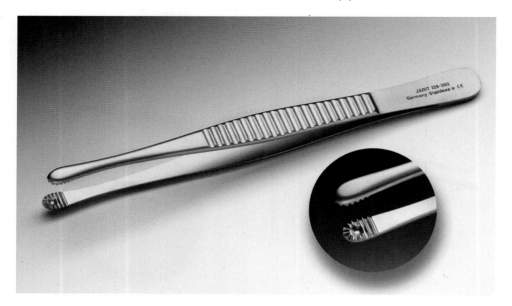

Instrument: RUSSIAN TISSUE FORCEPS
Other Names: Star, Russian star, Russians
Use(s): Used for grasping dense tissues and used during wound closure.

Description: Rounded tips with starburst pattern serrations.

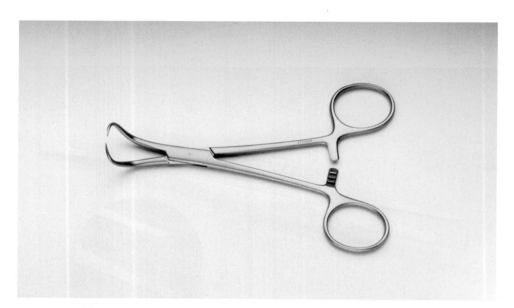

Instrument: TOWEL CLIP (PENETRATING)
Other Names: Backhaus towel clip, Roeder towel clip, Jones
Use(s): Used for holding towels in place when draping, when grasping tough tissue, and during reduction of small bone fractures.
Description: A ratcheted instrument with curved, sharp, tine-like jaws.
Instrument Insight: Used in all disciplines. Never use penetrating clips to attach the electro-surgical unit (ESU), suction, or any other item to

the drapes. This will perforate the drapes and compromise the sterile field.

⚠ **CAUTION:** When clipping towels together, be careful not to penetrate the patient's skin.

⚠ **CAUTION:** Exercise care when handling penetrating forceps. The sharp tips can easily compromise the integrity of your gloves, skin and those of the surgeon.

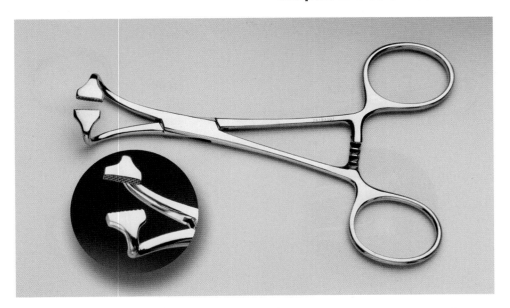

Instrument: NONPENETRATING TOWEL CLIP
Other Names: Atraumatic towel clamp
Use(s): Used for attaching Bovie and suction to the drapes.
Description: There are many different types of towel clamps; they may be metal or plastic and may have a variety of nonpenetrating tips.

⚠ **CAUTION:** Care should be taken not to clamp the patient's skin between the jaws when attaching accessory devices to the drapes.

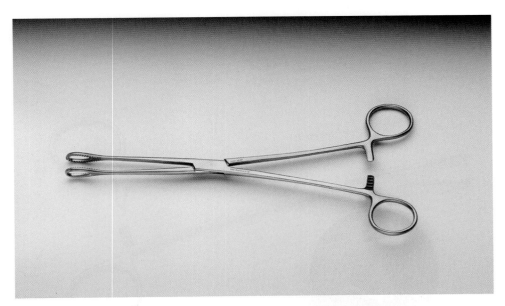

Instrument: FORESTER SPONGE FORCEPS
Other Names: Fletcher, sponge stick, ring forceps
Use(s): Used for creating a sponge stick, for grasping tissues such as the lungs, or for removing uterine contents.
Description: Can be curved or straight and has two round tips with horizontal serrations.

Instrument Insight: To assemble a sponge stick, fold a 4 × 4 Raytec in thirds and then in half and attach it to the ring forceps. A sponge stick can be used for the surgical preparation (painting), to absorb blood, or for blunt dissection in deep wounds.

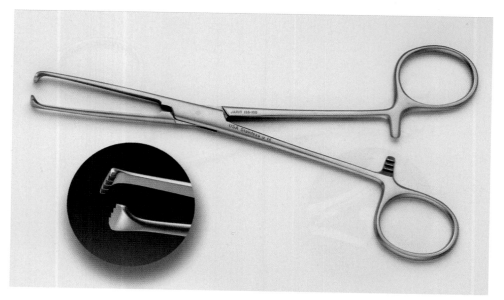

Instrument: ALLIS FORCEPS

Use(s): Used for lifting, holding, and retracting slippery dense tissue that is being removed. Commonly used for tonsils; for vaginal, breast, and thyroid tissues; or for grasping bowel during a resection.

Description: Curved or straight with multiple, interlocking fine teeth at the tip that reduce injury to the tissues.

Instrument Insight: It is important to ensure the teeth are properly aligned and in working order before use.

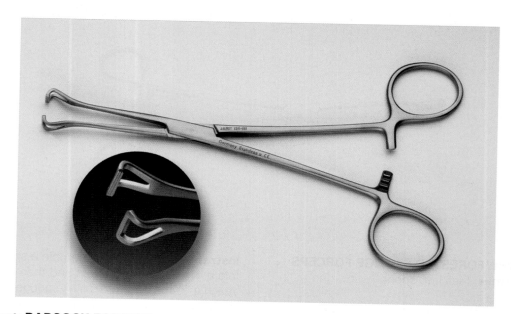

Instrument: BABCOCK FORCEPS

Use(s): Used for grasping and encircling delicate structures such as ureters, fallopian tubes, bowel, ovaries, and appendix.

Description: An atraumatic forceps with a flared, rounded, hollow end with smooth, flattened tips.

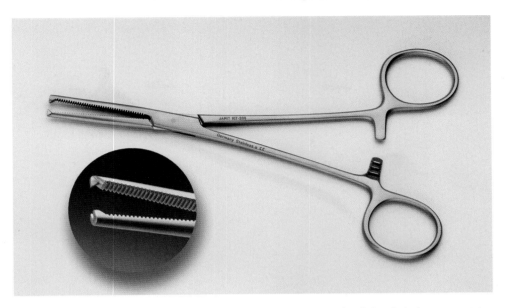

Instrument: KOCHER FORCEPS
Other Names: Koch, Ochsner
Use(s): Used for grasping tough, fibrous, slippery tissues such as muscle and fascia.
Description: The jaws have horizontal serrations and two to one large interlinking teeth at the tip.

Instrument Insight: It is important to ensure the teeth are properly aligned and in working order before use.

⚠ **CAUTION:** Exercise care when handling forceps with teeth. The sharp teeth can easily compromise the integrity of your gloves and those of the surgeon.

RETRACTING AND EXPOSING INSTRUMENTS

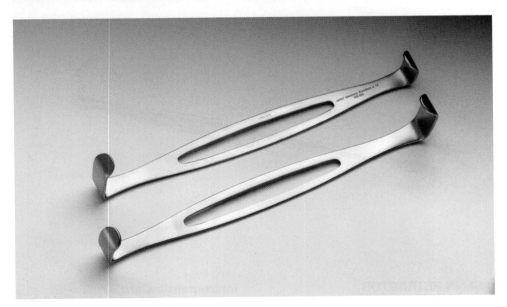

Instrument: ARMY-NAVY RETRACTOR
Other Names: Army's, Navy's, U.S. retractor
Use(s): Used for retraction of small superficial incisions to allow better exposure.
Description: A hand-held, double-ended retractor with an oval fenestration in the handle and a lateral curve to the blades on each end. One end is longer than the other so that it can be placed deeper into the wound.
Instrument Insight: Often packaged in pairs.

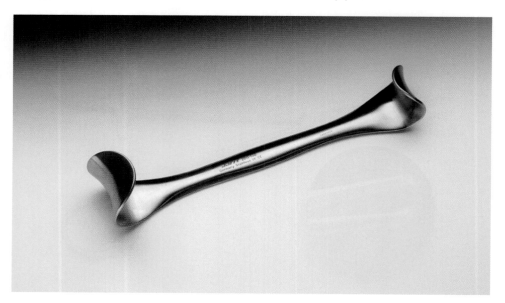

Instrument: GOELET RETRACTOR

Use(s): Used for retraction of small superficial incisions to allow better exposure.

Description: Handheld, double-ended retractor with smooth, cup-shape curved blades with a crescent-shaped lip. One end is longer than the other so that it can be placed farther into the wound. The size and shape never change.

Instrument Insight: Usually packaged in pairs.

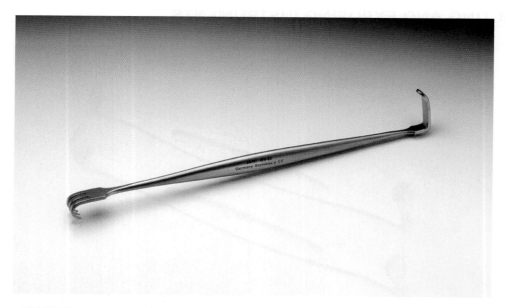

Instrument: SENN RETRACTOR

Other Names: Cat paw

Use(s): Used for retraction of skin edges and deeper tissues of small incisions.

Description: Double-ended, handheld retractor in which one end has three sharp or dull claws and the other end is a small, narrow, lateral-bent blade.

Instrument Insight: Usually come packaged in pairs. Always hand to the surgeon with the sharp claws facing downward.

⚠ CAUTION: Exercise care when handling retractors with sharp claws. The sharp claws can easily compromise the integrity of your gloves and skin.

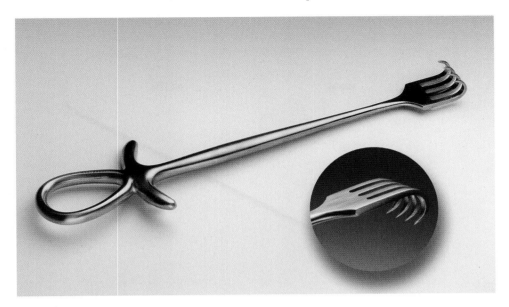

Instrument: **MURPHY RETRACTOR**
Other Names: Rake
Use(s): Used for superficial retraction of wound edges.
Description: The retractor has four claws that may be blunt or sharp. The handle has a teardrop opening with two prongs on each side.

Instrument Insight: Usually come packaged in pairs. Always hand this retractor to the surgeon with the sharp claws facing downward.

⚠ **CAUTION:** Be cognizant of the sharp claws. Sharp edges may puncture gloves and scratch the skin.

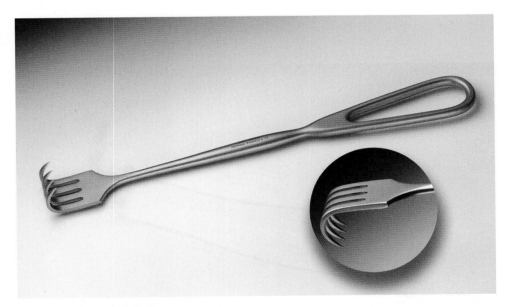

Instrument: **VOLKMAN RETRACTOR**
Other Names: Rake, Israeli
Use(s): Used for superficial retraction of wound edges.
Description: These may have two to six claws that may be blunt or sharp. The handle has a teardrop opening.

Instrument Insight: Usually come packaged in pairs. Always hand this retractor to the surgeon with the sharp claws down.

⚠ **CAUTION:** Be aware of the sharp claws. Sharp edges may puncture gloves and scratch the skin.

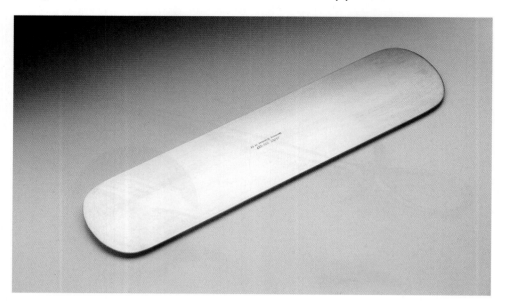

Instrument: RIBBON RETRACTOR
Other Names: Malleable
Use(s): Used for retraction of organs and intestines in a wound.

Description: A handheld, smooth, flat metal strip with rounded ends. These come in many different lengths and widths.
Instrument Insight: Can be bent or molded as needed for use.

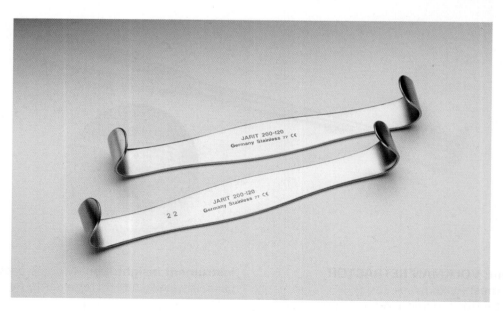

Instrument: PARKER RETRACTOR
Other Names: Park bench, nested right angle
Use(s): Used for retraction and exposure of a small or shallow wound.

Description: Handheld, double-ended with smooth, rounded ends.
Instrument Insight: Usually packaged in pairs.

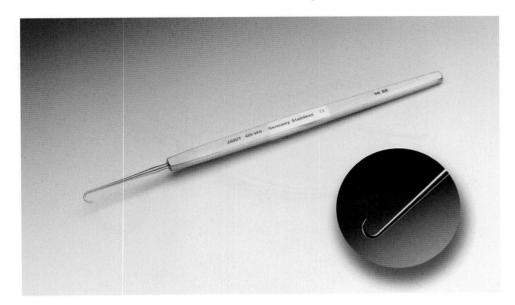

Instrument: SKIN HOOK
Other Names: Joseph, Gillies
Use(s): Used for retraction of the skin edges.
Description: A small hand-held instrument with one or two sharp hooks at one end.

Instrument Insight: Always hand instrument to the surgeon with the hook(s) down.

⚠ **CAUTION:** The hooks are very sharp. Exercise care when handling sharp instruments to avoid puncture to gloves and/or skin.

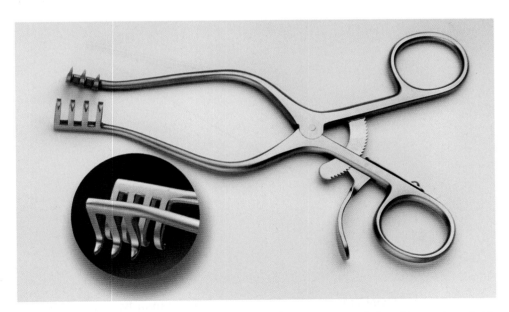

Instrument: WEITLANER RETRACTOR
Use(s): Holds wound edges open.
Description: Self-retaining finger-ringed instrument with a ratchet/release device on the shanks, which holds them open in the wound. The tip has three outward-curved prongs on one side and four on the other side that may be sharp or dull.

Instrument Insight: Always hand this retractor to the surgeon with the prongs down.

⚠ **CAUTION:** The prongs may be very sharp. Exercise care when handling sharp instruments to avoid puncture to gloves and/or skin.

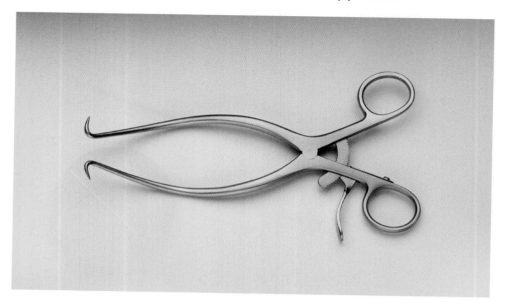

Instrument: GELPI RETRACTOR

Use(s): Provides wound exposure, ranging from superficial to deep depending on the wound depth.

Description: Self-retaining, ringed instrument with a ratchet/release device on the shanks and two outward-turned sharp prongs, one on each side.

Instrument Insight: Always hand this retractor to the surgeon with the prongs down.

⚠ **CAUTION:** The prongs are sharp and can puncture gloves and skin.

SUCTIONING AND ASPIRATING INSTRUMENTS

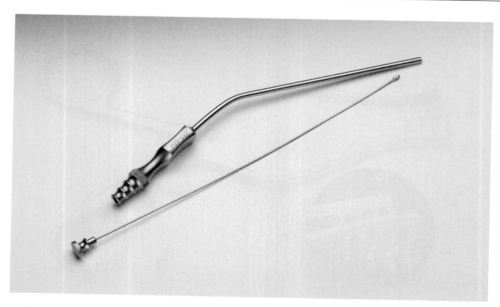

Instrument: FRAZIER SUCTION TIP

Use(s): Used for suctioning in confined spaces such as the nasal cavity, in lumbar and cervical procedures, or in craniotomies.

Description: An angled cylindrical tube with a relief opening/hole on the handgrip. The diameter of the suction tube is measured on the French (F) scale and ranges from 3F to 15F.

Instrument Insight: The Frazier suction tip is packaged with a thin wire stylet. This stylet fits inside the suction tip to push out any tissue, blood, or debris that gets trapped while suctioning. The suction is increased by the relief/opening.

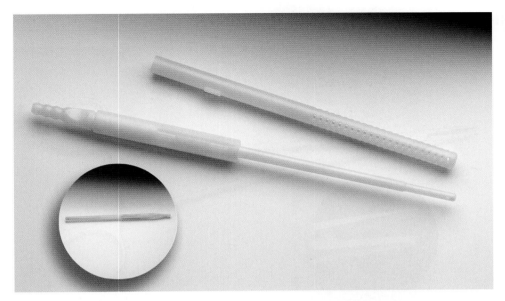

Instrument: POOLE SUCTION TIP
Other Names: Abdominal sucker
Use(s): Used for suctioning large amounts of blood and/or fluids from a body cavity. The inner cannula of this suction tip can be used to suction down the shaft of the femur during a total hip replacement procedure.

Description: This can be disposable or reusable and has two components: an outer sheath and an inner cannula.
Instrument Insight: Multiple fenestrations (holes) on the outer sheath allow for more suction. If less suction power is desired, the surgeon may use the inner cannula only.

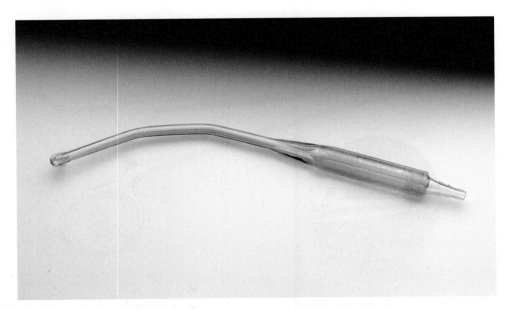

Instrument: YANKAUER SUCTION TIP
Other Names: Tonsil suction tip, oral
Use(s): Used for suctioning in all types of wounds. It allows for effective suctioning without aspiration damage to the surrounding tissue.

Description: A hollow plastic tube with a grip handle and a slightly bent shaft that terminates with a bulbous tip and large opening.
Instrument Insight: The disposable Yankauer is the most widely used suction tip.

SUTURING AND STAPLING INSTRUMENTS

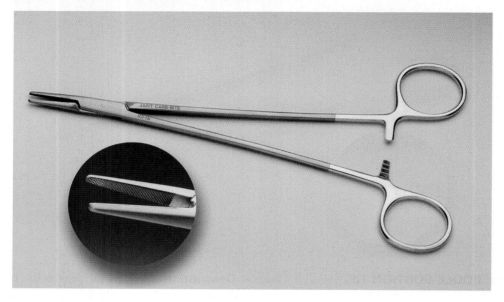

Instrument: CRILE-WOOD NEEDLE HOLDER
Other Names: Fine needle holder, fine needle driver
Use(s): Used for holding delicate to intermediate size needles when suturing.

Description: A narrow rounded tip with crisscross gripping pattern in the inner jaws.
Instrument Insight: The type of procedure and depth of the wound will determine the type and size needle holder.

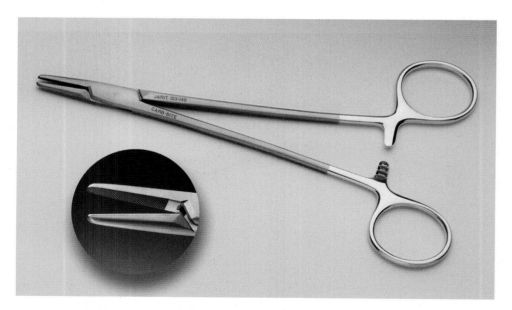

Instrument: MAYO-HEGAR NEEDLE HOLDER
Other Names: Heavy Needle driver
Use(s): Used for holding heavy needles when suturing.
Description: A broader jaw that is rounded at the tip with crisscross pattern on the inner jaws.

Instrument Insight: The type of procedure and depth of the wound will determine the type and size needle holder.

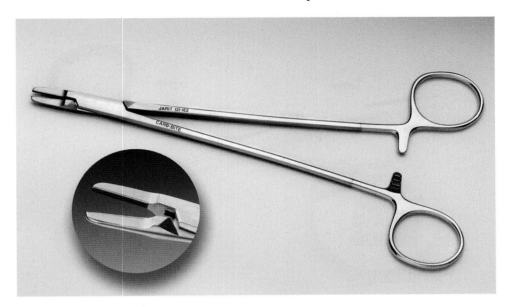

Instrument: RYDER NEEDLE HOLDER
Other Names: Ryder needle driver, fine needle drive
Use(s): Used for holding delicate to intermediate size needles when suturing. Often used for vascular procedures.

Instrument Insight: Never used for grasping large, heavy needles. The type and size of a needle holder to be use will be determined the type of procedure and the depth of the wound.

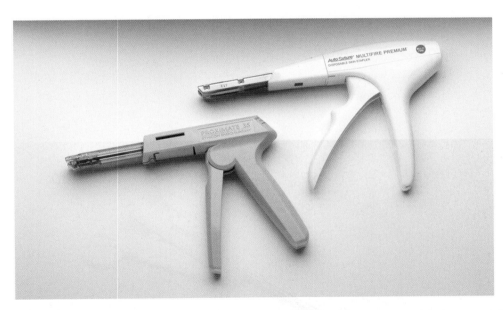

Instrument: SKIN STAPLER
Use(s): Used during wound closure for skin approximation.
Description: A sterile, single-patient use instrument; it is preloaded with stainless-steel rectangular staples that are used for approximation of the skin. There are many different manufacturers and models of staplers. It has a handle and a trigger that is squeezed to fire the staples; at the tip is an alignment arrow.
Instrument Insight: The arrow at the tip of the device is to align the stapler with the approximated skin edges for proper staple placement. Two persons often perform skin stapling. The surgeon or assistant uses two tissue forceps to grasp the skin edges and bring them together. The assistant or a surgical technologist positions the stapler over the wound, carefully aligning the arrow with the incision and squeezing the trigger until resistance is met. Once the staple is placed, remove the stapler and align it for the next firing until the wound is closed.

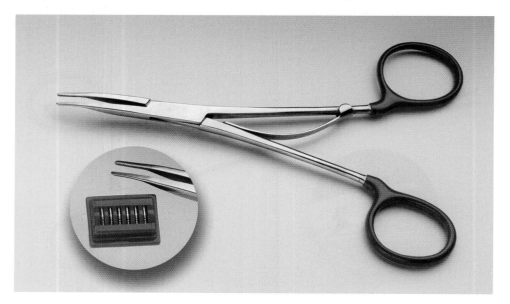

Instrument: HEMOCLIP APPLIER
Other Names: Clip applier
Use(s): Used for occluding vessels or other tubular structures.
Description: Angled tips with fine grooves in the inner jaws that slide over the clip to pick it up.

These are manufactured in various clip sizes and lengths in a color-coded cartridge for easy identification of clip size.
Instrument Insight: The size and type of clip have to match the appropriate clip applier.

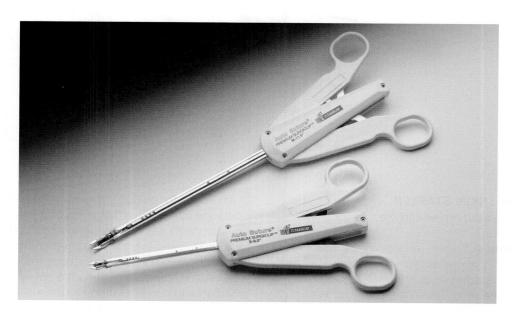

Instrument: SURGICLIP APPLIER
Other Names: Hemoclip, ligaclip
Use(s): Used for occluding vessels or other tubular structures.

Description: A sterile, single-patient use instrument, preloaded with clips. These are manufactured in various clip sizes and lengths.

3

General Instruments

ACCESSORY INSTRUMENTS

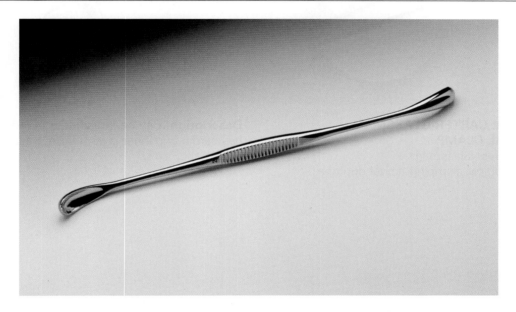

Instrument: FERGUSON GALLSTONE SCOOP
Other Names: Scoop, spoon
Use(s): Used for removing stones from the gallbladder.

Description: Double-ended, spoon-shaped, with one end larger than the other.
Instrument Insight: Usually small, medium, and large scoops in the set.

CLAMPING AND OCCLUDING INSTRUMENTS

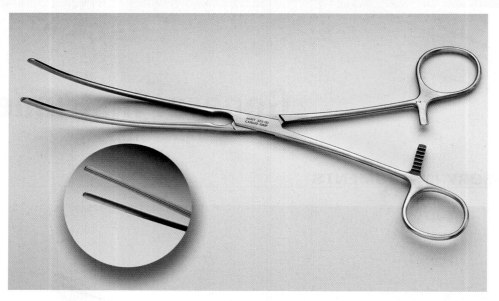

Instrument: CARTER-GLASSMAN INTESTINAL CLAMP
Other Names: Glassman
Use(s): Used for clamping bowel during a resection.

Description: Can be straight or curved and has cardio grip inner jaws, which grasp but are atraumatic.

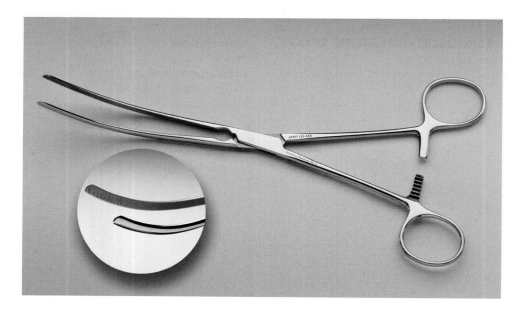

Instrument: DOYEN INTESTINAL CLAMP
Other Names: Doyen clamp
Use(s): Used for clamping bowel during a resection.
Description: Can be curved or straight; has smooth inner jaws.

Instrument Insight: The jaws of the Doyen are covered with rubber shods or shoelaces. Shoelaces are tubular woven cotton that slips over the entire jaws. Shods are rubber tubing that slides over the jaws. These help grip the intestine without causing trauma.

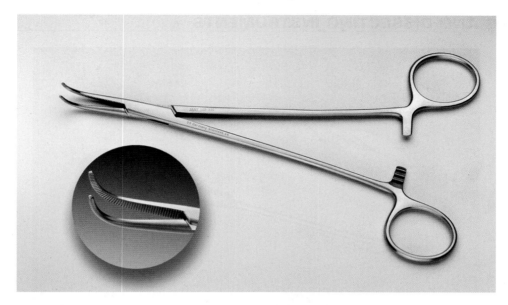

Instrument: GEMINI CLAMP
Other Names: Right angle, Lahey, Mixter
Use(s): Used for dissecting tissue planes, clamping vessels, and placing a tie or vessel loop under and around a tubular structure, such as a vessel or duct. This enables the surgeon to grasp the ligature or loop and pull it up and around the structure to either ligate or apply traction.

Description: A 90°-angle clamp with horizontal serrations that run the length of the jaws.
Instrument Insight: The gemini, right angle, Lahey, and Mixter are often referred to as the same instrument depending on the region of the country where they are being used, but they are in fact differentiated by the inner jaws.

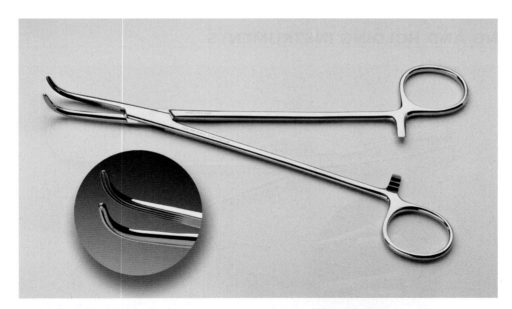

Instrument: LAHEY GALL DUCT FORCEPS
Other Names: Right angle, gemini, Mixter
Use(s): Used for dissecting tissue planes, clamping vessels, and placing a tie or vessel loop under and around a tubular structure, such as a vessel or duct.
Description: A 90°-angle clamp with vertical serrations that run the length of the jaws.

Instrument Insight: The gemini, right angle, Lahey, and Mixter are often referred to as the same instrument depending on the region of the country where they are being used, but they are in fact differentiated by the inner jaws.

CUTTING AND DISSECTING INSTRUMENTS

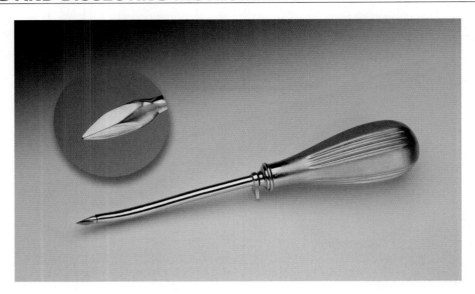

Instrument: GALLBLADDER TROCAR

Use(s): Used for draining the gall bladder of bile during an open cholecystectomy procedure.

Description: Two-pieced instrument that consists an outer sheath and a sharp obturator. The obturator fits inside the sheath.

Drainage is facilitated by pushing the sharp trocar into the gall bladder, then removing the obturator and attaching a syringe to aspirate the bile.

Instrument Insight: The obturator and sheath should be taken apart during the sterilization process. If it is inadvertently left together as one piece, the inside of the sheath and obturator would be considered unsterile and should be handed off the field as one piece. Do not separate the two pieces.

GRASPING AND HOLDING INSTRUMENTS

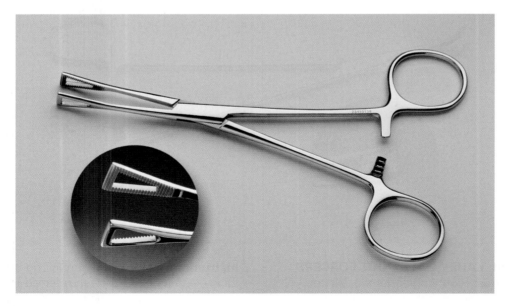

Instrument: PENNINGTON FORCEPS

Other Names: Duval, triangle, lung clamp

Use(s): Used for grasping tissue and organs during general procedures. Commonly used during intestinal and rectal procedures. Also used for grasping the uterine layers during closure of a cesarean section.

Description: Triangular tips with horizontal serrations.

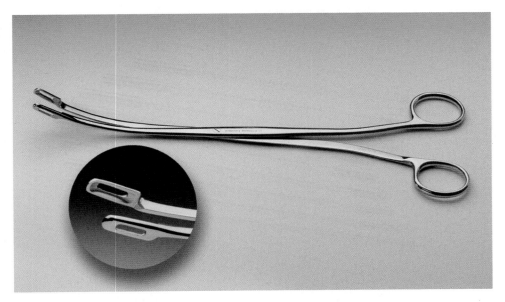

Instrument: DESJARDIN GALLSTONE FORCEPS

Other Names: Randall stone forceps

Use(s): Used for grasping polyps and stones in the common bile duct and gall bladder.

Description: A curved instrument with no ratchets, and the jaws work like scissors. The tips are oval cup-shaped with fenestrations.

PROBING AND DILATING INSTRUMENTS

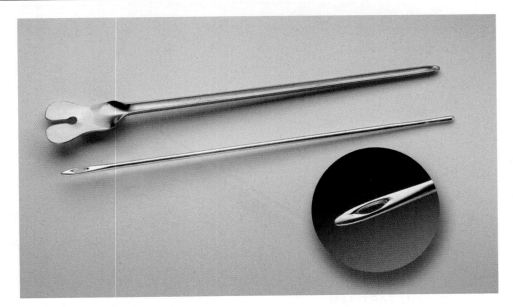

Instrument: PROBE AND GROOVED DIRECTOR

Use(s): Used to detect an obstruction in a tubular structure or determine the path and the extent of a fistula tract.

Description: The probe resembles a French eye blunt needle. The grooved director has a tongue-shaped handle and a concave channel, which guides the probe into the opening.

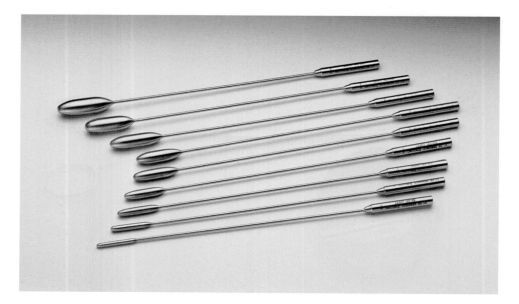

Instrument: BAKES COMMON DUCT DILATORS

Other Names: Common duct dilators

Use(s): Used to open and expand the common bile duct to allow passage of bile from the liver.

Description: Has an oval, solid stainless-steel tip that attaches to a narrowed stem, which extends to a solid, smooth handle.

Instrument Insight: Packaged as a set where each dilator graduates up in size. The stem is malleable and is often bent to allow passage into the duct.

RETRACTING AND EXPOSING INSTRUMENTS

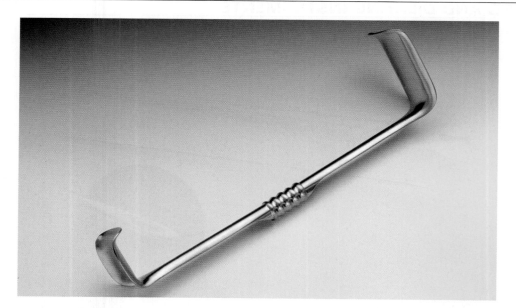

Instrument: RICHARDSON-EASTMAN RETRACTOR

Other Names: Double-ended Rich, Eastman, Big Rich

Use(s): Used for retraction of wound edges.

Description: A hand-held double-ended retractor with a lateral curvature of the blades. The bodies of the blades are concave with crescent-shaped lips that are laterally bent.

Instrument Insight: At initiation of the incision, the superficial end of the retractor is used; as the incision is deepened, the longer blade is used.

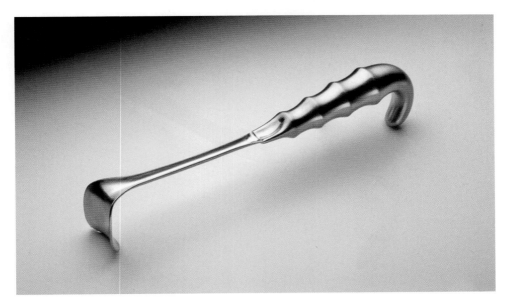

Instrument: RICHARDSON RETRACTOR
Other Names: Rich
Use(s): Used for retraction of wound edges.
Description: Has a hollow grip handle with a lateral curve to the blade. The body of the blade is concave with a crescent-shaped lip that is laterally bent.
Instrument Insight: These are often packaged in a set of three: small, medium, and large.

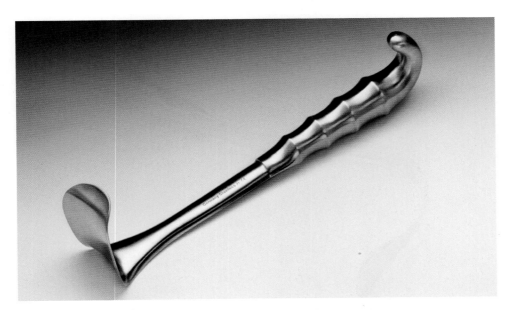

Instrument: KELLY RETRACTOR
Use(s): Used for retraction of wound edges.
Description: Has a hollow grip handle with a lateral right-angle curvature of the blade. The body of the blade is slightly dipped with a crescent-shaped lip that is slightly bent.
Instrument Insight: Often confused with a Richardson retractor, but the blades are distinctly different.

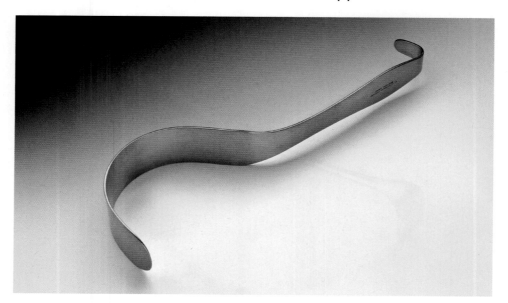

Instrument: DEAVER RETRACTOR

Use(s): Used for deep retraction of organs and viscera.

Description: A flat, stainless-steel strip that resembles a question mark. The width and length vary according to need.

Instrument Insight: Retraction with a Deaver sometimes can be awkward because of the flat shape of the handle. To aid in maintaining a grip, the handle should be placed in the palm of the hand and the hook should be placed over the top of the hand.

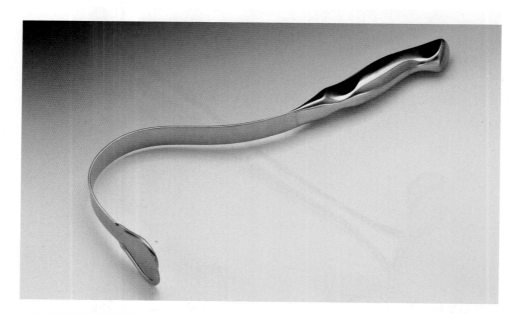

Instrument: HARRINGTON RETRACTOR
Other Names: Sweetheart, Harrington heart
Use(s): Used for retraction deep in an abdominal wound; often used to retract the liver and intestine.

Description: Has a grip handle that extends into a curved, flat, stainless-steel strip. The end of the blade enlarges into a heart shape. The heart-shaped portion is overlaid with a smooth ridge to decrease the chance of injury to an organ.

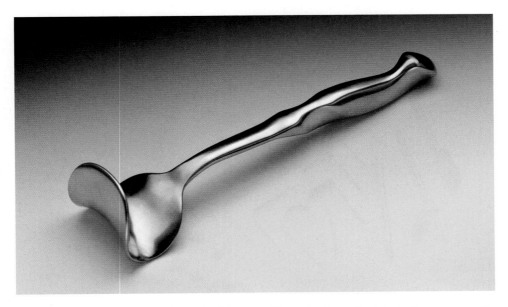

Instrument: MAYO ABDOMINAL RETRACTOR
Other Names: Abdominal wall
Use(s): Used for retraction of the abdominal wall.

Description: The blade has a smooth, cup-shape curve with a crescent-shape lip.

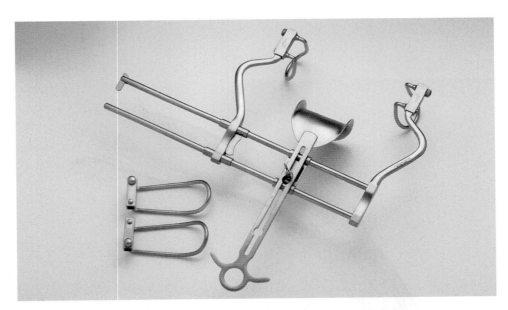

Instrument: BALFOUR RETRACTOR
Other Names: Self-retaining
Use(s): Used for retraction of a large abdominal wound.
Description: A self-retaining retractor with lateral wire blades and a wide center blade. A Balfour set includes the frame, four lateral sides, and two center blades, which are interchangeable according to the depth needed. The lateral blades may be solid, fenestrated, interchangeable, or fixed.
Instrument Insight: All the interchangeable pieces have to be counted separately (for example, one frame, four sides, and two blades). If the frame has any other removable parts, such as screws or wing nuts, these also need to be counted.

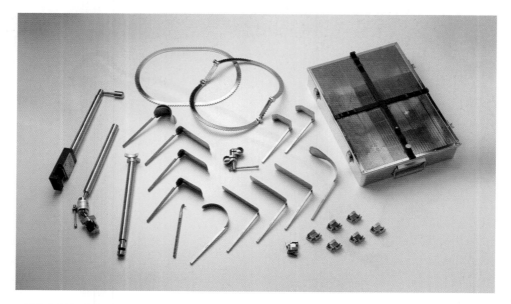

Instrument: BOOKWALTER
Other Names: Jaritrack retractor
Use(s): Used for retraction of large abdominal wounds.
Description: A large, self-retaining abdominal retractor that attaches to the operating table. It has blades in various sizes and shapes that attach to a frame to enhance visualization during the surgical procedure.
Instrument Insight: Each individual piece has to be counted.

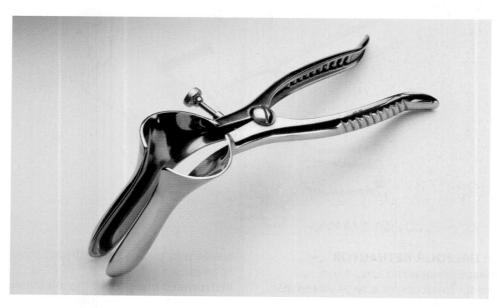

Instrument: PRATT RECTAL SPECULUM
Use(s): Used for providing exposure for visualization of the anus and rectum.
Description: A self-retaining speculum with rounded blades that open by squeezing the handles together. Turning the screw on the side will hold the blades open.
Instrument Insight: Apply copious amounts of lubrication to the blades to prevent tissue damage.

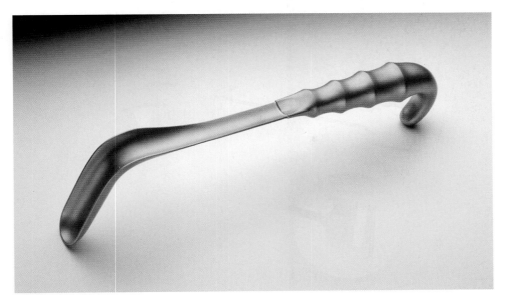

Instrument: SAWYER RECTAL RETRACTOR
Use(s): Used for providing exposure for visualization of the anus and rectum.
Description: A hand-held retractor with a right-angle convex blade that extends to a hollow grip handle.

Instrument Insight: Apply copious amounts of lubrication to the blade to prevent tissue damage.

SUTURING AND STAPLING INSTRUMENTS

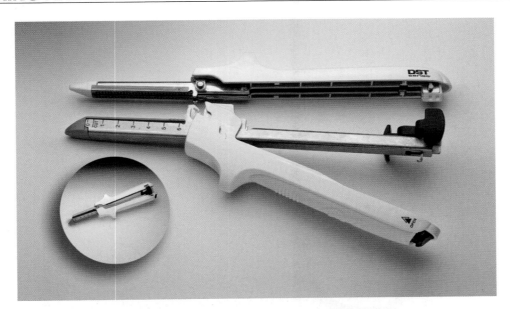

Instrument: LINEAR CUTTER-STAPLER
Other Names: GIA stapler
Use(s): Often used during gastric or bowel surgery for resection and reanastomosis. Also used to transect tissues in thoracic, gynecological, and pediatric procedures.
Description: Disposable, reloadable stapler that distributes two double-staggered rows of titanium staples while cutting the tissues between the rows. The length is determined by the tissue to be excised. This stapler comes in 60-mm, 80-mm, and 100-mm lengths.

Instrument Insight: Activation is accomplished by sliding the firing knob on the sides of the stapler forward until it stops completely. The manufacturer recommends that the stapler can be reloaded seven times for a total of eight firings. When reloading the stapler, make sure to wipe off the opposite side of the stapler to assure any staples left from the first firing are removed. Any staples left behind can cause the stapler to misfire or not to fire at all.

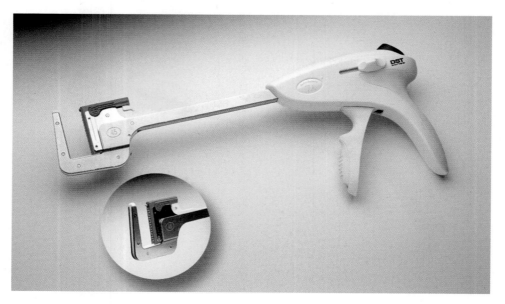

Instrument: **LINEAR STAPLER**

Other Names: TA stapler

Use(s): Used for transection and resection of tissues during abdominal, gynecological, pediatric, and thoracic surgeries.

Description: Disposable, reloadable stapler that distributes a double or triple (depending on model of stapler) staggered row of titanium staples. A scalpel is used to excise the tissue along the length of the staple line.

Instrument Insight: Activation of the linear stapler is done by squeezing the handles together, which compresses the tissues between the jaws and engages the staples. The manufacturer recommends that the stapler can be reloaded seven times for a total of eight firings.

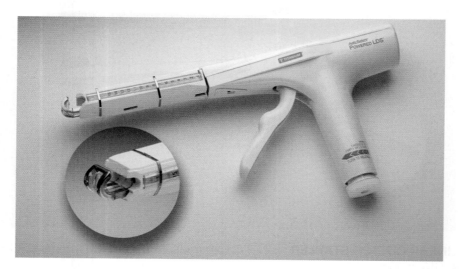

Instrument: **LIGATING AND DIVIDING STAPLER**

Other Names: LDS stapler

Use(s): Used for ligation and division of blood vessels and other tissues during abdominal, gynecological, and thoracic procedures. The LDS is often used in gastrointestinal surgery to ligate and divide the greater omentum and the mesentery.

Description: A disposable, single-use stapler that distributes two titanium staples within the jaw for ligation. A scalpel divides the tissue between the staples.

Instrument Insight: Activation is done by gripping the handles together. The stapler cartridge contains 15 pairs of staples. The remaining number of staples after each firing is indicated on the side panel of the cartridge.

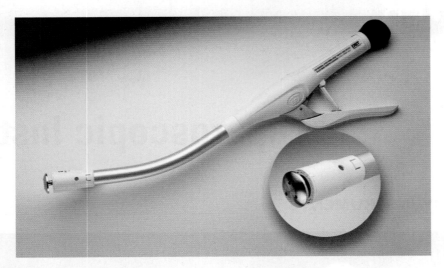

Instrument: INTRALUMINAL STAPLER
Other Names: CEEA stapler, EEA stapler, circular stapler
Use(s): Used for creation of end-to-end, end-to-side, or side-to-side anastomoses throughout the gastrointestinal tract. The stapler is used in both open abdominal and laparoscopic procedures.
Description: A disposable, single-use intraluminal stapler that places a circular, double-staggered row of titanium staples. Simultaneously following the staple formation, a circular knife blade cuts the excess tissue, creating a circular anastomosis.

Instrument Insight: The stapler is activated by compressing the handles together as far as they will allow. After the anastomosis, excess tissue that is transected needs to be inspected for completeness. There should be two complete circular rings of tissue, often called donuts. This is accomplished by turning the wing nut at the bottom of the handle counterclockwise, which causes the shaft to extend, allowing removal of the specimen.

Laparoscopic Instruments

ACCESSORY INSTRUMENTS

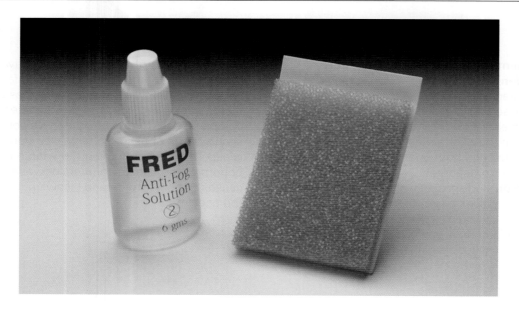

Instrument: ANTI-FOG SOLUTION
Other Names: Endo-fog, Fred, Dr. Fog
Use(s): Used for preventing the lens from fogging up during endoscopic procedures.
Description: Packaged with a bottle of solution and a sponge.

Instrument Insight: To use, remove paper backing from the sponge and place it on sterile drape of mayo stand. Remove the solution cap and place 5 or 6 drops of antifog solution onto the sponge. Wipe the end of the lens over the sponge and then blot with a sterile 4 × 4 sponge (do not wipe dry).

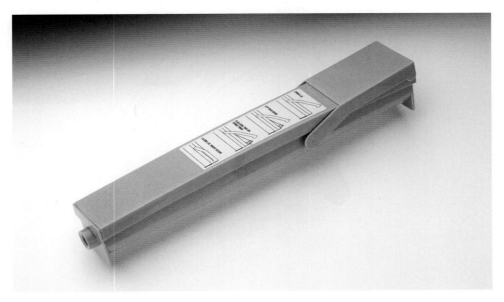

Instrument: LENS WARMER
Use(s): Used to warm the lens to body temperature to prevent condensation and fogging of the lens when entering the body cavity.
Description: The lens warmer that is pictured is disposable and comes in a sterile package.

To activate the warmer, lift the lid toward the rear of the device and squeeze the tagged area. This mixes the chemicals and causes warming.
Instrument Insight: There are many types of lens warmers and ways to warm a lens.

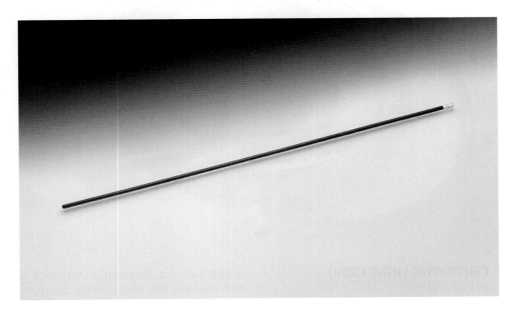

Instrument: ENDO KITTNER
Other Names: Endo kit, pusher, dissector, endo KD, Endo Peanut
Use(s): Used for blunt dissection of tissue plains during laparoscopic procedures. The tip may be used to apply direct pressure to bleeders.

Description: A 3-mm-long cylinder rod with a cotton gauze tip.
Instrument Insight: Can be inserted through a 5-mm or larger trocar.

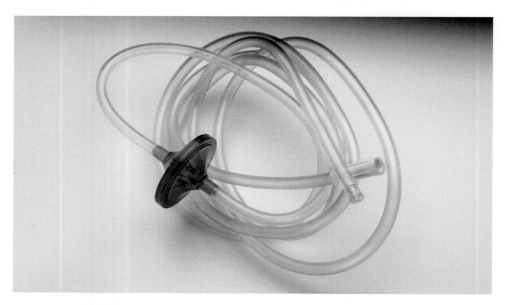

Instrument: INSUFFLATION TUBING

Use(s): Used for creating and maintaining a pneumoperitoneum; delivers carbon dioxide from the insufflator to the abdominal cavity.

Description: Synthetic tubing 10- to 12-feet long with a Luer-Lok connector at the proximal end and a micron filter approximately 16 to 24 inches from the distal standard connection end. The micron filter is designed to prevent cross-contamination between the patient and the insufflator.

Instrument Insight: The distal filter end is handed off the sterile field to be connected to the insufflator. Air should be purged from the tubing before it is connected to the abdominal cavity.

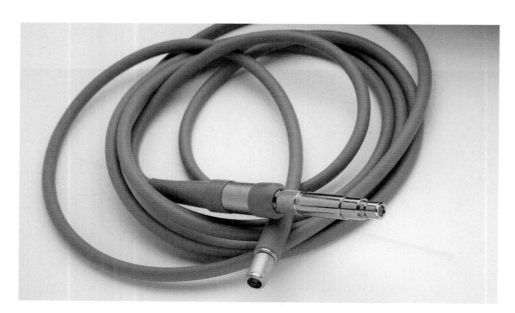

Instrument: FIBEROPTIC LIGHT CORD

Other Names: Light cord

Use(s): Used for illumination during endoscopic procedures; delivers high-intensity light through the endoscope.

Description: A 10-foot-long fiber optic cable with an endoscope adaptor at the proximal end and a light source adaptor at the distal end.

Instrument Insight: Exercise care when handling a fiber optic cord; it should never be placed under a heavy object, dropped, twisted, or kinked because the tiny fibers inside can be easily damaged.

⚠ **CAUTION:** When not in use, the light source must be placed on standby or turned off. The intense heat from the beam can cause the patient's drapes or any flammable vapors around the patient to ignite.

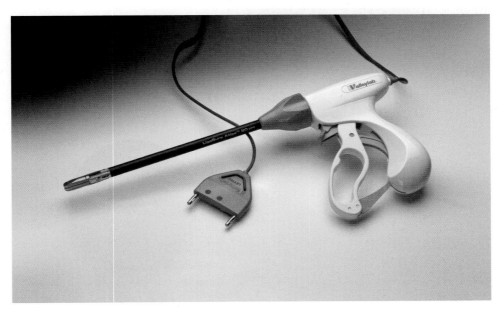

Instrument: LIGASURE™

Use(s): LigaSure works by applying a precise amount of bipolar energy and pressure to change the nature of the vessel walls. The collagen and elastin within the vessel walls fuse and reform into a single structure, obliterating the lumen, and creating a permanent seal.

Description: The system consists of a bipolar radio frequency generator and forceps. The instruments are designed to mimic standard surgical clamps. They are available in a 7-inch Pean-style clamp (LigaSure Standard), a 9-inch Heaney-style clamp (LigaSure Max) and a 5-mm laparoscopic Maryland-style grasper/dissector (LigaSure Lap).

Instrument Insight: Blood and tissue can build up on the jaws and may need to be removed periodically with a moistened sponge.

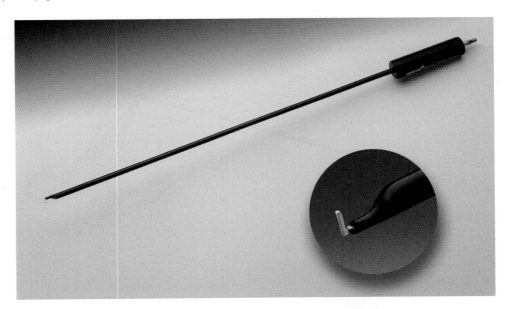

Instrument: L HOOK

Use(s): Used for electrosurgical dissection of tissues and cauterizing vessels.

Description: A long cylinder-insulated rod with an L-shaped monopolar tip. Depending on model and manufacturer, the electrode can be reusable or disposable and may attach to a monopolar cord or directly to the ESU pencil.

Instrument Insight: The electrode is insulated at the tip to ensure the current is directed to the targeted tissue. All monopolar electrodes require a dispersive pad on the patient because the electrical current passes through the patient's body. Before use, carefully inspect the instrument for any breaks in the insulation. Monopolar current travels from the generator to the active electrode and through the patient's body; it then is captured by the dispersive pad, which channels it back to the generator.

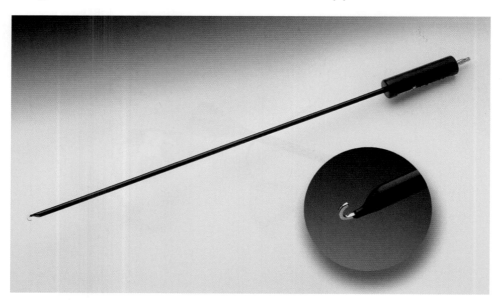

Instrument: J HOOK

Use(s): Used for electrosurgical dissection of tissues and cauterizing vessels during laparoscopic procedures.

Description: A long cylinder-insulated rod with a J-shaped monopolar tip. Depending on model and manufacturer, the electrode can be reusable or disposable and may attach to a monopolar cord or directly to the ESU pencil.

Instrument Insight: The electrode is insulated at the tip to ensure the current is directed to the targeted tissue. All monopolar electrodes require a dispersive pad on the patient because the electrical current passes through the patient's body. Before use, carefully inspect the instrument for any breaks in the insulation. Monopolar current travels from the generator to the active electrode and through the patient's body; it then is captured by the dispersive pad, which channels it back to the generator.

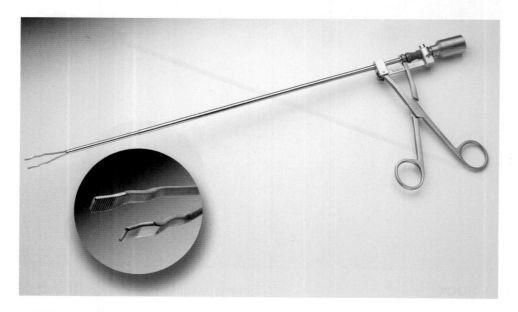

Instrument: KLEPPINGER BIPOLAR FORCEPS

Use(s): Used for coagulation of tissues and vessels during laparoscopic procedures.

Description: A paddle-tip forceps that attaches to a bipolar cord. The bipolar is activated by grasping the targeted tissues between the jaws and stepping on the foot pedal.

Instrument Insight: Bipolar forceps deliver current from one tip, through the tissue grasped to the opposite tip. The electrical current does not pass through the patient's body; therefore no dispersive pad is required.

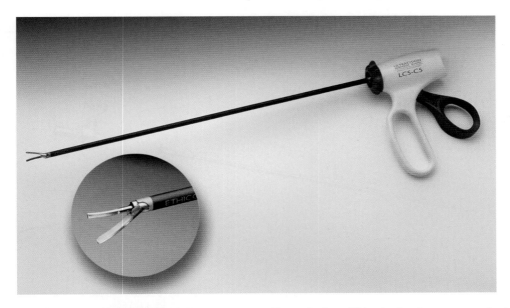

Instrument: ENDO HARMONIC SCALPEL
Other Names: Ultrasonic scalpel
Use(s): The harmonic scalpel is a coagulating instrument that delivers ultrasonic energy between the jaws to coagulate and divide tissue through low-temperature cavitation.

Description: This device has a manufacturer-packaged disposable hand piece. A nondisposable cord and wrench are also needed. These are packaged and sterilized by the facility.
Instrument Insight: Blood and tissue can build up on the jaws and may need to be removed periodically with a moist sponge.

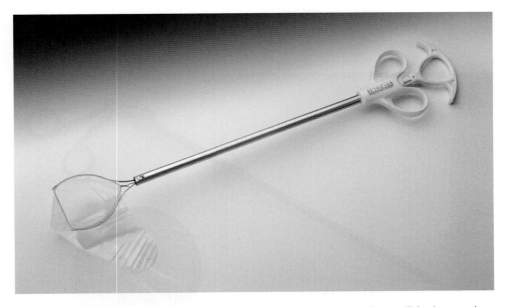

Instrument: ENDO CATCH
Other Names: Endo Pouch, Endosac
Use(s): Used to retrieve and contain specimens during endoscopic removal while minimizing spillage of contaminates into the abdominal cavity.
Description: A single-use specimen pouch that consists of a long cylindrical tube and a polyurethane pouch. The small pouch has a 2.5-inch opening and is 6 inches in depth; the large size pouch has a 5-inch opening and a 9-inch depth.
Instrument Insight: The small pouch is ideal for removal of tissues such as the gallbladder, appendix, ectopic pregnancies, ovaries, lymph nodes, lung resections, and other structures. The larger specimen retrieval bag is generally used for advanced procedures including, but not limited to, laparoscopic bowel resections, splenectomies, and nephrectomies.

CUTTING AND DISSECTING INSTRUMENTS

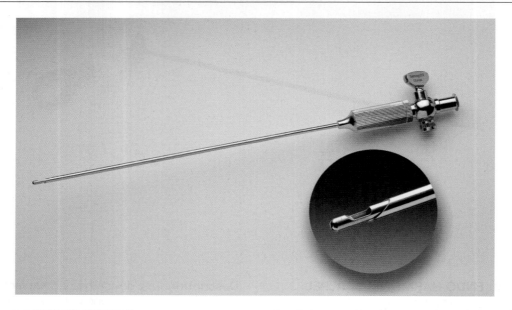

Instrument: VERRES NEEDLE
Other Names: Insufflation needle
Use(s): Used to enter the peritoneum and deliver carbon dioxide into the abdominal cavity to create a pneumoperitoneum.
Description: A hollow bore with a spring-loaded, retractable blunt stylet that extends beyond the tip of the needle. A stopcock at the proximal end is the connection site for the insufflation tubing.
Instrument Insight: The stylet retracts as the needle is pushed against tissue and will automatically advance upon entrance into the peritoneum.

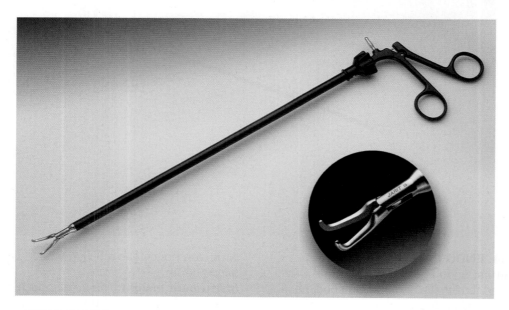

Instrument: ENDO RIGHT ANGLE FORCEPS
Other Names: Mixter
Use(s): Used for separating tissue planes and dissecting around tubular structures.
Description: A curved, right angle tip with cross-hatch serration running the length of the inner jaws.
Instrument Insight: Often dissectors have monopolar capabilities. The connection site for the cable is the gold stem at the handle end, and the current is activated with a foot pedal. As a general rule, dissectors do not have ratchet handles, but graspers do have ratchet handles.

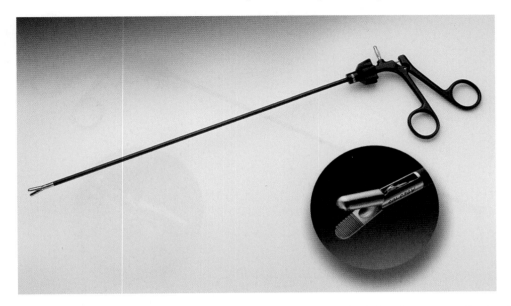

Instrument: BLUNT DISSECTOR
Use(s): Used for blunt dissection and separation of tissue planes.
Description: A straight rounded tip with horizontal serrations and a proximal recess.

Instrument Insight: As a general rule, dissectors do not have ratchet handles, but graspers do. Often dissectors have monopolar capabilities. The connection site for the cable is the gold stem at the handle end, and the current is activated with a foot pedal.

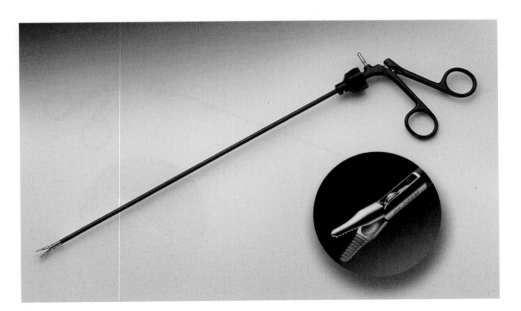

Instrument: DOLPHIN NOSE DISSECTOR
Use(s): Used for fine dissection and separation of thin adventitial tissue.
Description: Straight jaws that taper to a fine point with horizontal serrations and a proximal recess.

Instrument Insight: Often dissectors have monopolar capabilities. The connection site for the cable is the gold stem at the handle end, and the current is activated with a foot pedal. As a general rule, dissectors do not have ratchet handles, but graspers do.

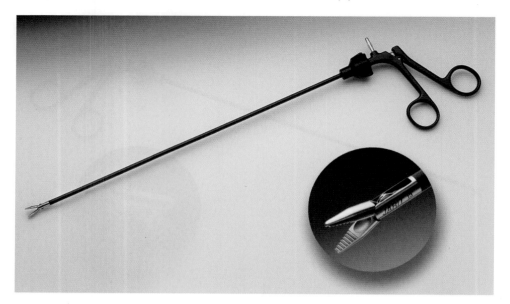

Instrument: CONE TIP DISSECTOR
Other Names: Bullet nose dissector
Use(s): Used for blunt dissection and separation of tissue planes.
Description: Bullet-shaped tapered jaws with horizontal serrations and a proximal recess

Instrument Insight: Often dissectors have monopolar capabilities. The connection site for the cable is the gold stem at the handle end, and the current is activated with a foot pedal. As a general rule, dissectors do not have ratchet handles, but graspers do.

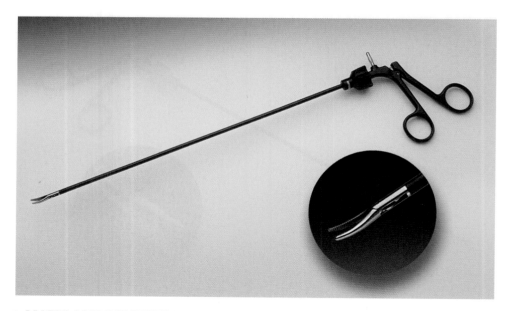

Instrument: MARYLAND DISSECTOR
Use(s): Used for fine dissection and separation of thin adventitial tissue.
Description: Curved, fine-tapered jaws with horizontal serrations running the length of the jaws.

Instrument Insight: Often dissectors have monopolar capabilities. The connection site for the cable is the gold stem at the handle end, and the current is activated with a foot pedal. As a general rule, dissectors do not have ratchet handles, but graspers do.

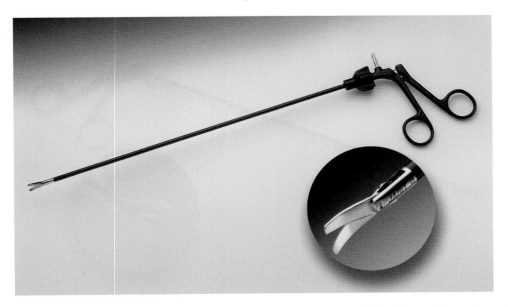

Instrument: ENDOSCOPIC SCISSORS
Other Names: Endo shears, coag scissors
Use(s): Cut and dissect tissues, ducts, vessels, and suture material.
Description: Rounded, blunt tip with curved blades.

Instrument Insight: Generally endo scissors have monopolar capabilities. The connection site for the cable is the gold stem at the handle end, and the current is activated with a foot pedal.

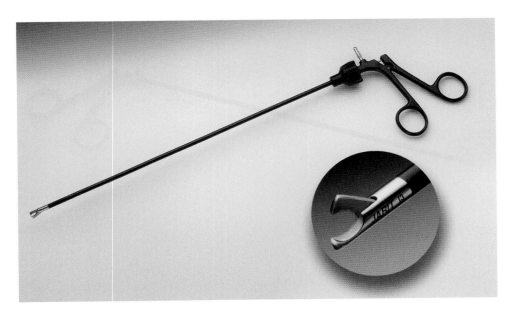

Instrument: ENDOSCOPIC HOOK SCISSORS
Use(s): Used to lift, isolate, and transect tissues such as ducts and vessels.
Description: Straight, squared-off blunt tip with concave arching of the inner cutting blades.

Instrument Insight: Generally endo scissors have monopolar capabilities. The connection site for the cable is the gold stem at the handle end, and the current is activated with a foot pedal.

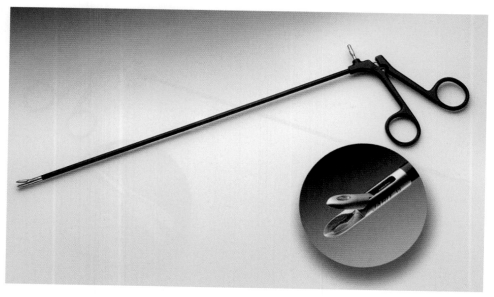

Instrument: ENDOSCOPIC BIOPSY FORCEPS
Use(s): Used for excision of small pieces of tissue for examination.
Description: Sharp, oval cup-shaped jaws that are fenestrated.

Instrument Insight: To prevent crushing or damaging the biopsy tissue, it can be swished in saline or pushed out with a fine needle through the fenestration in the jaws.

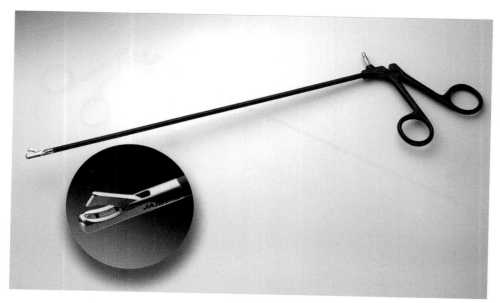

Instrument: ENDOSCOPIC BIOPSY PUNCH
Use(s): Used for excision of small pieces of heavy tissue for examination.
Description: Rectangular-shaped hollow jaws; the upper jaw has a sharp rim that fits inside

the serrated edge of the lower jaw when closed.
Instrument Insight: To prevent crushing or damaging the biopsy tissue, it can be swished in saline or pushed out with a fine needle.

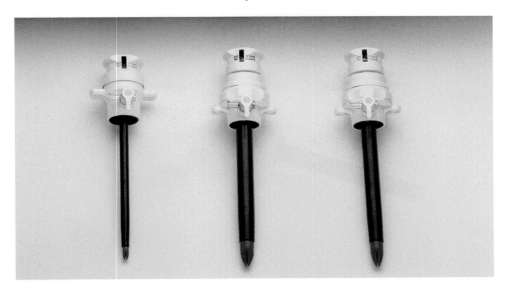

Instrument: VERSA PORT TROCARS

Use(s): Used to create an instrument port in which the endoscope and instruments can be introduced and exchanged through the cannula.

Description: A single-use, V-shaped, scalpel-bladed trocar with a spring-locking shield and a trocar cannula three-way stopcock. Versa port trocar sizes are 5 mm, 5-11 mm, and 5-12 mm. Rapid change continues to occur in the development and improvement of all trocars. Those pictured represent a few manufacturer variations.

Instrument Insight: Upon entrance into a cavity, the shield advances to cover the blade, reducing the potential for injury to internal structures. The trocar cannula has a self-adjusting seal that prevents pneumoperitoneal loss when exchanging instruments and a three-way stopcock for gas insufflation and rapid desufflation. The self-adjusting seal accommodates from 5 mm to 12 mm as appropriate.

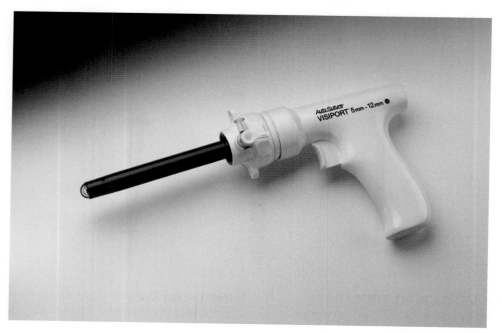

Instrument: VISIPORT
Other Names: Optical trocar
Use(s): Used to create an instrument port in which the endoscope and instruments can be introduced and exchanged through the cannula.
Description: A single-use, gun-like optical trocar that consists of a sheath with a blunt clear dome at the distal end that encases a crescent shaped knife blade. The pistol grip handle includes a trigger and an opening at the top that accommodates a 10-mm laparoscope, which allows for visualization through the clear dome as the sheath passes through the abdominal or thoracic body wall. When the trigger is squeezed, the blade extends approximately 1 mm beyond the dome and instantaneously retracts. This action allows for a controlled, sharp dissection through the tissue layers. The Visiport™ is available in 5 mm to 11 mm or 5 mm to 12 mm diameters.
Instrument Insight: When entering into a cavity, the clear dome shields the blade there by reducing the potential for injury to internal structures. The trocar cannula has a self-adjusting seal that prevents pneumoperitoneal loss when exchanging instruments and a three-way stopcock for gas insufflation and rapid desufflation. The self-adjusting seal accommodates 5 mm to 12 mm as appropriate.

GRASPING AND HOLDING INSTRUMENTS

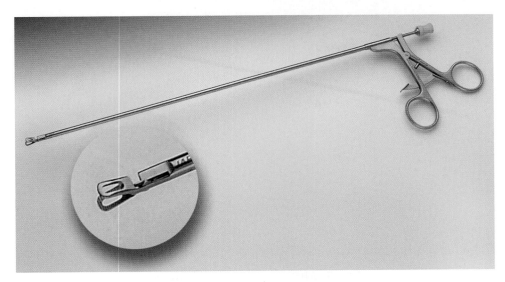

Instrument: ENDOSCOPIC CHOLANGIOGRAM FORCEPS

Other Names: Olsen clamp

Use(s): This forceps is used to grasp the cholangiogram catheter and guide it into the common bile duct for the injection of the contrast media.

Description: A long grasping forceps with a proximal port, which leads to rounded fenestrated and horizontal serrated jaws.

Instrument Insight: The cholangiogram catheter is fed through the proximal port until the tip extends just beyond the jaws forceps. The forceps is then closed, holding the catheter in place.

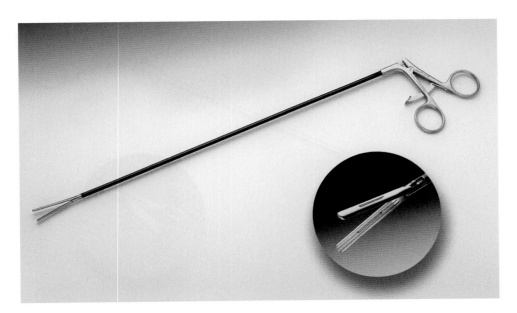

Instrument: ENDOSCOPIC DEBAKEY FORCEPS

Use(s): Used for grasping of tissues and organs without causing trauma.

Description: Fenestrated elongated jaws with a blunt tip with two parallel rows of fine serrations running the length of one of the jaws. The other jaw has one row of serrations in the center that interlocks when closed.

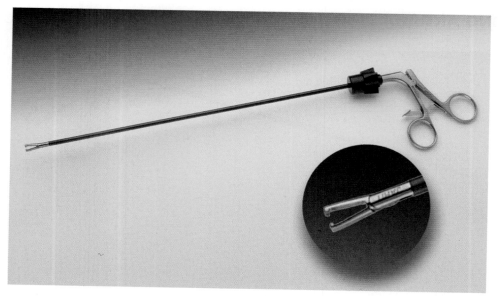

Instrument: ENDOSCOPIC ALLIS FORCEPS
Use(s): Lifts, holds, and retracts slippery dense tissue.

Description: Straight jaws with multiple, intertwining fine teeth at the tip.

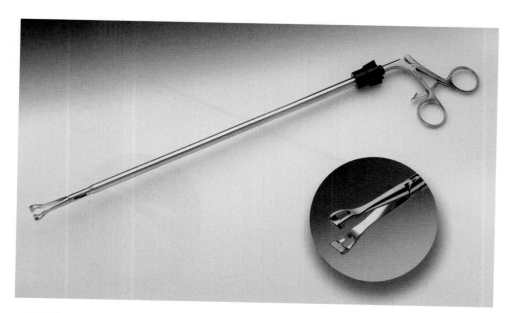

Instrument: ENDOSCOPIC BABCOCK FORCEPS
Use(s): Used for grasping and encircling delicate structures such as the ureters, fallopian tubes, ovaries, appendix, or bowel.

Description: Has a flared, rounded end with smooth, flattened tips. Comes in both 5-mm and 10-mm sizes and can be either disposable or nondisposable.

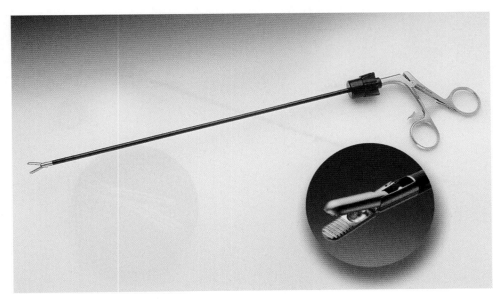

Instrument: BLUNT GRASPER

Use(s): Used for grasping and manipulating tissues and organs, causing minimal trauma. These graspers are often used on tissue that is to be removed.

Description: A straight, rounded tip with horizontal serrations and a proximal recess.

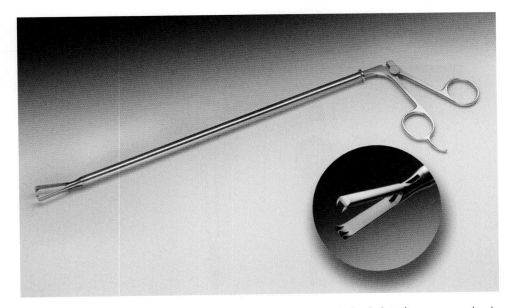

Instrument: CLAW GRASPER

Other Names: Mother-in-law

Use(s): Used for penetrating and holding excised organs and tissues for extraction from the abdominal cavity.

Description: Wide, elongated spring-loaded jaws with 2 × 3 heavy interlocking teeth.

Instrument Insight: As a general rule, graspers have ratcheted handles, but dissectors do not.

⚠ CAUTION: Exercise care when handling penetrating forceps. The sharp tips can easily comprise the integrity of gloves or skin.

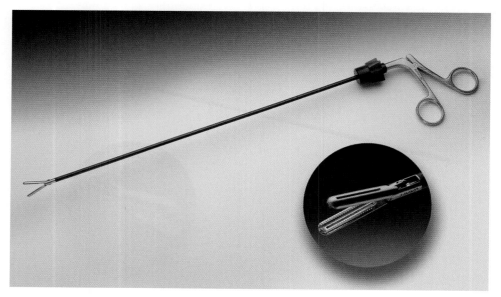

Instrument: HUNTER BOWEL GRASPER
Use(s): Used for atraumatic grasping and manipulating delicate tissues, such as the bowel and stomach.

Description: Fine, long jaws with rounded tips and DeBakey-style serrations.

PROBING AND DILATING INSTRUMENTS

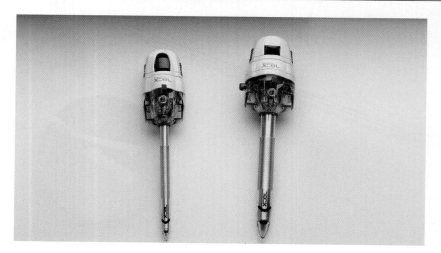

Instrument: XCEL TROCARS
Use(s): Used to create an instrument port in which the endoscope and instruments can be introduced and exchanged through the cannula.
Description: Optic tip bladeless trocar with a universal sealed sheath and a three-way stopcock.

Instrument Insight: After the creation of a pneumoperitoneum, a small skin incision is made at the port site. A downward twisting motion causes the tissue to separate, eliminating the need for the tissue to be cut. The optic tip allows the surgeon to place the laparoscope inside the trocar to view the tissue layer during insertion.

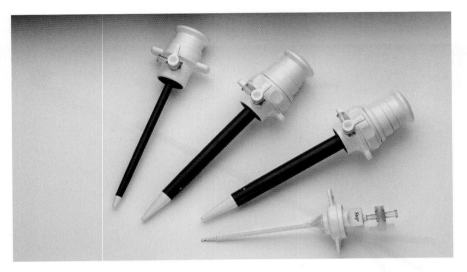

Instrument: VERSA STEP TROCARS

Use(s): Used to create an instrument port in which the endoscope and instruments can be introduced and exchanged through the sheath or cannula.

Description: A radial-dilating trocar system, which includes an expandable mesh sleeve, an insufflation/access needle, a blunt-tip fascial obturator and sheath, and a three-way stopcock. Rapid change continues to occur in the development and improvement of trocars. Those pictured represent a few manufacturer variations.

Instrument Insight: After the creation of a pneumoperitoneum, a small skin incision is made at the port site. The expandable mesh sleeve is loaded over the access needle and introduced into the peritoneum. After removing the needle, the blunt-tip obturator loaded into the sheath is passed through the mesh sleeve into the peritoneum. The obturator is removed, and the sheath is left for introduction of instruments.

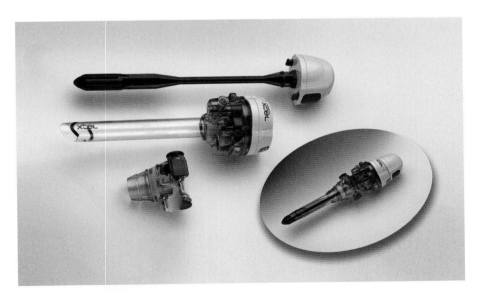

Instrument: BLUNT TROCAR

Other Names: Hasson, Xcel blunt port, blunt tip

Use(s): Placed in a variety of areas but most often at the umbilical site for creation of a pneumoperitoneum; a blunt trocar is often the port used for the laparoscope.

Description: A 5-mm to 12-mm trocar with a blunt obturator, self-sealing sheath or cannula with three-way stopcock, and a grip-anchoring device to secure it in place.

Instrument Insight: The blunt trocar is used for the open or "Hasson" technique. This is accomplished by making a small incision at the umbilical area into the peritoneum. The blunt trocar is then placed and anchored down (usually with suture), and insufflation takes place. This is another technique to first visualize the abdominal cavity before placing a sharp trocar, therefore preventing tissue or organ damage.

RETRACTING AND EXPOSING INSTRUMENTS

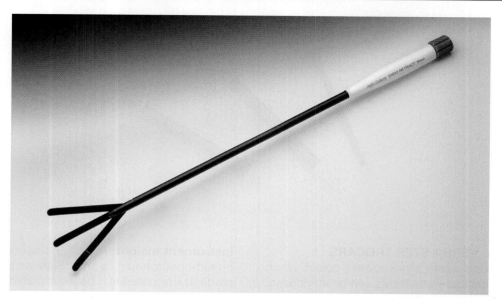

Instrument: ENDO FAN RETRACTOR
Other Names: Fan finger retractor, Peacock retractor
Use(s): Used for elevation, retraction, and mobilization of organs and tissues, providing optimal visualization of the surgical field.
Description: A single-use retractor with three or five telescoping atraumatic blades,

Instrument Insight: The finger blades should be fully closed upon insertion and removal from the cannula. The blades are closed by turning the proximal teal knob counterclockwise and are deployed by turning the knob clockwise.

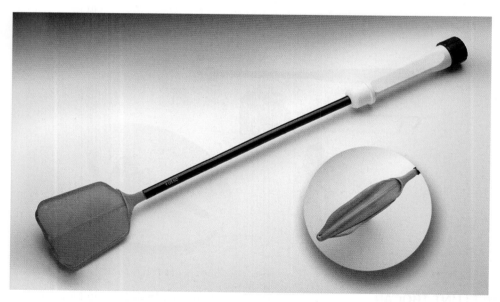

Instrument: ENDO PADDLE RETRACTOR
Use(s): Used for elevation, retraction, and mobilization of organs and tissues, providing optimal visualization of the surgical field.
Description: A single-use retractor with a nylon-covered paddle frame, introducer sheath with seal housing, and black rotation knob.
Instrument Insight: To retract the paddle, turn the rotation knob clockwise until the paddle is fully closed. Push the white seal housing

forward until the paddle is completely housed inside the introducer sheath. Grasp the seal housing, and insert the retractor through the trocar cannula. After it is inserted through the cannula, pull the seal housing back completely, exposing the paddle. Turn the rotation knob counterclockwise to deploy the paddle within the body cavity. The paddle must be fully retracted and housed in the introducer sheath before removal.

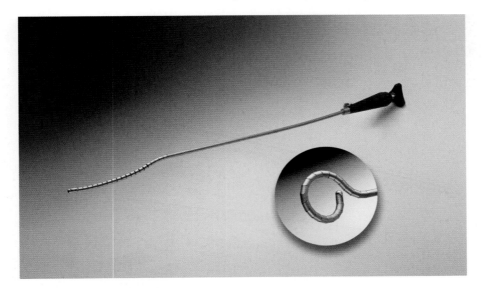

Instrument: ENDOFLEX RETRACTOR
Other Name: Snake retractor, Diamond-flex
Use(s): Used for elevation, retraction, and mobilization of abdominal organs providing optimal visualization during endoscopic procedures. Commonly used for retraction of the liver in complex upper GI procedures, such as fundoplication and gastric bypass.
Description: The device originates as snake-like, malleable, hollow, 5-mm metal tubes with small individual sections at the working end that are threaded over internal tension cables that are affixed at the tip. Each individual tubular section is cut obliquely so that when the inner metal cables are tightened by turning the knob on the handle, the retractors conform into its designated shape.
Instrument Insight: Normally, the retractor is inserted loose and flexible though a 5-mm port and articulated after being placed within the abdominal cavity to form the retractor.

SUCTIONING AND ASPIRATING INSTRUMENTS

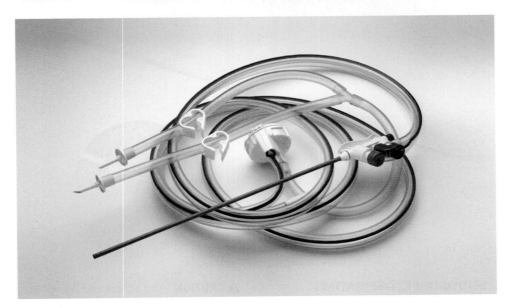

Instrument: SUCTION IRRIGATOR
Use(s): Used to irrigate and aspirate fluid and debris from the surgical site.
Description: Long, straight, hollow suction tube attached to a combination tubing that has a suction valve and an irrigation valve.
Instrument Insight: There are many types and manufacturers of suction irrigators, such as gravity, pump, or battery operated.

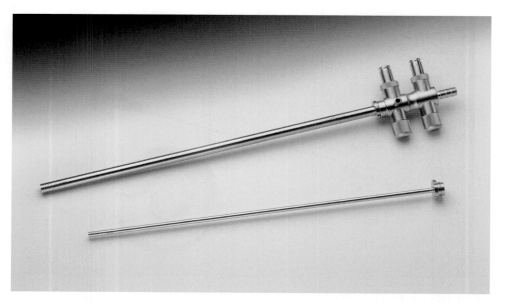

Instrument: NEZHAT-DORSEY SUCTION TIPS
Use(s): This suction tip is used for irrigating and aspirating fluid and debris from the surgical site.

Description: A long, hollow suction tip with a bivalve. One is for suction and the other for irrigation.

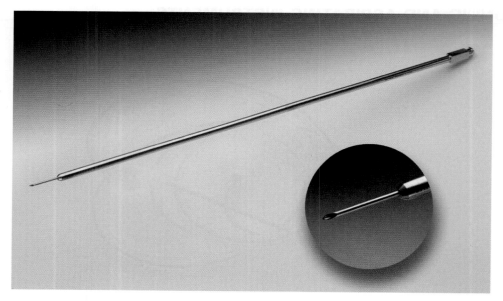

Instrument: ENDOSCOPIC ASPIRATING NEEDLE
Use(s): This needle is used for aspiration of body fluids and cysts.
Description: The proximal end is a Luer-Lok fitting that is attached to a long 5-mm hollow tube with a 19-gauge needle tip.

⚠ CAUTION: The tip should be within the vision of the operator at all times when in the abdominal cavity. The aspiration is accomplished by attaching a syringe or suction.

SUTURING AND STAPLING INSTRUMENTS

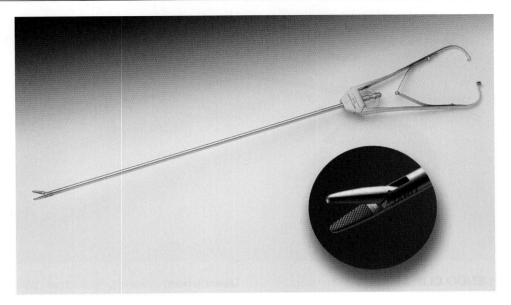

Instrument: APPLE NEEDLE HOLDER

Use(s): Used to securely grasp the needle during suturing.

Description: Tapered straight, curved, or angled tip with cross-hatch carbon-bite inner jaws and a leaf-spring mechanism handle for ease in release and closure.

Instrument Insight: The apple needle holder is designed for grasping 5–0 and smaller needles.

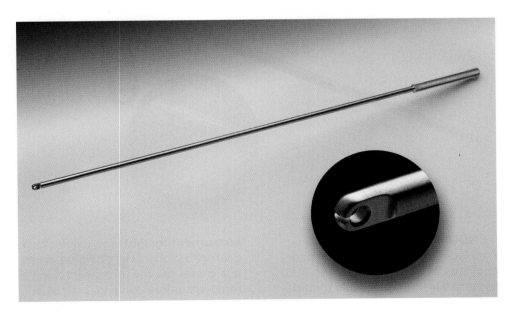

Instrument: KNOT PUSHER

Use(s): Guides knots from outside of the trocar cannula to the suture site. This technique is known as extracorporeal suturing.

Description: A long cylinder rod with a round hole towards the end and a transverse slot at the very tip.

Instrument Insight: The throw of the suture is placed into the open slot and slid into the round hole; it is then guided through the cannula to the suture site, which sets the knot. This action is repeated until the knot is secure.

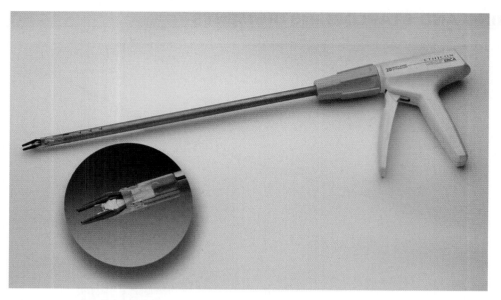

Instrument: ENDO CLIP APPLIER
Other Names: Hemoclip, clip
Use(s): Used for occluding vessels or other tubular structures.

Description: A sterile, individual patient-use instrument, preloaded with clips. These are manufactured in various titanium clip sizes from 5 mm to 10 mm and different lengths.

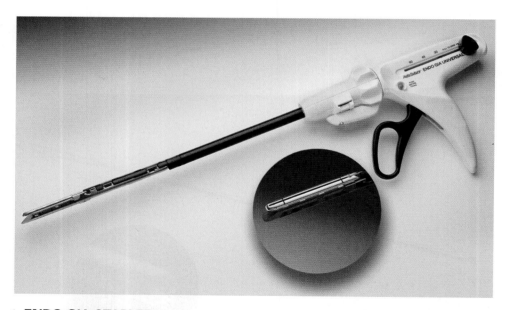

Instrument: ENDO GIA STAPLER
Use(s): Often used during laparoscopic appendectomy and gastric and bowel resections. Also used to transect tissues in endoscopic thoracic or gynecological procedures.
Description: A single patient-use, reloadable articulating and rotating stapler that distributes two triple, staggered rows of titanium staples while cutting the tissues between the rows. The length is determined by the tissue to be excised. This stapler is available in 30-mm, 45-mm, and 60-mm sizes.

Instrument Insight: The stapler loads come packaged with a bright-colored plastic safety guard over the row of staples that needs to be removed before handing it to the surgeon. Activation is accomplished by sliding forward the firing knob on the side of the stapler until it stops completely. The manufacturer recommends the stapler can be reloaded up to 25 times for a total of 25 applications.

VIEWING INSTRUMENTS

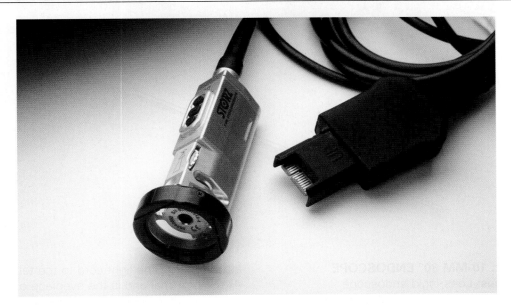

Instrument: ENDOSCOPIC CAMERA

Use(s): Used for the transmission of images from the rigid or flexible endoscope to the video monitor.

Description: At the distal end of the camera is the coupler that attaches the camera to the eyepiece of the rigid scope. The coupler is attached to the camera head, which provides the image quality. Attached to the camera head is a cord, which relays the images back to the video system.

Instrument Insight: Most camera failures are related to a damaged cord. Care should be exercised when handling the camera and cord. They should never be placed under a heavy object or dropped, twisted, or kinked. Also keep the distal end covered until it is ready to be plugged into the unit.

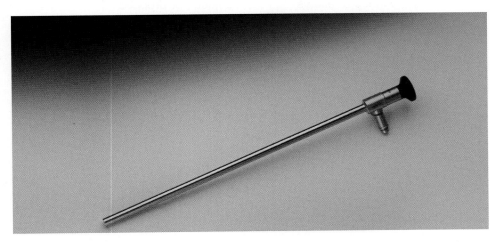

Instrument: 10-MM 0° ENDOSCOPE

Other Names: Lens, rigid endoscope

Use(s): Provide visualization of body cavities and content, which may include internal organs and structures, through an orifice or surgical opening.

Description: A rigid, stainless-steel, 10-mm endoscope containing an optical chain of precisely aligned glass lenses and spacers. The objective lens is located at the distal tip of the scope. This determines the viewing angle. The stainless-steel cylinder rod is called the optical element or the telescope, providing both images and light. The light connector allows attachment of the light cord to the telescope. At the proximal end is the eyepiece or ocular lens; this attaches to the camera coupler, or the surgeon may directly view the cavity.

Instrument Insight: 10 mm indicates the diameter of the scope, and 0° is the forward angle in which the objective lens views. Endoscopes are expensive and fragile. Care should be exercised when handling an endoscope; it should never be picked up by the distal telescope end, placed under heavy objects, or dropped.

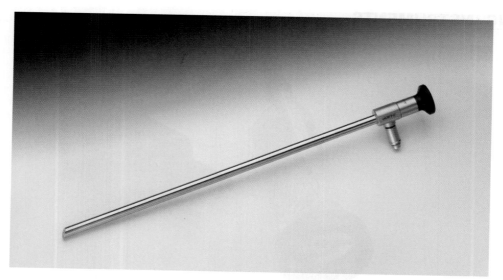

Instrument: 10-MM 30° ENDOSCOPE
Other Names: Lens, rigid endoscope
Use(s): Used for visualization of body cavities, internal organs, and structures through an orifice or surgical opening.
Description: A nonflexible, stainless-steel, 10-mm endoscope containing an optical chain of precisely aligned glass lenses and spacers. The objective lens is located at the distal tip of the scope. This determines the viewing angle. The stainless-steel cylinder rod is called the optical element or the telescope, providing both images and light. The light connector allows attachment of the light cord to the telescope. At the proximal end is the eyepiece or ocular lens; this attaches to the camera coupler, or the surgeon may directly view the cavity.

Instrument Insight: 10 mm indicates the diameter of the scope, and 30° is the oblique angle in which the objective lens views.

⚠ CAUTION: Endoscopes are expensive and fragile. Care should be exercised when handling an endoscope; it should never be picked up by the distal telescope end, placed under heavy objects, or dropped.

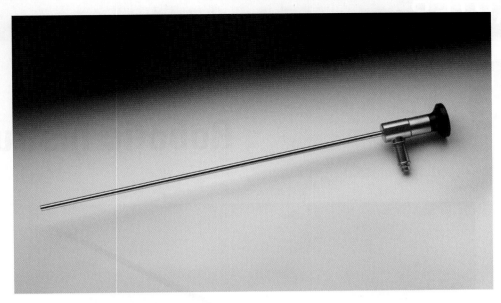

Instrument: 5-MM 0° ENDOSCOPE

Other Names: Lens rigid endoscope

Use(s): Used for visualization of body cavities, internal organs, and structures through an orifice or surgical opening.

Description: A nonflexible, stainless-steel, 5-mm endoscope containing an optical chain of precisely aligned glass lenses and spacers. The objective lens is located at the distal tip of the scope. This determines the viewing angle. The stainless-steel cylinder rod is called the optical element or the telescope, providing both images and light.

The light connector allows attachment of the light cord to the telescope. At the proximal end is the eyepiece or ocular lens; this attaches to the camera coupler, or the surgeon may directly view the cavity.

Instrument Insight: 5 mm indicates the diameter of the scope, and 0° is the forward angle in which the objective lens views.

⚠ **CAUTION:** Endoscopes are expensive and fragile. Care should be exercised when handling an endoscope; it should never be picked up by the distal telescope end, placed under heavy objects, or dropped.

5

Robotic Instruments

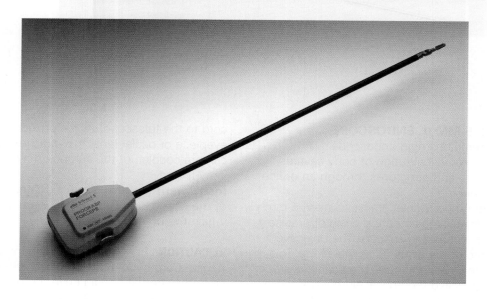

Instrument: *ENDOWRIST*

Use(s): The *EndoWrist* instruments are modeled after the human wrist and fasten to the electromechanical arms of the da Vinci System. These instruments offer full range of motion and natural dexterity that represents the surgeon's right and left hand when preforming intricate tissue manipulation and dissection through minute ports. The da Vinci System is commonly used for but not limited to gynecological, urological, general, cardiovascular, and otorhinolaryngology specialties.

Description: The EndoWrist tips are characterized by instruments that are commonly used by the surgeons in open and minimally invasive surgeries; these include scissors, forceps, retractors, scalpels, electrocautery, and others that are commonly used devices. These are approximately 5 to 8 mm in diameter and between 49 and 51 cm in length.

Instrument Insight: EndoWrist instruments are called "smart disposables" because they are resterilized and reused for a distinct number of procedures. An internal computer chip confirms the manufacturer, the type and function of the instrument, and the number of past uses. The chip will not allow the instrument to be used if it has exceeded the approved number of procedures. This assures proper performance of the instrument during every procedure.

ACCESSORY INSTRUMENTS

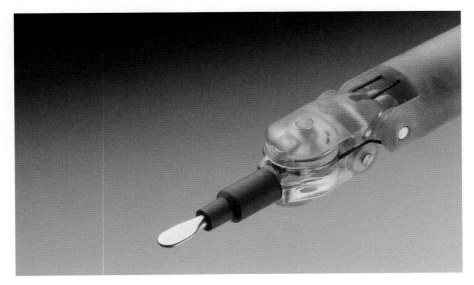

Instrument: PERMANENT CAUTERY SPATULA
Other Names: Bovie, cautery
Use(s): Coagulates tissues and maintains hemostasis and aids in blunt dissection.

Description: A monopolar cautery device with a long paddle blade.
Instrument Insight: All of the EndoWrist instruments that have electrosurgical capabilities have an amber colored insulation at the wrist joint.

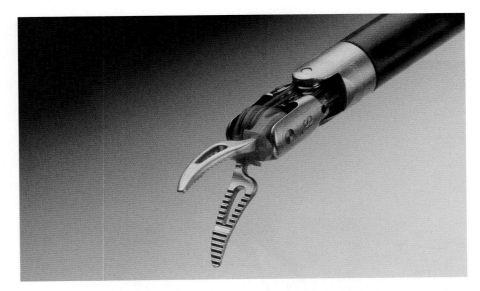

Instrument: MARYLAND BIPOLAR FORCEPS
Other Names: Bipolar, Maryland
Use(s): Used for grasping, dissecting, and coagulating tissues.
Description: A bipolar device with curved tapered jaws and triangular fenestration at the base.

Instrument Insight: All of the EndoWrist instruments that have electrosurgical capabilities have amber colored insulation at the wrist joint.

CUTTING AND DISSECTING INSTRUMENTS

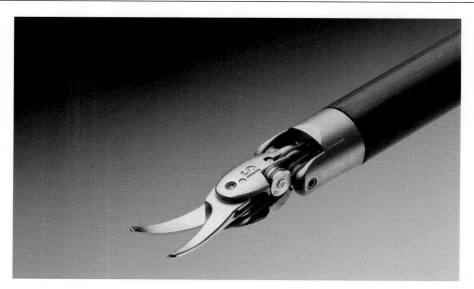

Instrument: CURVED SCISSORS
Other Names: Shears
Use(s): Used for precision cutting and sharp and blunt dissection of tissue.

Description: Curved, beveled blades with tapered atraumatic tips.

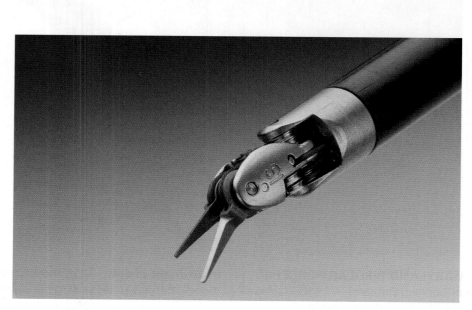

Instrument: POTTS SCISSORS
Use(s): Used for the creation of an arteriotomy for coronary anastomosis.

Description: Straight, fine, tapered, beveled blades.

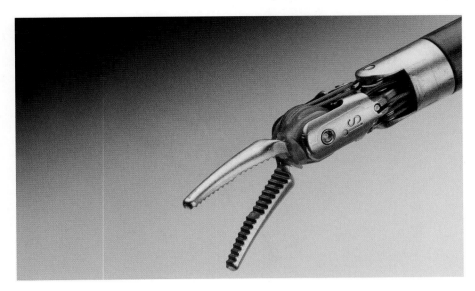

Instrument: PK DISSECTING FORCEPS
Other Names: PK
Use(s): This is used for grasping, coagulating, and cutting tissues.
Description: The PK has curved and tapering outer jaws with horizontal serration that runs the length of the inner jaws.

Instrument Insight: The PK provides radiofrequency energy to seal, transect, and mobilize tissues at low temperature, which minimizes tissue sticking, charring, and plume.

All of the EndoWrist instruments that have electrosurgical capabilities have amber colored insulation at the wrist joint.

GRASPING AND HOLDING INSTRUMENTS

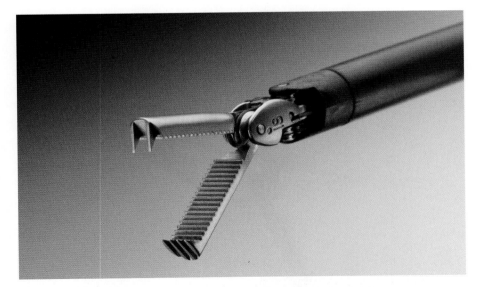

Instrument: COBRA GRASPER
Other Names: Biter, Toothed grasper, Cobra
Use(s): The cobra is used for grasping and retracting dense tissues. Commonly used for grasping the pelvic fascial layers during cuff closure in a hysterectomy.

Description: Straight jaws with horizontal serration running the length. At the tip, one jaw has two sharp teeth and the other has four, and when closed they interlock.

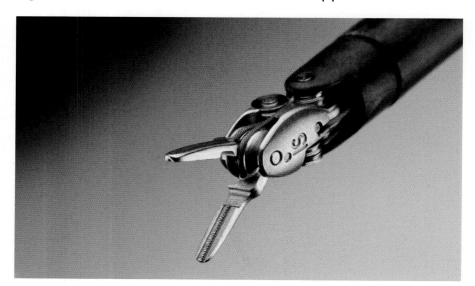

Instrument: DEBAKEY FORCEPS

Use(s): Facilitates atraumatic tissue handling.

Description: Straight smooth forceps with an elongated, narrowed blunt tip. A set of parallel fine serrations runs the length of one jaw with a center row of serrations on the opposite side that interlocks to grip when closed.

Instrument Insight: Considered a vascular tissue forceps, but commonly used in all specialty areas because of its ability to securely grip without causing damage to tissues.

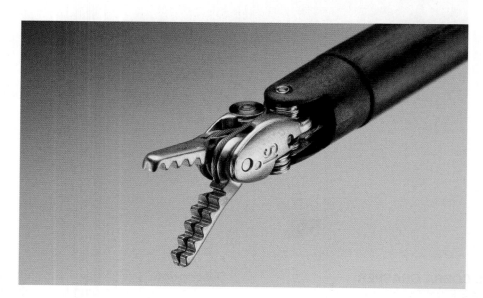

Instrument: RESANO FORCEPS

Other Names: Shark forceps

Use(s): Facilitates firm but atraumatic handling of valve and arterial tissues.

Description: Smooth, straight outer jaws with blunt triangular serration that interlock when closed.

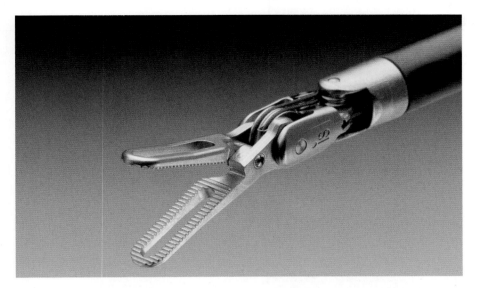

Instrument: PROGRASP™ FORCEPS
Other Names: Delicate Grasper, Fenestrated
Use(s): Used to grasp and retract delicate tissues. Commonly used to grasp and retract bowel during abdominal procedures.

Description: Smooth, flattened wide outer jaws with an oval fenestration in the middle and horizontal serration running the length of the inner jaws.

RETRACTING AND EXPOSING INSTRUMENTS

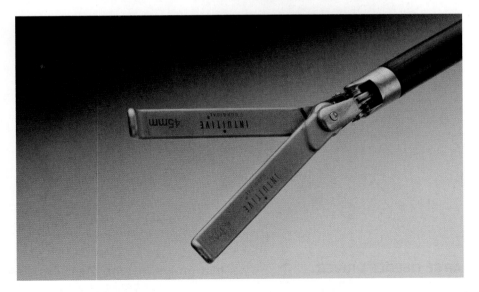

Instrument: ARTERIAL RETRACTOR
Other Names: Fan retractor, finger retractor
Use(s): The arterial retractor provides exposure of the mitral valve and atrial retraction. Often used during a mitral valve repair.

Description: Two straight atraumatic blades with a slight curve at the end.
Instrument Insight: The two blades of the arterial retractor draw in on one another to resemble one blade, which facilitates insertion in a tiny port.

SUTURING AND STAPLING INSTRUMENTS

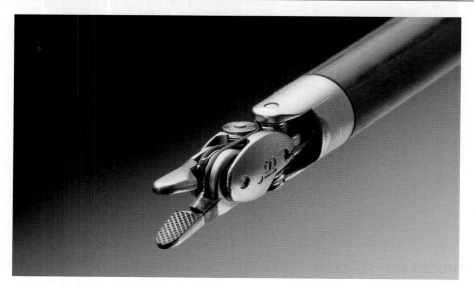

Instrument: SUTURECUT NEEDLE DRIVER
Use(s): Used for grasping needles and cutting suture. Often used when placing interrupted suture; also used when closing the vaginal cuff during a hysterectomy.

Description: Tapered, smooth outer jaws with cross-hatch serration on the inner and scissor blades at the base.
Instrument Insight: Suturing and cutting with one instrument reduces instrument exchange and saves time.

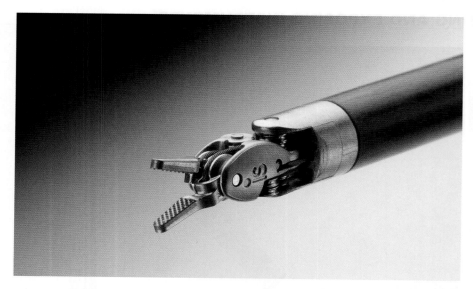

Instrument: LARGE NEEDLE DRIVER
Other Names: Large needle holder
Use(s): Used for securing the needle while suturing tissues.
Description: A straight, smooth, tapering outer jaw with diamond pattern carbide inserts in the inner jaw.

Instrument Insight: The carbide inserts give the needle holder better griping properties to secure the needle.

Obstetrics and Gynecologic Instruments

6

ACCESSORY INSTRUMENTS

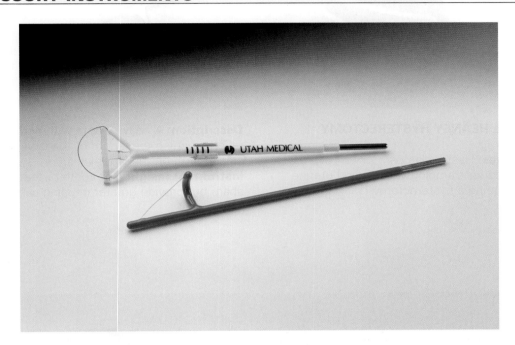

Instrument: LEEP LOOP ELECTRODE
Other Names: Loop
Use(s): Used for removing abnormal cervical cells electrosurgically for further pathological examination.
Description: This procedure is often called a hot cone biopsy. Most loops have an insulated shaft and crossbar to prevent accidental thermal injury with a stainless steel or tungsten wire of the loop that is approximately 0.2 mm thick.
Instrument Insight: The size and shape of the loop will be determined by the amount of cervical dysplasia and surgeon preference.

CLAMPING AND OCCLUDING INSTRUMENTS

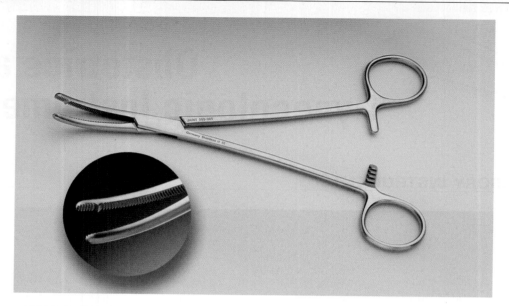

Instrument: HEANEY HYSTERECTOMY FORCEPS
Other Names: Hyster clamps
Use(s): Used for clamping vessels and uterine ligaments during a hysterectomy.

Description: A heavy clamp with horizontal serrations running the length of the jaws and with a single tooth on the inner jaws.
Instrument Insight: The tooth or teeth are not sharp but provide greater gripping capabilities.

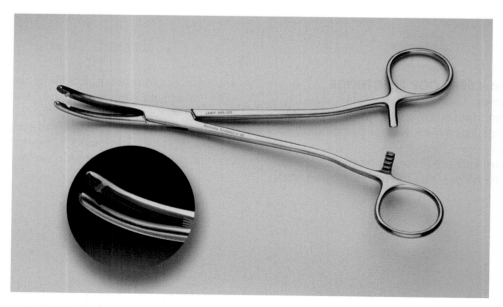

Instrument: HEANEY-BALLENTINE HYSTERECTOMY FORCEPS
Other Names: Heaney clamp, Masterson
Use(s): Used for clamping vessels and ligaments during a hysterectomy.
Description: A heavy clamp with vertical serrations running the length of the jaws and with a single or double tooth on the inner jaws; can have either straight or curved jaws.
Instrument Insight: The tooth or teeth are not sharp but provide greater gripping capabilities.

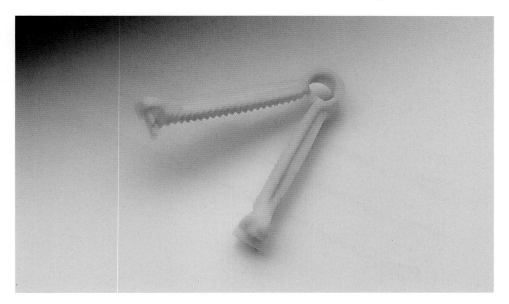

Instrument: CORD CLAMP
Use(s): The cord clamp is used to clamp the cord of the neonate; the cord remains attached to the newborn following separation from the placenta.

Description: A plastic disposable clamp with horizontal serrations running the length of the jaws.
Instrument Insight: The cord clamp is a single-use device and should not be closed before use because this can damage its reliability.

CUTTING AND DISSECTING INSTRUMENTS

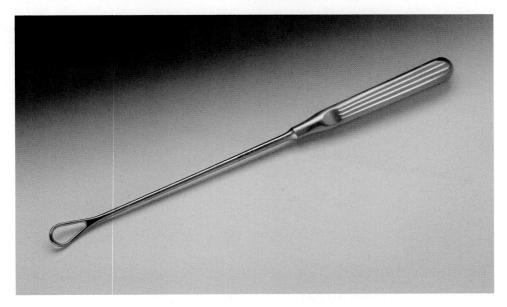

Instrument: THOMAS UTERINE CURETTE
Other Names: Blunt curette
Use(s): Used for bluntly removing uterine contents after sharp curetting.

Description: A hollow grip handle that extends to a malleable shaft and a blunt looped tip.

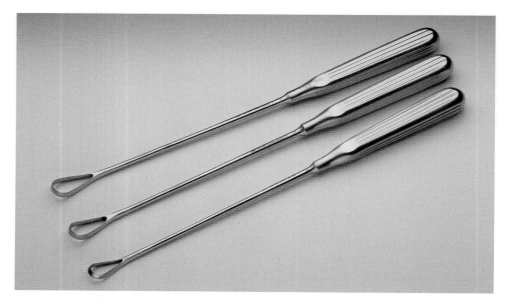

Instrument: SIMS UTERINE CURETTE
Other Names: Sharp curettes
Use(s): Used for scraping the endocervical and endometrial lining of the uterus during a dilation and curettage (D&C) procedure.

Description: A hollow grip handle that extends to a malleable shaft and a sharp looped tip.
Instrument Insight: The shaft is malleable so that the surgeon can bend it to the angle needed to scrape the uterus.

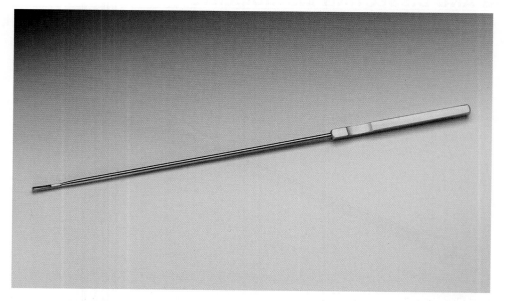

Instrument: KEVORKIAN ENDOCERVICAL CURETTE
Other Names: Endocervical curette, box curette
Use(s): Used for obtaining cervical scrapings or biopsies.

Description: A grip handle that extends to a narrow and sharp rectangular tip.

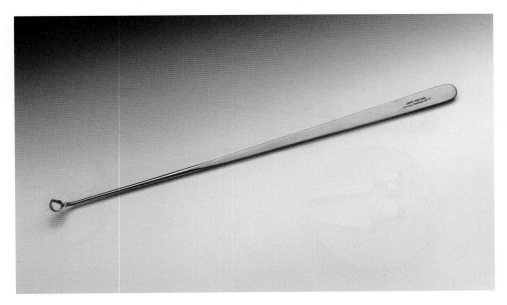

Instrument: HEANEY UTERINE BIOPSY CURETTE
Use(s): Used for obtaining uterine scrapings.
Description: A flattened handle that extends to a sharp, serrated looped tip.

⚠ **CAUTION:** The serrations are sharp and can easily compromise the integrity of your gloves, skin and those of the surgeon.

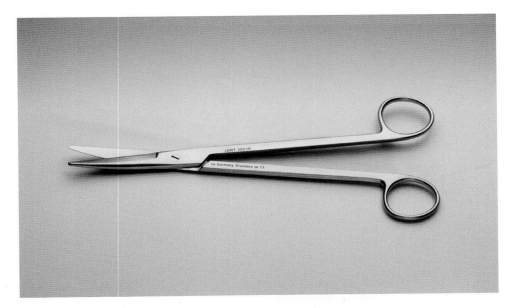

Instrument: MAYO UTERINE SCISSORS
Other Names: Uterine scissors
Use(s): Used for cutting the heavy uterine ligaments and vessels during a total abdominal hysterectomy.

Description: Long heavy scissors with curved or straight blades. The straight blades are usually used for cutting suture and the curved blades for cutting tissue.

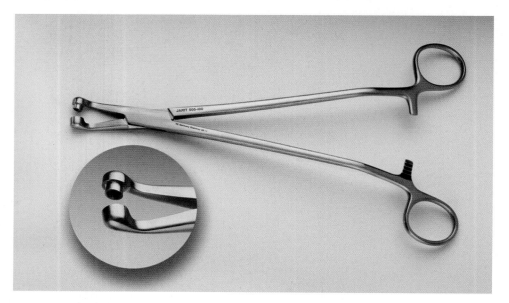

Instrument: THOMAS-GAYLOR UTERINE BIOPSY FORCEPS
Other Names: Gaylor punch
Use(s): Used for taking small bites of uterine tissue for examination.

Description: A ringed instrument with a curved cup tip. The cup tips are sharp, and as they are closed they bite into tissues.

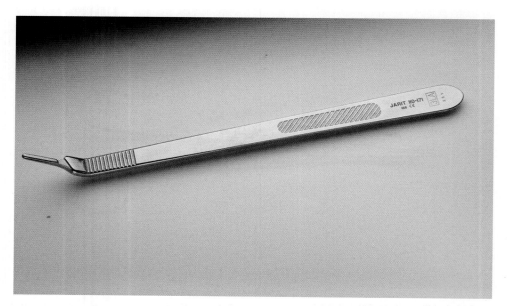

Instrument: LONG ANGLED #3 KNIFE HANDLE
Other Names: Cold cone knife
Use(s): Used for removing abnormal cervical tissues during a cold conization of the cervix.

Description: A long #3 handle that is angled at the blade end.
Instrument Insight: Generally for a conization procedure, the handle is loaded with a #11 blade.

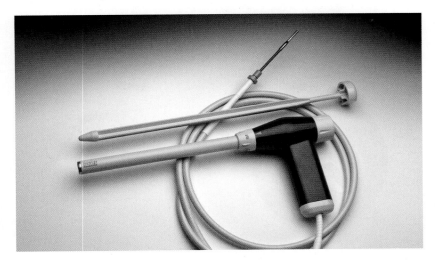

Instrument: GYNECARE MORCELLEX
Other Names: Morcellator
Use(s): The Morcellex is used for cutting, coring, and extracting the uterus and other tissues through a port during a laparoscopic supracervical hysterectomy.
Description: A single patient use device that is packaged with multiple components these are assembled progressively during use. The components are a blade housing assembly, obturator, reducer cap, and detachable handle with attached drive cord. When assembled the device resembles a gun.
Instrument Insight: The steps for assembling the Morcellex: The obturator is inserted into the central lumen of the blade housing assembly. Align the latches and apply pressure until an audible "click" is heard. The assembly will then be inserted under direct visualization through an incision. The obturator is removed by squeezing the latches and pulling it out from the central lumen. The blade housing assembly may be used as an instrument port until the time of tissue morcellation. When morcellation is required, slide the detachable handle into the grooves on the blade housing assembly until it seats firmly. The cord and air tube will be attached to the drive unit. The Morcellex can be activated via foot pedal or by the use of the trigger on the handle based on surgeon's preference.

⚠ **CAUTION:** Do not press the activation trigger during handle attachment.

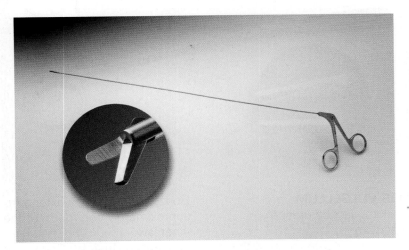

Instrument: HYSTEROSCOPE SCISSORS
Other Names: Hysteroscopic scissors
Use(s): Used for excising tissues and taking biopsies from internal uterus through the hysteroscope.
Description: These scissors have right-angle finger rings at the proximal end that lead to a long flexible wire that turns into straight scissor blades on the distal end. These are very small and will fit through the working channel on the hysteroscope.
Instrument Insight: These are delicate and should be handled with care; the wire portion should not be kinked, and heavy items should never be placed on top of them.

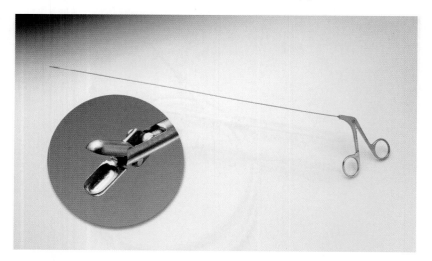

Instrument: HYSTEROSCOPE BIOPSY FORCEPS

Other Names: Biopsy forceps

Use(s): Used for excising tissues and taking biopsies from internal uterus through the hysteroscope.

Description: These forceps have right-angle finger rings at the proximal end that lead to a long flexible wire that turns into a rounded sharp-cup forceps on the distal end. These are very small and will fit through the working channel on the hysteroscope.

Instrument Insight: These are delicate and should be handled with care; the wire portion should not be kinked, and heavy items should never be placed on top of them.

GRASPING AND HOLDING INSTRUMENTS

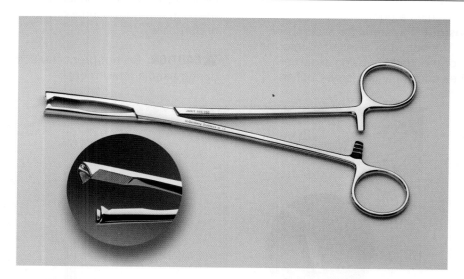

Instrument: JACOBS VULSELLUM

Other Names: Vulsellum, Jacobs uterine forceps, Jacobs tenaculum

Use(s): Used for grasping the anterior lip of the cervix for manipulation. The sharp teeth penetrate the fibrous tissue for greater control. Commonly used during vaginal procedures such as D&C or vaginal hysterectomy.

Description: A curved or straight heavy forceps with a flat, squared tip. Each inner jaw contains two heavy sharp teeth at the outer edge that interlock over each other when compressed. Horizontal serrations extend from the teeth to approximately one fourth of the way down the inner jaw.

Instrument Insight: Because of penetration of the tissue, after removal of the forceps the site should be assessed for bleeding. Hemostasis can be achieved with silver nitrate sticks, cautery, or Monsel solution.

⚠ **CAUTION:** Care should be taken when handling this instrument because the sharp teeth can easily puncture gloves and/or skin.

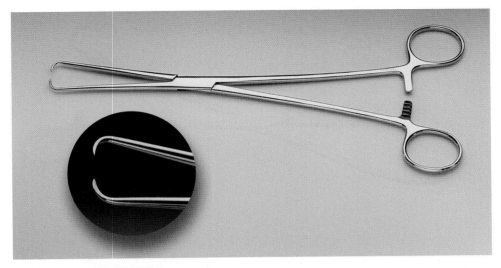

Instrument: SCHROEDER TENACULUM
Other Names: Single-tooth tenaculum, Braun tenaculum
Use(s): Used for grasping the anterior lip of the cervix for manipulation. The sharp prongs on each jaw penetrate the fibrous tissue for greater control. Commonly used during vaginal procedures such as D&C, vaginal hysterectomy, or abdominal hysterectomy.
Description: Smooth round jaws that extend to sharp, inward-curved prongs.

Instrument Insight: Because of penetration of the tissue, after removal of the forceps the site should be assessed for bleeding. Hemostasis can be achieved with silver nitrate sticks, cautery, or Monsel solution.

⚠ **CAUTION:** Care should be taken when handling this instrument because the sharp prongs can easily puncture gloves and/or skin.

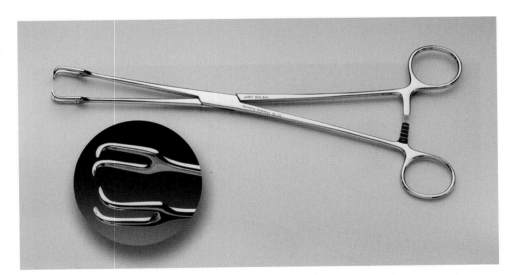

Instrument: SCHROEDER UTERINE VULSELLUM
Other Names: Double-tooth tenaculum
Use(s): Used for grasping the anterior lip of the cervix for manipulation. The sharp prongs on each jaw penetrate the fibrous tissue for greater control. Commonly used during vaginal procedures such as D&C or vaginal hysterectomy.
Description: Curved or straight forceps with smooth, round jaws that bifurcate into two sharp, cupped prongs.

Instrument Insight: Because of penetration of the tissue, after removal of the forceps the site should be assessed for bleeding. Hemostasis can be achieved with silver nitrate sticks, cautery, or Monsel solution.

⚠ **CAUTION:** Care should be taken when handling this instrument because the sharp prongs can easily puncture gloves and/or skin.

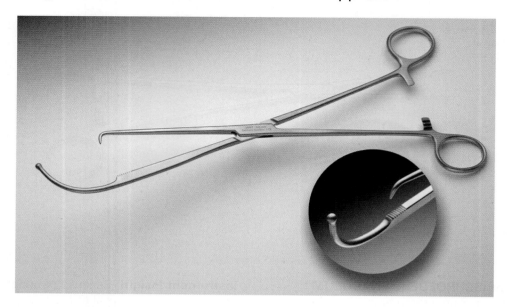

Instrument: HULKA TENACULUM
Other Names: Uterine manipulator
Use(s): Used to manipulate the uterus and thereby facilitate visualization of and access to pelvic structures during laparoscopic procedures. The probe tip is inserted into the cervical os and the sharp prong penetrates the anterior cervical lip.
Description: One of the jaws has a long ball-tip probe extending to heavy horizontal serrations.

The other side is shorter and has smooth, round jaws that extend to a sharp, inward-curved prong. The heavy serrations and the curved prong interlock when compressed.

⚠ **CAUTION:** Care should be taken when handling this instrument because of the sharp prong that can easily puncture gloves and skin.

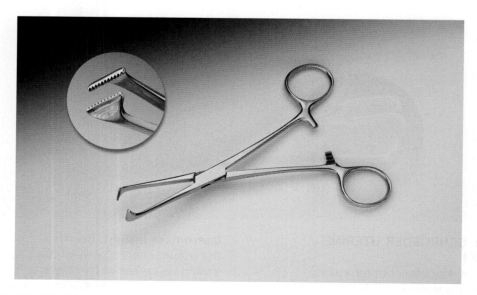

Instrument: ALLIS-ADAIR
Other Names: Big Allis
Use(s): Used for lifting, holding, and retracting slippery dense tissue that is being removed. In OB/GYN procedures, it is commonly used to grasp vaginal tissue during an anterior and posterior repair.

Description: Wide heavy tip with multiple, interlocking fine teeth at the tip that reduce injury to the tissues. The jaws are much wider and heavier than a regular Allis.
Instrument Insight: Will often need multiple forceps to grasp the excess tissue in A&P repair.

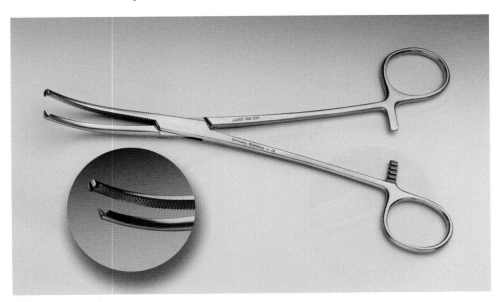

Instrument: CURVED OCHSNER FORCEPS
Other Names: Curved Kocher
Use(s): Used for grasping tough, fibrous, slippery tissues.
Description: The curved inner jaws have transverse serrations that run the length of the jaws. At the tip of the jaws are three large interlinking teeth. This instrument is available with both straight and curved jaws.

⚠ **CAUTION:** Care should be taken when handling this instrument because the sharp teeth can easily puncture gloves and skin.

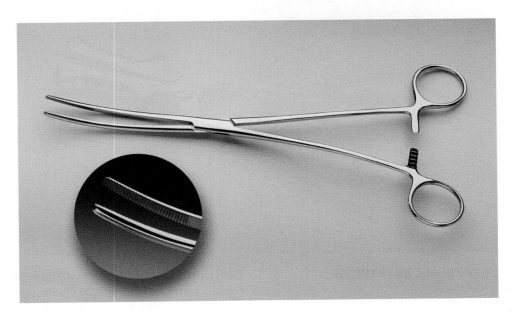

Instrument: BOZEMAN UTERINE DRESSING FORCEPS
Other Names: Dressing forceps, packing forceps
Use(s): Used for placing vaginal packing in the vagina after vaginal procedures.
Description: Long curved forceps with horizontal serrations running one fourth of the way down the inner jaws.

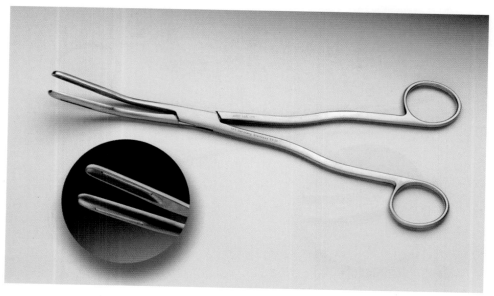

Instrument: OVERSTREET ENDOMETRIAL POLYP FORCEPS
Other Names: Polyp forceps
Use(s): Used for removal of endometrial polyps and other intrauterine tissue.

Description: Curved or straight forceps with two fenestrated, oval-cupped tips.

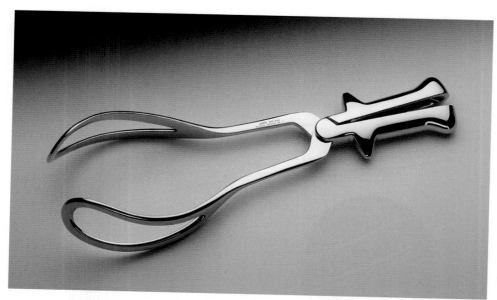

Instrument: SIMPSON OBSTETRICAL FORCEPS
Other Names: Tongs, forceps
Use(s): Used for facilitating fetal descent and delivery when the fetus is lodged in the birth canal. The blades are placed properly around the fetal head, and pulling the handle will aid in fetal descent.

Description: Two large, curved, teardrop-shaped blades that extend into two shafts that interlock at the handle. The interlocking handle is not fixed; therefore the two sides can be completely separated for ease in placement.

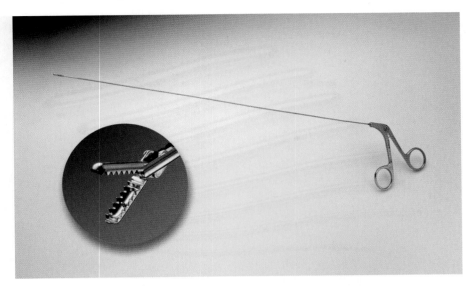

Instrument: HYSTEROSCOPE GRASPING FORCEPS

Other Names: Graspers

Use(s): Used for grasping tissues in the internal uterus when excising or taking biopsies through the hysteroscope.

Description: These graspers have right angle finger rings at the proximal end that lead to a long flexible wire that turns into a rounded tip forceps with multiple interlocking teeth on the distal end. These are very small and will fit through the working channel on the hysteroscope.

Instrument Insight: These are delicate and should be handled with care; the wire portion should not be kinked, and heavy items should never be placed on top of them.

PROBING AND DILATING INSTRUMENTS

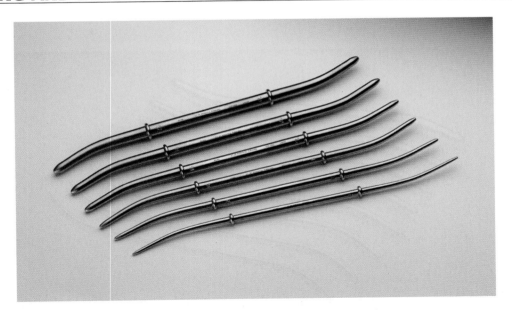

Instrument: HANK DILATORS

Other Names: Uterine dilators, cervical dilators

Use(s): Used for progressive dilation of the cervical os for intrauterine procedures, such as dilatation and curettage (D&C), suction and curettage (S&C), dilatation and evacuation (D&E), or hysteroscopy.

Description: Double-ended probe with an elevated cuff designed to limit uterine penetration.

Hank dilators are sized from 9–10 French to 19–20 French with one end of the dilator larger than the other.

Instrument Insight: Arrange dilators in a line from smallest to largest on the back table. Place the middle of the dilator in the surgeon's hand like a pencil with the smaller end facing the field.

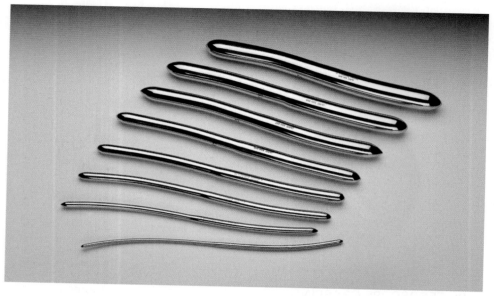

Instrument: HEGAR DILATORS
Other Names: Uterine dilators, cervical dilators
Use(s): Used for progressive dilation of the cervical os for intrauterine procedures, such as D&C, S&C, D&E, or hysteroscopy.
Description: Double-ended heavy probe; sized from 1–2 mm to 17–18 mm with one end of the dilator larger than the other.

Instrument Insight: Arrange dilators in a line from smallest to largest on the back table. Place the middle of the dilator in the surgeon's hand like a pencil with the smaller end facing the field.

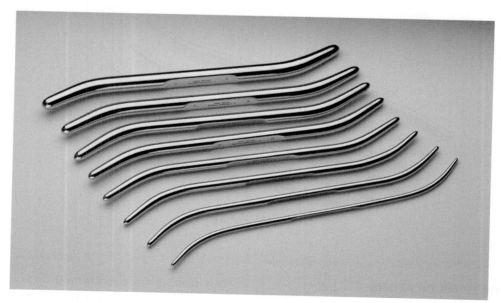

Instrument: PRATT UTERINE DILATORS
Other Names: Uterine dilators, cervical dilators
Use(s): Used for progressive dilation of the cervical os for intrauterine procedures, such as D&C, S&C, or hysteroscopy.
Description: Double-ended probe that graduates up by 2 French from 13–15 French to 41–43 French with one end of the dilator larger than the other.

Instrument Insight: Arrange dilators in a line from smallest to largest on the back table. Place the middle of the dilator in the surgeon's hand like a pencil with the smaller end facing the field.

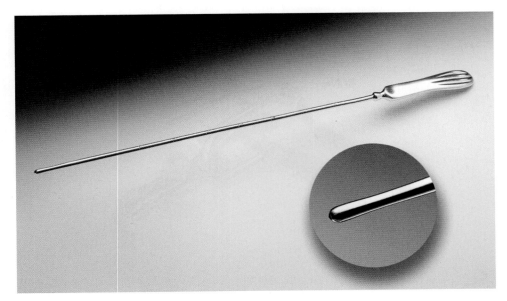

Instrument: SIMS UTERINE SOUND
Other Names: Sound, depth gauge
Use(s): This instrument is inserted into the cervical os to measure the depth of the uterus from the cervix to the back of the uterus or the fundus. The purpose for measuring the uterus is to prevent perforation of the uterus while curetting of the endometrial lining during a D&C.
Description: A long narrow probe that is malleable and is calibrated in inches or centimeters.

RETRACTING AND EXPOSING INSTRUMENTS

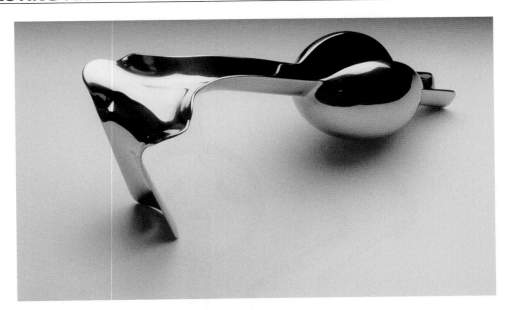

Instrument: AUVARD WEIGHTED VAGINAL SPECULUM
Other Names: Weighted speculum
Use(s): Used for retraction of the posterior vaginal wall. The blade is placed into the vaginal vault, and the weight of the speculum allows it to hang in place.
Description: A self-retaining retractor with angled concave blades that extend to a widened oblong lip. From this lip, there is a concave channel that leads to the bottom. At approximately two thirds of the way down the channel is the round weighted ball.
Instrument Insight: The average weight of this retractor is 2.5 pounds. A sterile glove may be placed over the bottom of the retractor to catch any fluid.

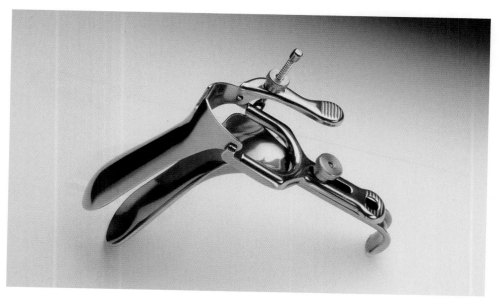

Instrument: GRAVES VAGINAL SPECULUM
Other Names: Duckbill, Bivalve Speculum
Use(s): Used for retraction of the anterior and posterior vaginal walls.
Description: Self-retaining retractor with inner upper and lower concave blades that are held open by a nut screw mechanism.

Instrument Insight: This speculum is available in different sizes; the size to be used is determined by the size of the patient.

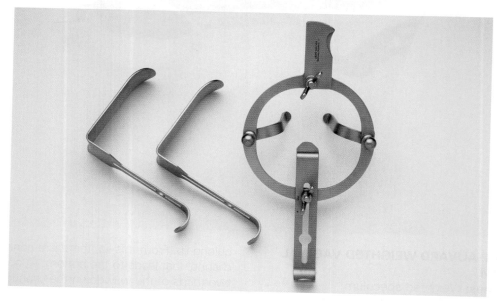

Instrument: O'SULLIVAN-O'CONNOR RETRACTOR
Other Names: Irish, O'Sullivan, O'Connor
Use(s): Used for retraction of the abdominal wall during open abdominal and pelvic procedures.

Description: A ring frame self-retaining retractor with attached lateral blades and interchangeable upper and lower blades.
Instrument Insight: Each individual piece of the retractor is included separately as part of the count.

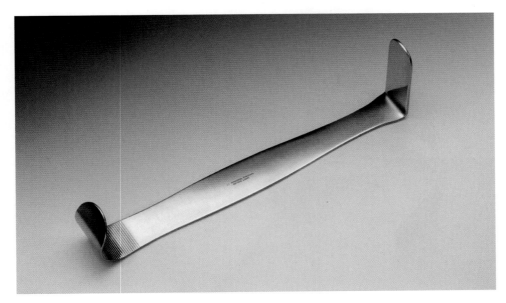

Instrument: HEANEY RETRACTOR
Other Names: Lateral retractor, right angle retractor
Use(s): Used for retraction of the anterior vaginal wall.

Description: A 90° angle flat blade that extends to a curved hook on the handle end.
Instrument Insight: The retractor is placed in the palm of the hand with the hook up and over the top of the hand for easier holding.

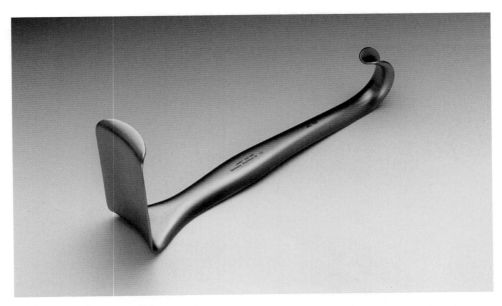

Instrument: EASTMAN RETRACTOR
Other Names: Lateral retractor
Use(s): Used for retracting the anterior vaginal wall.
Description: Has a hook-end handle that extends to a widened, lateral, right-angle blade that is slightly concave with a downward bent, crescent-shaped lip.
Instrument Insight: The retractor is placed in the palm of the hand with the hook up and over the top of the hand for easier holding.

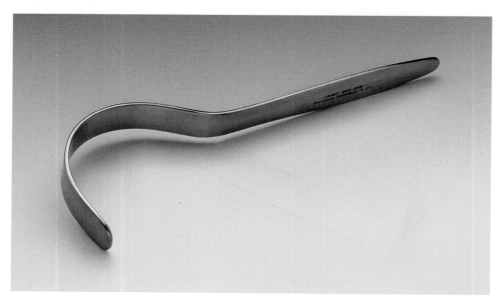

Instrument: BABY DEAVER RETRACTOR
Other Names: Small Deaver
Use(s): Used for retraction of the anterior vaginal wall. Also used for pediatric abdominal procedures.

Description: A flat, narrow, stainless-steel strip that resembles a question mark.

SUCTIONING AND ASPIRATING INSTRUMENTS

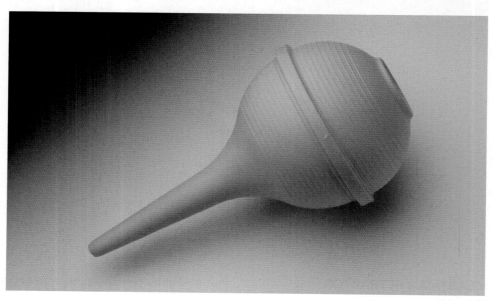

Instrument: BULB SYRINGE
Other Names: Baby sucker, ear syringe
Use(s): Used for aspiration of mucus and fluid from the mouth and nose of a neonate.

Description: A disposable, pliable hollow bulb that extends to a soft pliable tube.
Instrument Insight: Have readily available upon birth of a neonate.

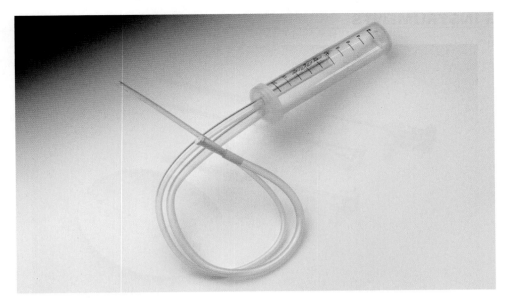

Instrument: DELEE SUCTION
Other Names: Mucous trap
Use(s): Used for aspiration of mucus and fluid from the mouth, nose, and throat of a neonate during a cesarean delivery.
Description: An oral or mechanical suction device with a 20-mL canister that has a mucous trap and filter. This prevents the mucus or fluid from entering the baby's mouth. On the canister lid is a 10F flexible suction catheter and a suction tube.
Instrument Insight: This should be immediately available upon delivery of the fetal head.

⚠ **CAUTION:** Do not hook the suction device to a regulator on full suction because this would be too strong.

SUTURING AND STAPLING INSTRUMENTS

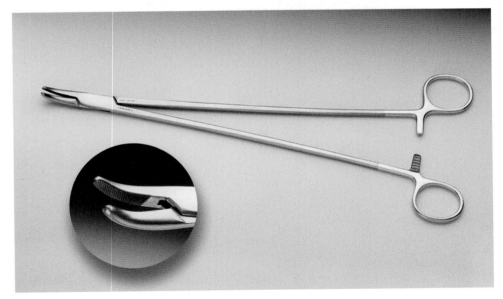

Instrument: HEANEY NEEDLE HOLDER
Other Names: Curved needle holder, Heany needle driver, Curved needle driver
Use(s): Used for proper placement of a suture needle when suturing around curved structures and in confined spaces, such as during a vaginal hysterectomy.
Description: A curved heavy needle holder with a carbide cross-hatch pattern of serrations on the inner jaws.
Instrument Insight: The needle should be positioned on the jaws of the needle holder with its curve toward the swaged end of the suture.

VIEWING INSTRUMENTS

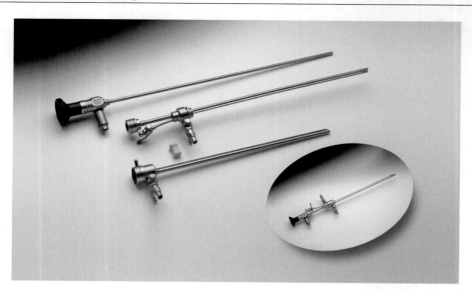

Instrument: HYSTEROSCOPE

Use(s): Hysteroscope is a sheath and telescope that is inserted into the uterus via the vagina and cervix to visualize the internal structures of the uterus and the tubal orifices, endocervical canal, cervix, and vagina. Hysteroscopy can be performed for diagnostic or therapeutic indications.

Description: The hysteroscope consists of a telescope lens, outer sheath, and an inner sheath. The outer is a hollow metal tube with a stopcock on the side for the inflow of irrigation at the proximal end and a rounded angled tip at the distal end. The inner sheath is a smaller hollow tube that at the proximal end accepts the telescope lens. It also has a stopcock on the side for the inflow of irrigation and a working channel on the other side in which instruments are inserted. The working channel is fitted with a reducer cap to prevent fluid from leaking out during insertion and removal of instruments.

Instrument Insight: The stopcocks should be closed before irrigation is opened. If the handle of the stopcock is aligned with the port, the stopcock is open. If the handle is up or down, the stopcock is closed. The port on the working channel should have a reducer cap and the stopcock closed to control the leakage of irrigation.

7

Genitourinary Instruments

ACCESSORY INSTRUMENTS

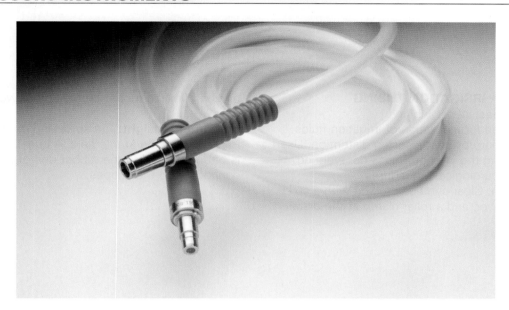

Instrument: FIBEROPTIC LIGHT CORD
Other Names: Light cord
Use(s): Used for delivering high-intensity light to the endoscope for illumination of the interior bladder.
Description: A 10-foot fiberoptic cable with an endoscope adaptor at the proximal end and a light source adaptor at the distal end.
Instrument Insight: Care must be exercised when handling a fiberoptic cord. It should never be placed under a heavy object, dropped, twisted, or kinked; the tiny glass fibers inside can be easily damaged.

⚠ **CAUTION:** When not in use, the light source should be turned off. The intense beam can cause ignition of the drapes or any flammable vapors; it can also burn through the drapes and injure the patient.

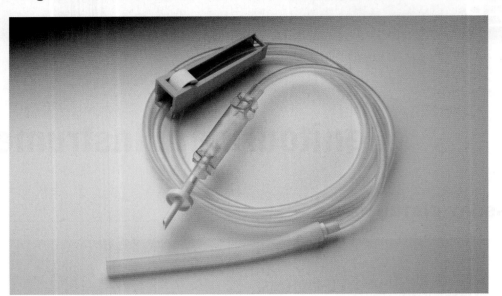

Instrument: IRRIGATION TUBING
Other Names: Water Tubing
Use(s): Used for instillation of irrigation fluids into the urinary bladder, causing distention. Used for visualizing the interior. This is done during endoscopic urological procedures.
Description: Clear synthetic tubing with a spike, a drip chamber, and a roller clamp at the distal end and flexible rubber tubing on the working end.

Instrument Insight: The spike end of the tubing is handed off the sterile field. A Luer-Lok adaptor is often attached to the rubber end of tubing for connection to the scopes.

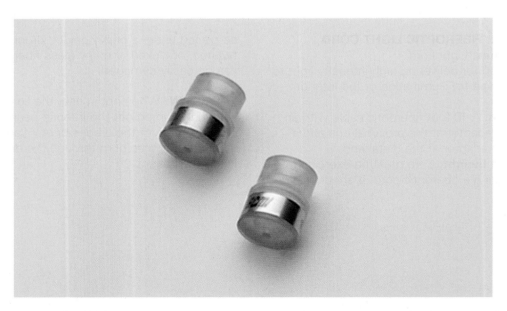

Instrument: REDUCER CAPS
Other Names: Seals
Use(s): Reduce leakage of irrigation when inserting a device into the working channels of bridges, the catheter-deflecting element, and flexible scopes.

Description: Reusable flexible caps with a small hole on the working end. Reducers are available in different sizes depending on the size of the device to be used.
Instrument Insight: The seals are stretched over the opening of the working channels.

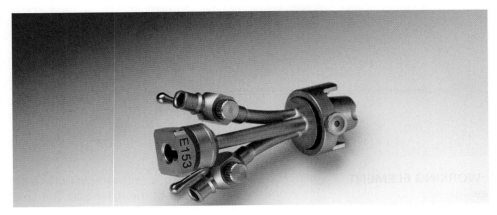

Instrument: TELESCOPE BRIDGE

Other Names: Bridge

Use(s): Used to adapt the telescope lens to fit into the cystoscope sheath and may allow insertion of one or two accessories. These would include guidewires, ureteral catheters, stents, and other flexible devices.

Description: The proximal end accepts the telescope and has a working channel on each side. The distal end is the connection to the cystoscope sheath. Bridges are available in several styles. They can be an adaptor only or be manufactured with one or two working ports.

Instrument Insight: The lens will not fit into the cystoscope sheath without a bridge. The ports on bridges are covered with a reducer cap and have stopcocks to control the leakage of irrigation. If the handle of the stopcock is aligned with the port, the stopcock is open. If the handle is up or down, the stopcock is closed.

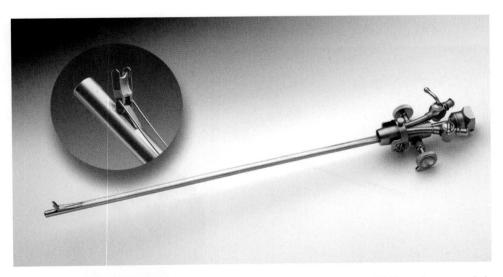

Instrument: CATHETER DEFLECTING ELEMENT

Other Names: Cath element, deflecting bridge

Use(s): This device allows the surgeon to aim the tip of the accessory at a specific area or anatomical structure. A deflecting element is commonly used during a cystoscopy for retrograde pyelograms to direct the catheter into the ureteral orifice.

Description: The proximal end accepts the telescope lens, which is slid through the hollow tube to the end for viewing. There are working channels on each side in which the ureteral catheter is inserted. Below the channels are thumb wheels to manipulate the "lid" or tip up and down. The deflecting element fits into the cystoscope sheath for use.

Instrument Insight: To prevent damage to the urethra and the lid apparatus, it is important to remember to return the lid to the neutral position before handing the catheter deflecting element to the surgeon. The ureteral catheter is inserted into the side port and pulled down to the lid at the tip of the sheath. The lid is lowered and the element is inserted into a cystoscope for use. Once inside the bladder, the lid is manipulated to guide the catheter into the ureteral orifice.

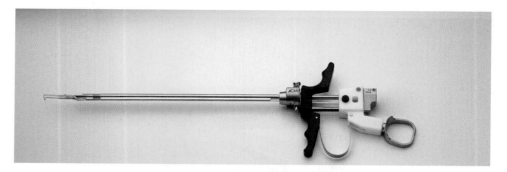

Instrument: WORKING ELEMENT

Other Names: Iglesias

Use(s): Used with a resectoscope, telescope, and electrode to resect tissue and coagulate bleeders during a transurethral resection of the prostate or a bladder tumor.

Description: The proximal end accepts the telescope, which is slid through the sheath to the working end for viewing. The handle has a spring mechanism that draws the electrode back into the resectoscope sheath. Attaching the electrode is accomplished by sliding the wire end through the guide below the telescope sheath and into the handle where it is seated. The small black button on the side releases the electrode. It is not necessary to depress the button to seat the electrode. The small hole next to the black button is for active cord connection. The small silver button at the top of the sheath will release the working element from the resectoscope sheath.

Instrument Insight: A 30° telescope is loaded into the working element, and this enables the electrode to be seen during the procedure. Activation of the working element is accomplished when the surgeon steps on the foot pedal and compresses the handle, which draws the electrode through the tissue and back into the resectoscope sheath.

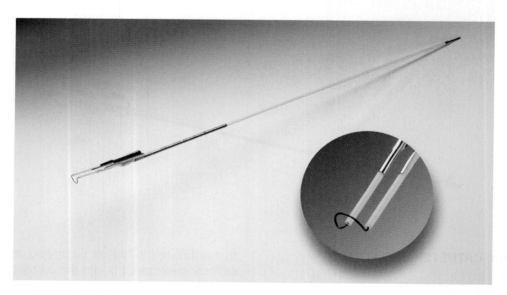

Instrument: LOOP ELECTRODE

Other Names: Loop

Use(s): Commonly used for resection and coagulation of prostatic and bladder tissues during transurethral procedures. A loop electrode vaporizes the tissue in its immediate area as it resects a piece of tissue. Bleeders may also be coagulated simultaneously or individually.

Description: An insulated wire that bifurcates at the working end and leads to a metal crescent-shaped wire between the two prongs.

Instrument Insight: The electrode is seated into the working element by sliding the proximal end through the small hollow tube under the telescope sheath and into the handle. The small trough lies on top of the electrode and slides over the sheath, securing it to the working element. The electrodes are color-coded to fit the proper size resectoscope.

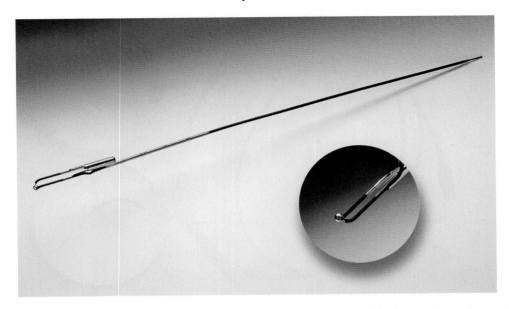

Instrument: BALL LOOP ELECTRODE

Use(s): Used for coagulation of a larger surface area of the bladder.

Description: An insulated wire that bifurcates at the working end and leads to a metal roller ball at the working end.

Instrument Insight: The electrode is seated into the working element by sliding the proximal end through the small hollow tube under the telescope sheath and into the handle. The small trough lies on top of the electrode and slides over the sheath, securing it to the working element. The electrodes are color-coded to fit the proper size resectoscope.

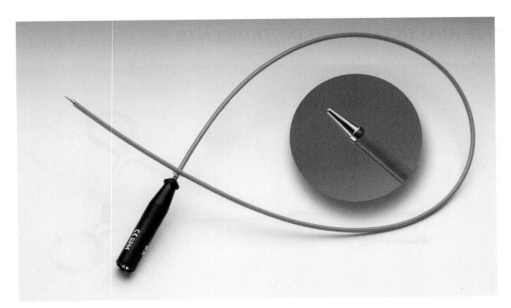

Instrument: BUGBEE ELECTRODE

Use(s): Used for coagulating small areas, usually after a bladder biopsy.

Description: The Bugbee is a flexible monopolar cautery electrode available in various diameters and lengths.

Instrument Insight: The Bugbee is a reusable electrode that is generally packaged with the cord that attaches to the generator.

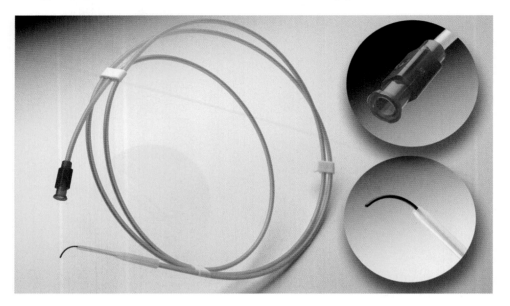

Instrument: GUIDEWIRE
Other Names: Glidewire
Use(s): Used for guiding stents, dilatators, baskets, and other devices into the ureters.
Description: A long, thin wire with a curved or straight flexible tip. Depending on the manufacturer, the wire will be constructed of a metal or synthetic material, which may be covered with a lubricous coating to ease insertion. The wire is a single-use item that comes packaged inside a hard plastic coil that has an irrigation port at the proximal end and an insertion guide at the working end.

Instrument Insight: Moistening the guidewire will ease the insertion through the working channel of the scope. This can be accomplished by injecting water through the irrigation port on the plastic coil or by dipping the wire itself in a basin of water.

CLAMPING AND OCCLUDING INSTRUMENTS

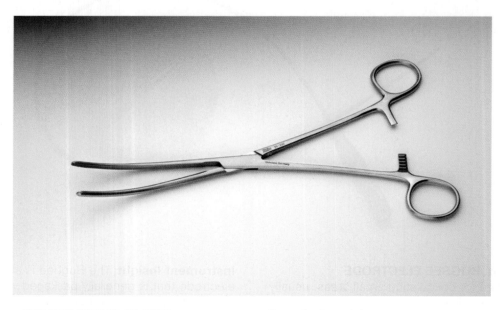

Instrument: YOUNG RENAL CLAMP
Use(s): Used for clamping heavy tissues and the pedicles during open kidney procedures.

Description: A long, heavy, curved clamp with longitudinal serrations and with cross-serrations at the tip.

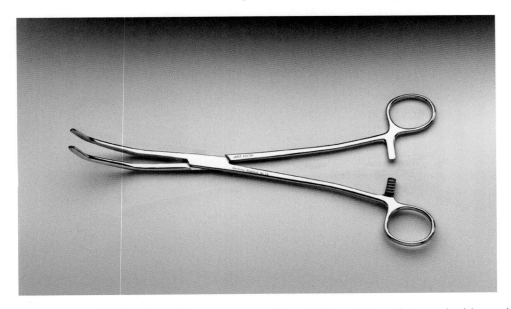

Instrument: HERRICK KIDNEY CLAMP
Other Names: Pedicle clamp
Use(s): Used for clamping heavy tissues and the pedicles during open kidney procedures.

Description: A long, heavy, double-angle clamp with longitudinal serrations.

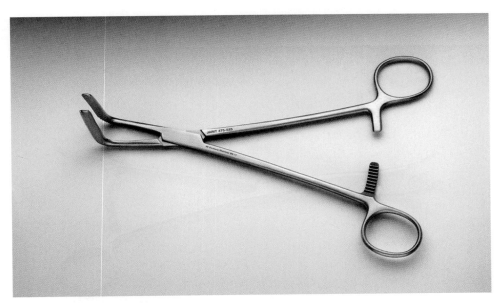

Instrument: WERTHEIM-CULLEN PEDICLE CLAMP
Other Names: Pedicle clamp
Use(s): Used for clamping heavy tissues and the pedicles during open kidney procedures.

Description: Broad right angle clamp with longitudinal serrations that run from the tip to the curvature.

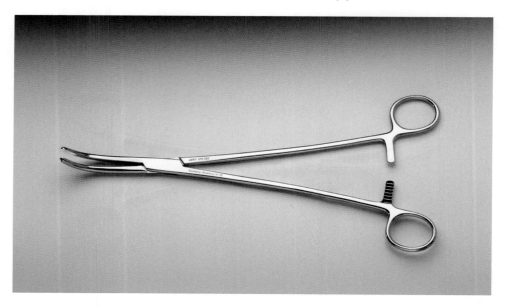

Instrument: WERTHEIM CLAMP
Use(s): Used for clamping heavy tissue and vessels during open urological procedures.

Description: A long, heavy, curved clamp with horizontal serrations running the length of the jaws.

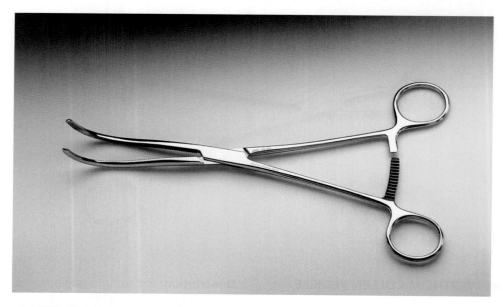

Instrument: MAYO-GUYON VESSEL CLAMP
Use(s): Used for clamping heavy tissue and vessels during open urological procedures.

Description: A heavy clamp with long, curved jaws and horizontal serrations running the length of the jaws.

CUTTING AND DISSECTING INSTRUMENTS

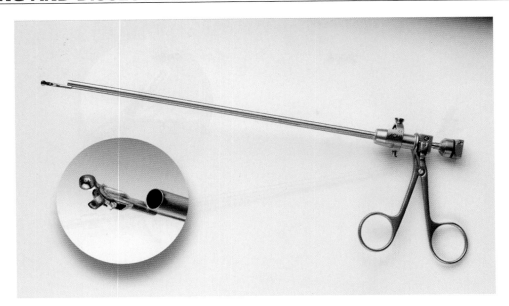

Instrument: BIOPSY FORCEPS

Use(s): To remove small bites of tissue in the bladder for examination.

Description: The proximal end accepts the telescope lens, and the finger rings open and close the cup-shaped jaws at the working end. The biopsy forceps attaches to the cystoscope sheath.

Instrument Insight: To prevent crushing or damaging the biopsy tissue, it can be swished in saline or pushed out of the jaws with a fine needle.

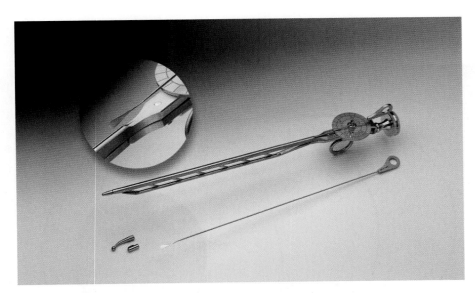

Instrument: OTIS URETHROTOME

Use(s): Used to perform a blind urethrotomy for strictures.

Description: This has two pieces: Urethrotome and a blade. The Urethrotome is straight dilator that is expanded open when the round knob on the distal end is turned. The dial below the knob allows the surgeon to determine the amount of dilatation that is occurring when the knob is turned. The blade fits down into the dilating rod and is pushed upward as the dilator is opened. When the dilator is expanded to the appropriate diameter, the surgeon will pull the blade out, cutting the stricture.

Instrument Insight: Otis Urethrotome is inserted into the urethra and is dilated to the desired width. The blade is pulled out and cuts the stretched urethra, releasing the strictures.

⚠ **CAUTION:** When loading the blade onto urethrotome always use the handle on the blade to do so. The blade is very sharp and can cut through your gloves and skin.

GRASPING AND HOLDING INSTRUMENTS

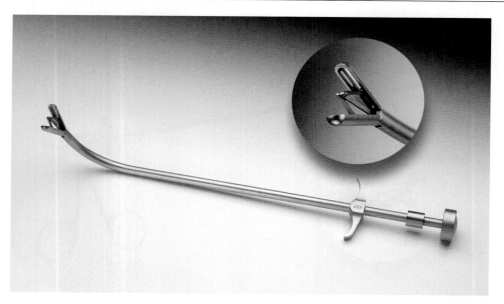

Instrument: LOWSLEY PROSTATIC TRACTOR
Use(s): Used for manipulating the prostate downward in the direction of the perineum during a perineal prostatectomy.
Description: A slender, curved instrument with cupped blades at the tip that open and close by rotation of the handle at the proximal end.

Instrument Insight: The Lowsley is passed through the urethra into the bladder and then opened; therefore, it should be handed to the surgeon with the blades closed.

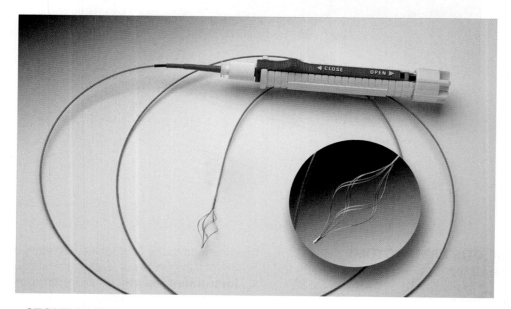

Instrument: STONE BASKET
Use(s): Used for entrapping and removing renal calculi via a ureteroscope or a cystoscope.
Description: A single-use device that consists of a plastic handle with a thumb slide mechanism for opening and closing the basket, a catheter sheath, and a wire catheter with expandable

wire basket. These devices are available in a variety of lengths, tip designs, and basket configurations depending on the manufacturer.
Instrument Insight: When the thumb slide on the handle is slid forward, the basket collapses into the outer sheath and when pulled backward the basket is expanded.

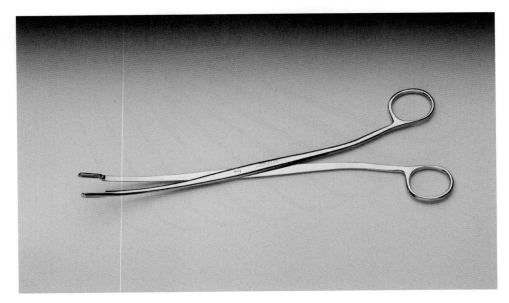

Instrument: RANDALL STONE FORCEPS
Use(s): Used for grasping renal stones.
Description: A curved, nonratcheted grasping forceps with fenestrated, oval-cup jaws with horizontal serrations. The Randall forceps are available in different intensities of curvature, ranging from one fourth, one half, and three fourths of a curve to a full curve.

PROBING AND DILATING INSTRUMENTS

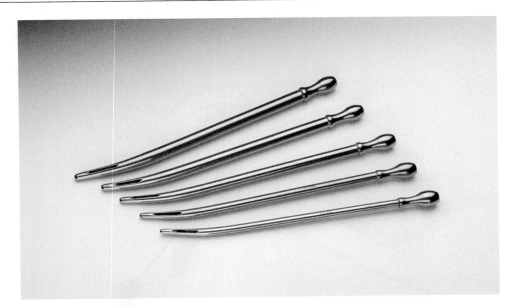

Instrument: WALTHER FEMALE URETHRAL SOUNDS
Other Names: Female sounds, female dilators, urethral dilators
Use(s): Provide gradual dilation of the female urethra. Often used before the placement of the cystoscope or resectoscope to ease insertion. The female sounds can also be used to obtain a urine specimen or drain the bladder.

Description: A stainless-steel tube with a narrowed, curved tip and oval drainage lumen. The sound size is measured on the French scale with even numbers only that range from 12F to 38F.
Instrument Insight: The sounds should be arranged on the back table from smallest to largest.

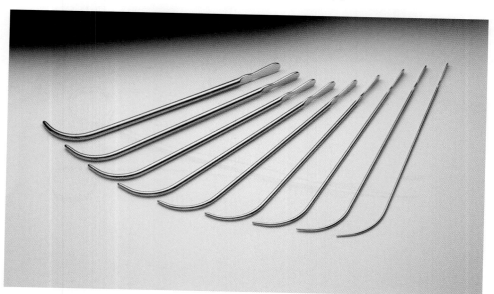

Instrument: VAN BUREN URETHRAL SOUNDS

Other Names: Male sounds, Van Buren, urethral dilators

Use(s): Provide gradual dilation of the male urethra. Often used before the placement of the cystoscope or resectoscope to ease insertion.

Description: A long stainless-steel rod with a narrowed, curved tip. The sound size is measured on the French scale with even numbers only that range from 8F to 40F.

Instrument Insight: The sounds should be arranged on the back table from smallest to largest.

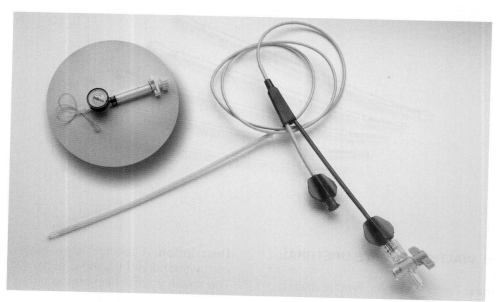

Instrument: BALLOON DILATOR

Use(s): Used for dilatation of ureteral strictures.

Description: A long plastic ureteral catheter with a high-pressure balloon tip on the distal end. At the proximal end is a balloon inflation port with stopcock and a guidewire insertion port.

Instrument Insight: The balloon is inflated with a contrast media solution for visualization by fluoroscopy.

RETRACTING AND EXPOSING INSTRUMENTS

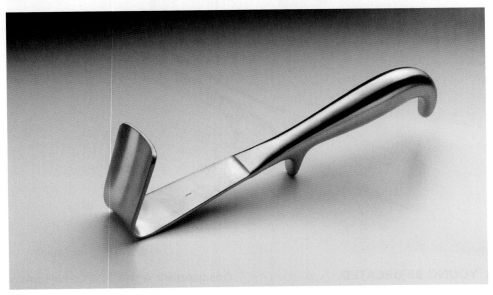

Instrument: YOUNG ANTERIOR RETRACTOR
Other Names: Anterior prostate retractor
Use(s): Used for retracting muscles and tissues during a radical perineal prostatectomy.

Description: A smooth, concave, anterior-bent blade with a solid grip handle.

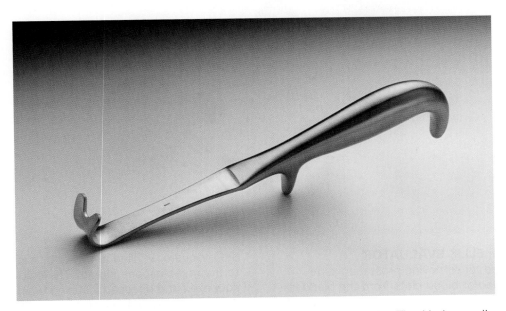

Instrument: YOUNG BULB RETRACTOR
Other Names: Notched retractor, bulb retractor
Use(s): Used for retracting muscles and tissues during a radical perineal prostatectomy.
Description: A short bent blade with a U-shaped notch at the end and a solid grip handle.

Instrument Insight: The U shape allows the catheter to be placed at the notch to prevent bending or crushing of the catheter.

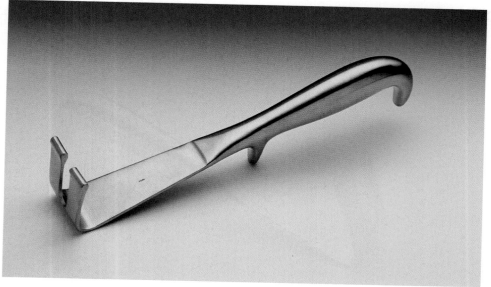

Instrument: YOUNG BIFURCATED RETRACTOR
Other Names: Bifurcated prostate retractor
Use(s): Used for retracting muscles and tissues during a radical perineal prostatectomy.

Description: A smooth, lateral-bent retractor with a U-shaped bifurcation in the blade and a solid grip handle.
Instrument Insight: The U shape allows the catheter to be placed at the notch to prevent bending or crushing of the catheter.

SUCTIONING AND ASPIRATING INSTRUMENTS

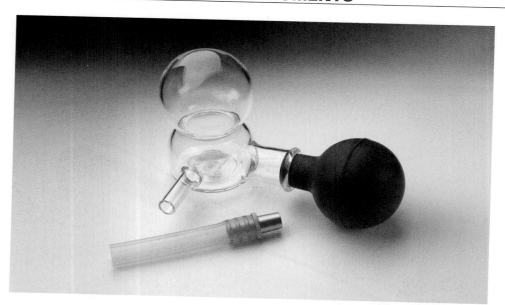

Instrument: ELLIK EVACUATOR
Use(s): Used for removing prostatic tissue segments and/or blood clots from the bladder.
Description: A double-glass bowl and bulb with adaptor tip. The silicone tubing slides over the glass arm of the bowl. The adaptor is required to connect the evacuator to the inner sheath of the resectoscope.
Instrument Insight: All air must be eliminated from the bulb and glass bowl before use. After

the evacuator is filled with water, it is attached to the resectoscope sheath. The bulb is squeezed and released, causing whirling action of the water in and out of the bladder. The tissue pieces are trapped in the bottom portion of the glass bowl. To avoid reintroduction of the tissue back into the bladder, the tissue should be removed between uses.

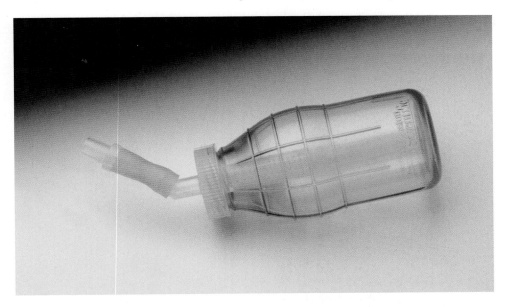

Instrument: MICROVASIVE EVACUATOR
Other Names: Disposable evacuator
Use(s): Used for removing tissue segments and/or blood clots from the bladder.
Description: A pliable plastic container with a screw on the lid that has a filter mechanism attached to the inside and an adaptor arm on the exterior. The adaptor fits inside the inner sheath of the resectoscope.

Instrument Insight: All air must be removed from the container before use. After the evacuator is filled with water, it is attached to the resectoscope sheath. The container is squeezed and released, causing a whirling action of the water in and out of the bladder. The filter mechanism inside the container traps the specimen, which allows for reuse without removing the tissue.

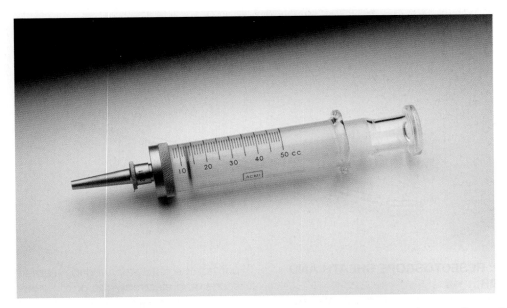

Instrument: TOOMEY SYRINGE
Use(s): Used for aspirating specimens and blood clots from the bladder. Often used to check for bleeding after a transurethral resection; this is done by injecting irrigation through the urethral catheter and aspirating it back out, checking the color of the return.

Description: A glass syringe calibrated in milliliters with a stainless steel catheter adaptor tip.
Instrument Insight: When assembling the Toomey syringe, wetting the plunger portion will ease the insertion into the barrel. A Toomey syringe may also be a single patient use that is entirely made of plastic.

VIEWING INSTRUMENTS

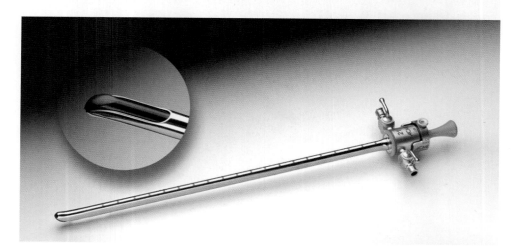

Instrument: CYSTOSCOPE SHEATH AND OBTURATOR

Use(s): Used for visual examination of the urethra, bladder, and ureteral orifices. The cystoscope is used for retrograde pyelograms, bladder biopsies, ureteral stone manipulation, stent placement, and other endoscopic urological procedures. The obturator is used to ease initial insertion of the cystoscope into the bladder.

Description: The cystoscope sheath is a hollow tube with a rounded tip and mouth at the distal end. The proximal end is the insertion port for the obturator, bridge, telescope, deflecting mechanism, biopsy forceps, and other devices. It also has a stopcock on each side for the inflow of irrigation. The size of the cystoscope is measured according to the French (F) scale. A 21F cystoscope is the most widely used. The obturator is a removable core that has a rounded end that protrudes to the far opening of the sheath.

Instrument Insight: Cystoscope sheaths and obturators are color-coded to assist with proper assembly. Each company has its own color code, but if you spend time working with these instruments, it is beneficial to commit the colors to memory.

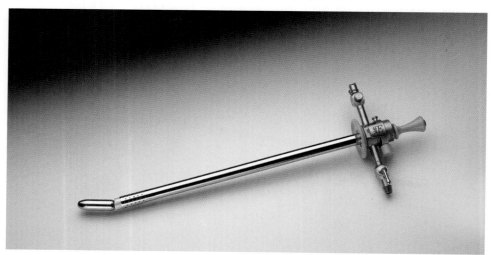

Instrument: RESECTOSCOPE SHEATH AND OBTURATOR

Use(s): The outer sheath is used with the working element, telescope, and electrode to resect tissues and coagulate bleeders during a transurethral resection of the prostate or bladder tumor. The obturator is used to ease initial insertion of the resectoscope into the bladder.

Description: The resectoscope sheath is a hollow stainless-steel tube with a beveled ceramic tip at the distal end. The proximal end is an insertion port for the obturator, working element, telescope, and electrode; the proximal end also has a stopcock on each side for the inflow of irrigation. The obturator is a removable core that has a bullet-shaped end that protrudes through and beyond the far opening. The resectoscope is available in two sizes: 25F and 27F.

Instrument Insight: Resectoscope sheaths and obturators are color coded to assist with proper assembly.

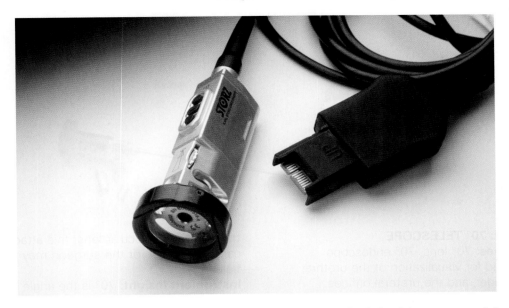

Instrument: ENDOSCOPIC CAMERA
Use(s): Used for transmission images from the rigid telescope to the video monitor.
Description: At the distal end of the camera is the coupler that attaches the camera to the eyepiece of the rigid scope. The coupler is attached to the camera head, which provides the image quality. Attached to the camera head is the cord, which relays images back to the video system.

Instrument Insight: Most camera failures are related to a damaged cord. Care should be exercised when handling the camera and cord. They should never be placed under a heavy object, dropped, twisted, kinked, or immersed in water or any liquid.

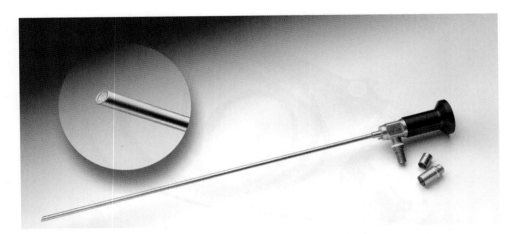

Instrument: 30° TELESCOPE
Other Names: 30° lens, 30° endoscope
Use(s): Used for visualization of the urethra, interior bladder, and the ureteral orifices.
Description: A rigid stainless-steel tube containing an optical chain of precisely aligned glass lenses and spacers. The objective lens is located at the distal tip of the scope. This determines the viewing angle. The stainless-steel cylinder rod is called the optical element of the telescope, providing both images and light. The light connector allows attachment of the light cord to the telescope. At the proximal end is the eyepiece or ocular lens; this attaches to

the camera coupler, or the surgeon may view the field directly.
Instrument Insight: 30° is the angle in which the objective lens views. The 30° lens is the most often used in urology because it delivers the best panoramic view and allows for visualization of the urethra and the trigone area in the bladder.

⚠ **CAUTION:** Endoscopes are expensive and fragile. Care should be exercised when handling an endoscope; it should never be picked up by the distal telescope end, placed under heavy objects, or dropped.

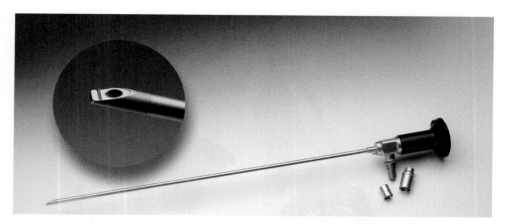

Instrument: 70° TELESCOPE

Other Names: 70° lens, 70° endoscope

Use(s): Used for visualization of the urethra, interior bladder, and the ureteral orifices.

Description: A rigid stainless-steel tube containing an optical chain of precisely aligned glass lenses and spacers. The objective lens is located at the distal tip of the scope. This determines the viewing angle. The stainless-steel rod cylinder is called the optical element of the telescope, providing both images and light. The light connector allows attachment of the light cord to the telescope. At the proximal end is the eyepiece or ocular lens; this attaches to the camera coupler, or the surgeon may view the field directly.

Instrument Insight: 70° is the angle in which the objective lens views. The 70° lens is often used to inspect the bladder walls.

⚠ **CAUTION:** Endoscopes are expensive and fragile. Care should be exercised when handling an endoscope; it should never be picked up by the distal telescope end, placed under heavy objects, or dropped.

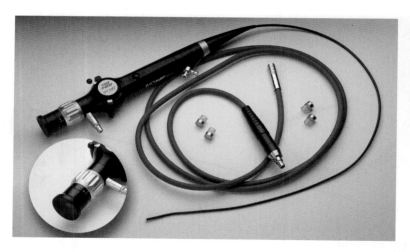

Instrument: FLEXIBLE URETEROSCOPE

Use(s): Used for visual examination of the urinary tract, including the ureters and the renal pelvis. Ureteroscopy is commonly performed for removal of ureteral or renal calculi. It also can be used for other urological procedures such as diagnosis, fulguration of bleeders, removal of neoplasm, and retrieval of migrated stents.

Description: The proximal end is comprised of the eyepiece, the light connection post, a deflecting control knob (which operates the bending section, the suction, and air/water valves), and the biopsy port. The central body is attached to an insertion tube, which is a flexible tube that contains channels for suction, biopsy, irrigation, and fiberoptic light and image bundles. At the distal end is a bending section, which contains the objective lens and light lens and can be manipulated in various directions within the internal structures.

Instrument Insight: When using a flexible ureteroscope, it should never be placed under a heavy object, dropped, twisted, or kinked because the tiny glass lens and fibers inside can be easily damaged.

8

Ophthalmic Instruments

ACCESSORY INSTRUMENTS

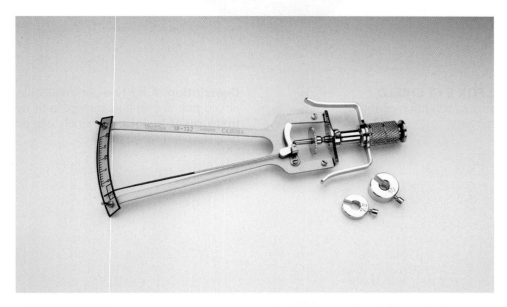

Instrument: TONOMETER
Other Names: Schiotz tonometer
Use(s): Used for measuring intraocular pressure of the eye by recording the resistance of the cornea to weight.
Description: The distal working end is a concave plunger, which is gently placed onto the cornea.

A small, round weight is slid into the center section of the tonometer, which pushes down on the plunger and flattens the cornea. The needle on the proximal end moves to register the pressure. Weights of 5.5, 7.5, and 10 grams are used.

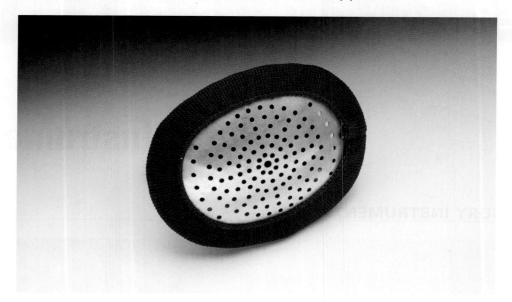

Instrument: FOX EYE SHIELD
Use(s): Used for protection of the eye after ophthalmic surgery.

Description: A lightweight, malleable, metal eye shield that is oval and convex to fit over the eye.
Instrument Insight: Generally placed over the dressing and taped in place.

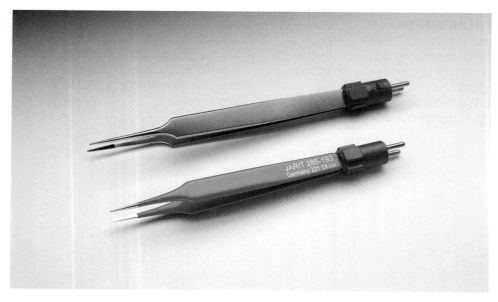

Instrument: JEWELER'S BIPOLAR FORCEPS
Use(s): Used for coagulating small blood vessels of the eye and the eyelids.
Description: Resembles a tissue forceps, is either insulated or noninsulated, and has straight forceps with fine tips.

Instrument Insight: There are many different types of bipolar forceps that can be used in eye procedures.

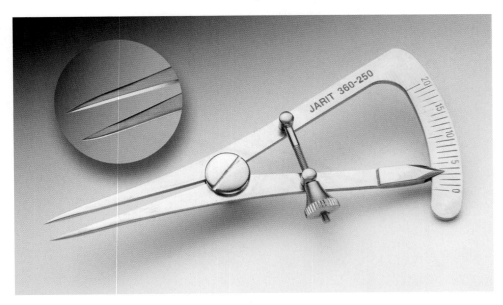

Instrument: CASTROVIEJO CALIPER
Use(s): Used for precise measuring of eye structures such as the cornea, lens, pupils, or lids.

Description: The proximal end measures from 0 to 20 mm in 1-mm increments. When the screw device is tightened or loosened, the smooth narrowed tips open or close.

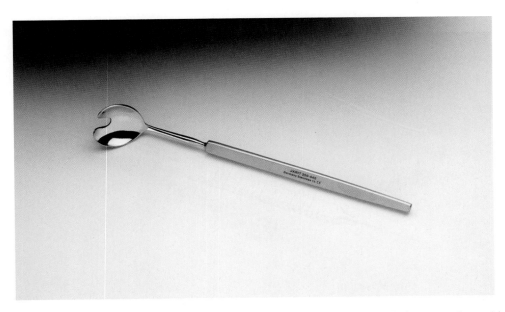

Instrument: WELLS ENUCLEATION SPOON
Use(s): Used for lifting the globe upward to dissect the optic nerve during enucleation.

Description: An angled spoon-shaped instrument with a rounded notch at the distal end.

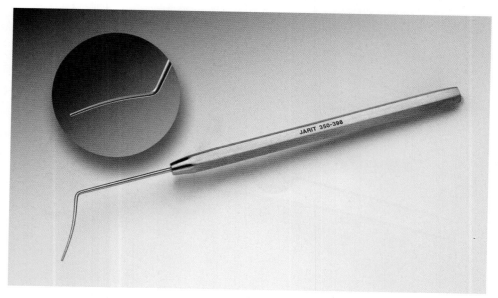

Instrument: BARRAQUER IRIS SPATULA
Other Names: Iris spatula
Use(s): Used for repositioning the iris.

Description: A blunt angled tip with a gently curved flat blade and a short hexagonal handle.

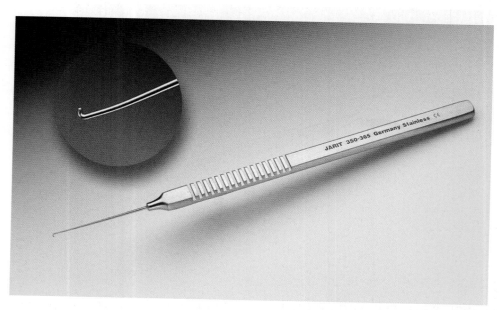

Instrument: SINSKEY HOOK
Use(s): Used for manipulating the lens.

Description: A blunt right angle hook with a flattened handle.

CLAMPING AND OCCLUDING INSTRUMENTS

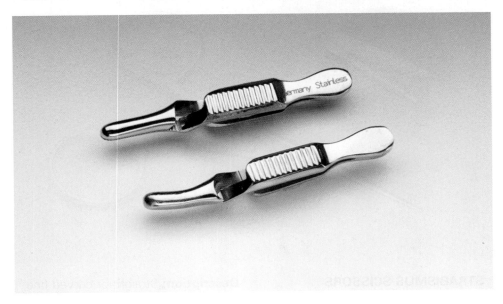

Instrument: SERREFINE CLAMPS
Use(s): Used to tag and hold bridle or fine sutures.
Description: Spring-action clamp with curved or straight jaws with horizontal serrations and a blunt tip.

Instrument Insight: These are also used in vascular surgery to occlude small vessels.

CUTTING AND DISSECTING INSTRUMENTS

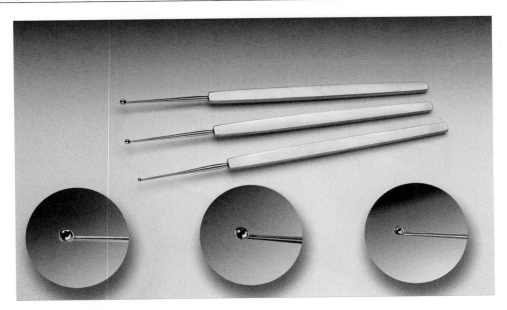

Instrument: MEYHOEFFER CHALAZION CURETTES
Use(s): Used for removing Chalazion contents by scraping.

Description: Small, sharp, scoop-shaped tips with a flattened handle.
Instrument Insight: Tips range from 1 to 3.5 mm in diameter.

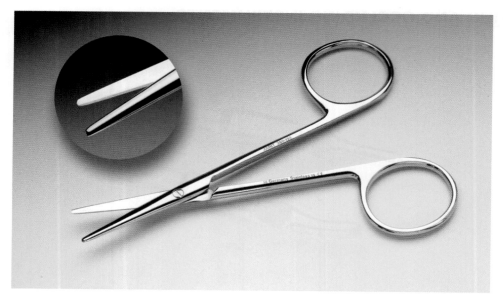

Instrument: STRABISMUS SCISSORS
Use(s): Used for dissecting the lateral and medial muscles during recession and resection.

Description: Straight or curved fine, blunt-tip scissors.

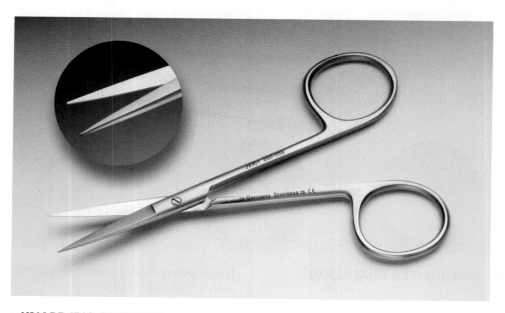

Instrument: KNAPP IRIS SCISSORS
Use(s): Used for incising and dissecting the iris.

Description: Straight or curved sharp, fine-tip scissors.

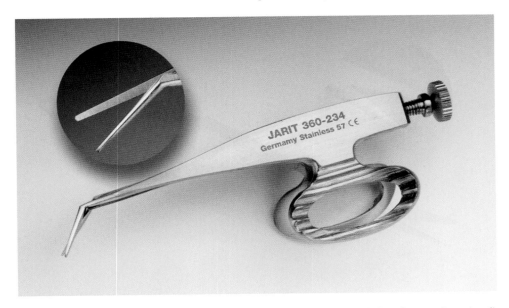

Instrument: BARRAQUER IRIS SCISSORS
Use(s): Used for incising and dissecting the iris.
Description: Micro scissors with oval fingertip pads and angled, blunt-tip blades.

Instrument Insight: Squeezing the finger pads between the thumb and forefinger will close these scissors.

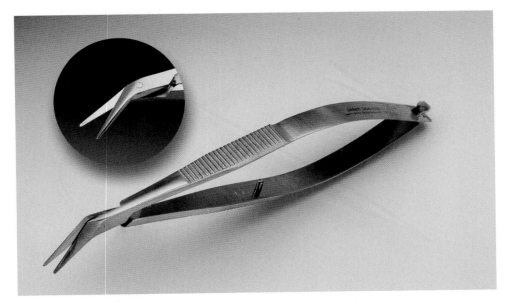

Instrument: CASTROVIEJO CORNEAL SCISSORS
Other Names: Castro's
Use(s): Used for incising and dissecting the cornea. During a corneal implant procedure, these scissors are commonly used to complete the trephination.
Description: Microsurgical spring-action scissors with angled blades.

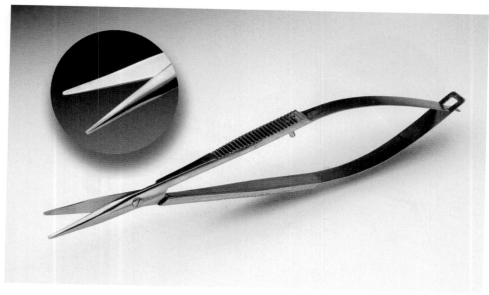

Instrument: WESTCOTT TENOTOMY SCISSORS

Use(s): Used for incising the cornea, sclera, and iris and for dividing eye muscles.

Description: Spring-action scissors with fine, narrowed, blunt tips that can be curved or straight.

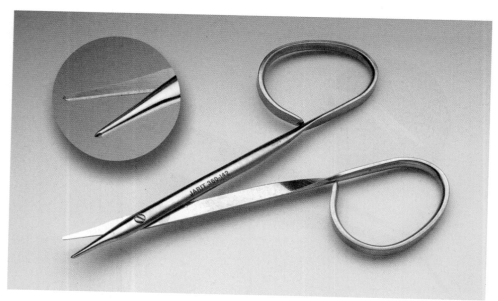

Instrument: STEVENS TENOTOMY SCISSORS

Other Names: Stevens scissors

Use(s): Used for dividing and dissecting the muscles and tendons of the eye. These are commonly used for dividing the lateral and medial tendons and muscles of the eye during recession and resection for strabismus.

Description: Small, fine scissors that can have curved or straight blades that narrow to blunt tips.

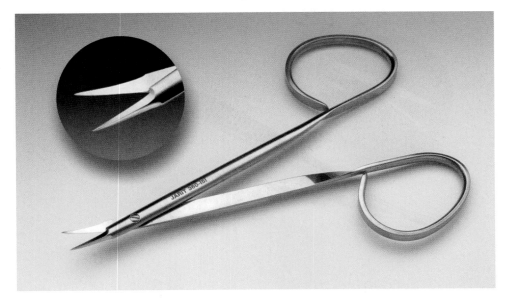

Instrument: EYE SUTURE SCISSORS
Use(s): Cut fine eye sutures.
Description: Small, fine scissors with straight beveled blades that taper to sharp tips.

Instrument Insight: These scissors should be used to cut suture only.

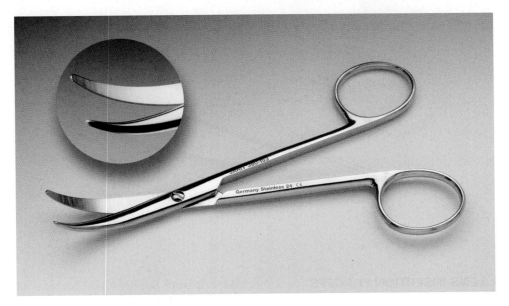

Instrument: ENUCLEATION SCISSORS
Use(s): Used to free the globe from the orbit and transect the optic nerve.

Description: Extremely curved scissors that narrow to a blunt tip.

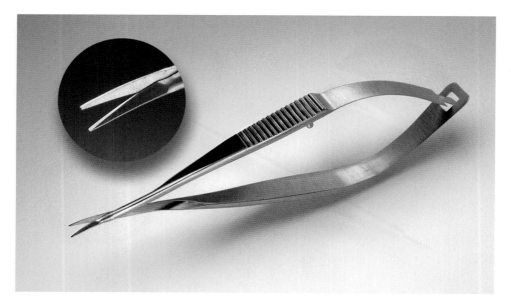

Instrument: VANNAS CAPSULOTOMY SCISSORS
Other Names: Vannas

Use(s): To incise into the capsule tissue.
Description: Spring-action micro scissors with fine curved or straight blunt-tip blades.

GRASPING AND HOLDING INSTRUMENTS

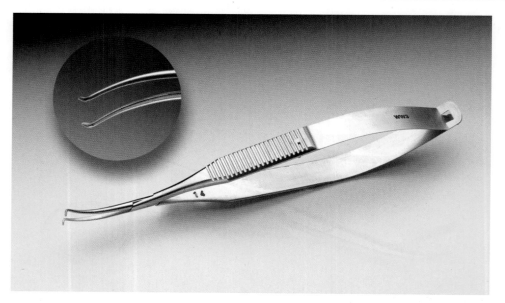

Instrument: LENS INSERTION FORCEPS
Other Names: Clayman lens forceps, lens inserter
Use(s): Used for grasping, inserting, and positioning an intraocular lens implant.

Description: Spring-action forceps with smooth, curved jaws and angled tips.

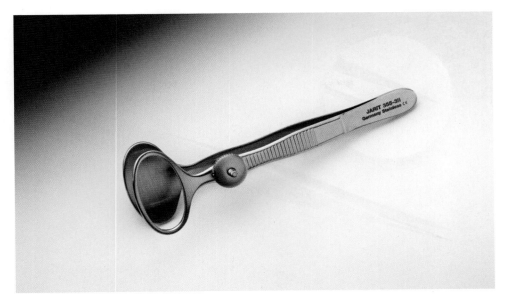

Instrument: DESMARRES CHALAZION CLAMP

Other Names: Oval chalazion clamp

Use(s): Used to stabilize and evert the eyelid to expose the chalazion.

Description: Forceps with a flattened oval plate at the end of one arm and a matching open oval ring on the other arm with a screw-locking device that holds the clamp in place.

Instrument Insight: This clamp provides hemostasis and a rigid surface against which the cyst can be incised.

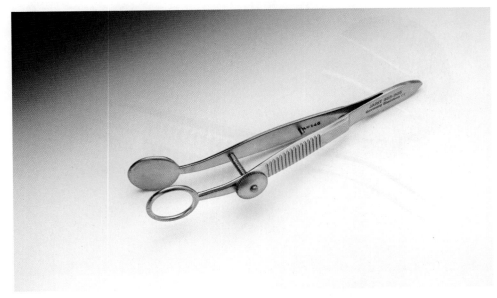

Instrument: HUNT CHALAZION CLAMP

Other Names: Round chalazion clamp

Use(s): Used to stabilize and evert the eyelid to expose the chalazion.

Description: Forceps with a flattened round plate at the end of one arm and a matching open ring on the other arm with a screw-locking device that holds the clamp in place.

Instrument Insight: This clamp provides hemostasis and a rigid surface against which the cyst can be incised.

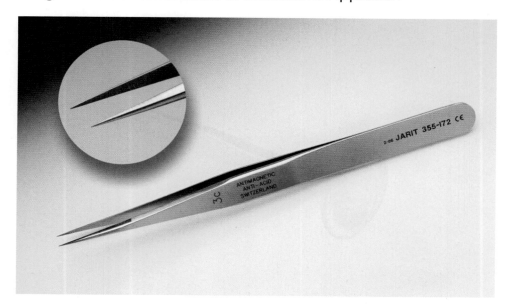

Instrument: JEWELER'S FORCEPS
Use(s): Used for grasping the intraocular lens.
Description: Smooth forceps with narrowed, pointed tips.

Instrument Insight: The tips are very sharp and can easily puncture gloves or drapes.

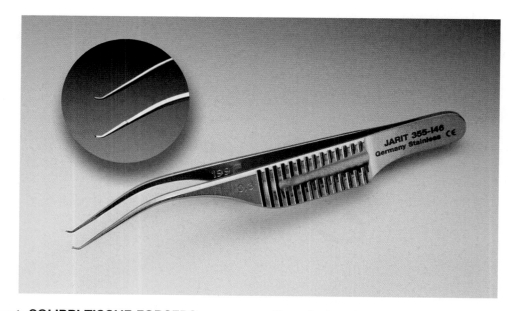

Instrument: COLIBRI TISSUE FORCEPS
Use(s): This forceps is designed for several functions. The tooth at the tip is used for holding the cornea or the sclera edge when suturing. The platform behind the tip allows for tying suture. It can also be used to grasp the iris.

Description: Long, thin, downward curving jaws with angled, toothed tips and a smooth platform behind the tips.
Instrument Insight: *Colibri* means *bird* in Italian and refers to the design of the forceps. The long thin body assures optimal viewing during surgical procedures.

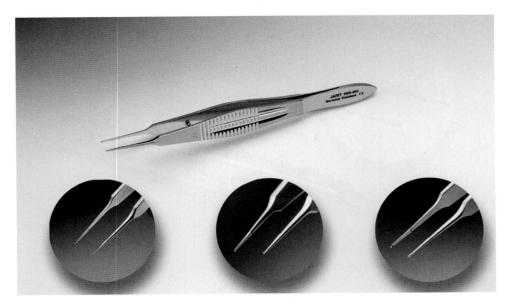

Instrument: CASTROVIEJO SUTURING TISSUE FORCEPS 0.12 MM, 0.3 MM, 0.5 MM
Use(s): Used to grasp and manipulate tissues and tie fine sutures.
Description: Small, fine tissue forceps with long, thin jaws that have smooth tying platforms and three interlocking teeth at the tips.

Instrument Insight: The area of the eye on which surgery is performed determines the size of the tissue forceps that will be used.

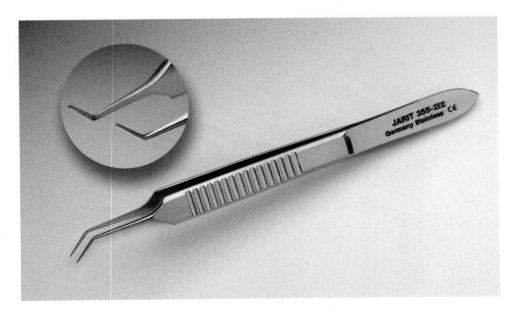

Instrument: McPHERSON TYING FORCEPS
Use(s): Designed for tying fine suture; commonly used in corneal grafting and cataract surgery.

Description: Small, fine tissue forceps that can have angled or straight jaws with smooth tying platforms.
Instrument Insight: This should not be used for grasping tissues because it will crush them.

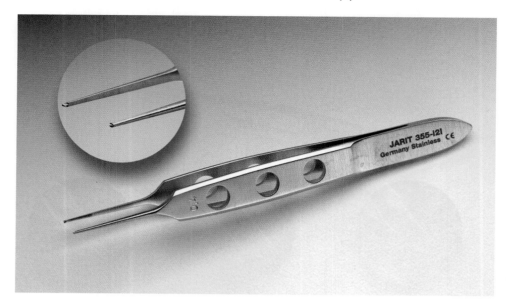

Instrument: BISHOP-HARMON IRIS TISSUE FORCEPS
Use(s): Used for grasping tissue in and around the eye.

Description: Small, fine tissue forceps with long, thin jaws and three interlocking teeth at the tips.

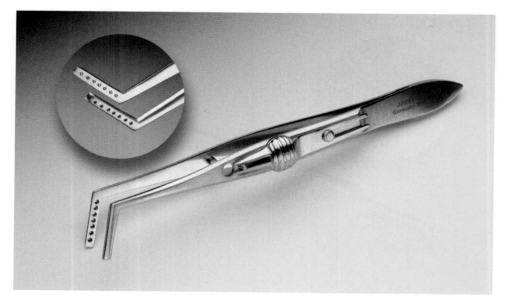

Instrument: JAMESON FORCEPS
Other Names: Muscle clamp
Use(s): Used to clamp and hold the extrinsic muscle and provide hemostasis during strabismus procedures.

Description: A flat serrated handle with a side lock and a right-angle shaft with six 1-mm teeth on one jaw that fit into the holes on the other jaw.

PROBING AND DILATING INSTRUMENTS

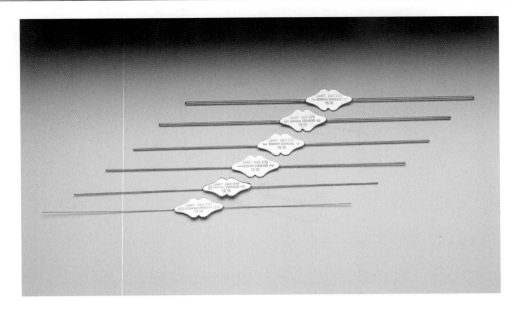

Instrument: BOWMAN LACRIMAL PROBE
Other Names: Lacrimal dilators, duct probes
Use(s): Used for probing and gradually dilating the lacrimal duct. This instrument is also used to dilate the salivary duct opening under the tongue.

Description: A thin wire on each side of a diamond-shaped plate, with the wire on one side larger than that on the other. The plate is designed to grasp and steady the probe.
Instrument Insight: Processed in sets of six.

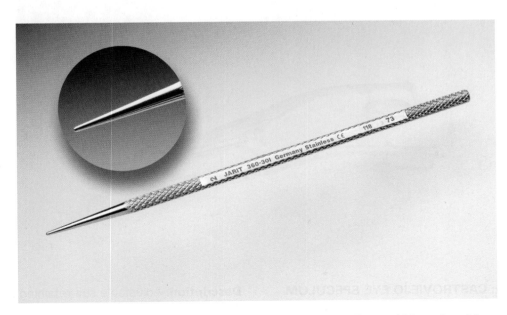

Instrument: WILDER LACRIMAL DILATOR
Other Names: Punctal lacrimal dilator
Use(s): Used for dilating the lacrimal punctum.

Description: Tapered blunt tip with round, rough handle.

RETRACTING AND EXPOSING INSTRUMENTS

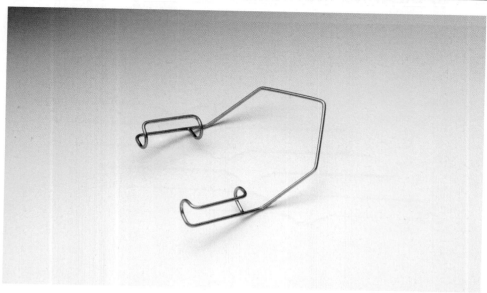

Instrument: BARRAQUER EYE SPECULUM
Other Names: Paper clip, wire speculum
Use(s): Holds open the upper and lower eyelids. Commonly used for cataract extraction.

Description: A rigid wire frame with open, curved blades.

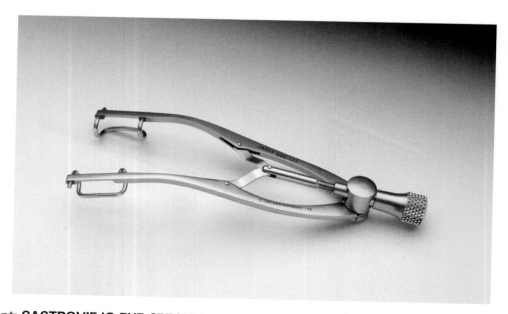

Instrument: CASTROVIEJO EYE SPECULUM
Use(s): Used for wide retraction of the upper and lower eyelids. Often used in strabismus and enucleation procedures in which wide retraction of the lids is needed.

Description: Adjustable self-retaining retractor with curved, open blades.

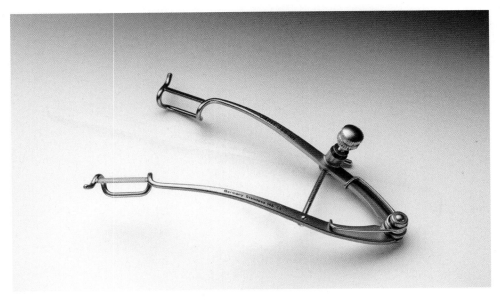

Instrument: WILLIAMS EYE SPECULUM
Use(s): Used for wide retraction of the upper and lower eyelids. Often used in strabismus and enucleation procedures in which wide retraction of the lids is needed.

Description: Adjustable self-retaining retractor with curved, open blades.

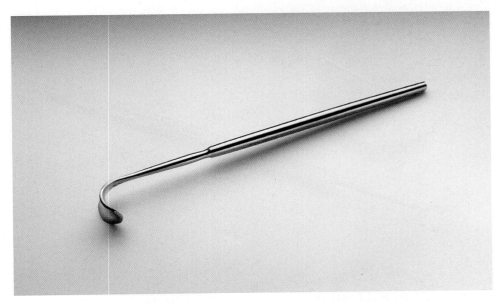

Instrument: DESMARRES LID RETRACTOR
Use(s): Used for retraction of the eyelids.

Description: Hand-held retractor with a concave curved blade and a round, smooth handle.

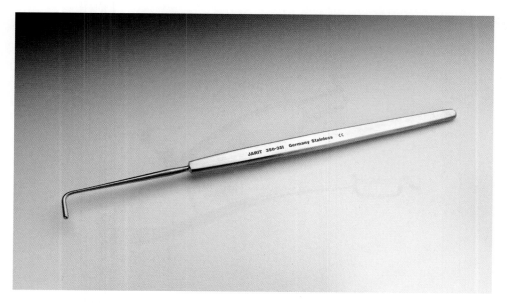

Instrument: VON GRAEFE STRABISMUS HOOK

Other Names: Muscle hook

Use(s): Used for lifting and freeing the extrinsic eye muscles from the sclera during strabismus procedures.

Description: A blunt right-angled hook with a flattened smooth handle.

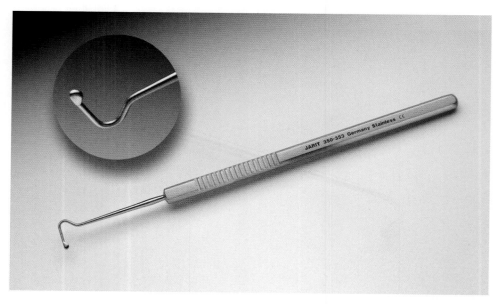

Instrument: JAMESON MUSCLE HOOK

Use(s): Used for lifting and retracting the extrinsic eye muscles during strabismus procedures.

Description: An acute-angle hook with a round tip and a flattened handle.

SUTURING AND STAPLING INSTRUMENTS

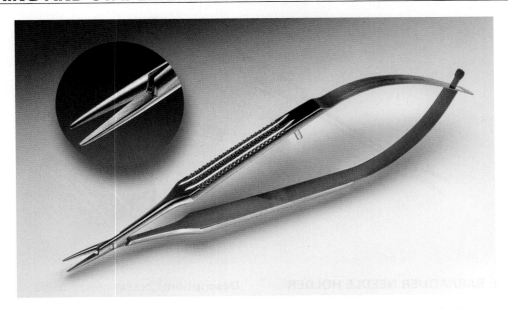

Instrument: CASTROVIEJO NEEDLE HOLDER
Use(s): Used for holding fine suture needles in eye procedures.

Description: These can be a locking or nonlocking needle holder with narrowed blunt jaws.

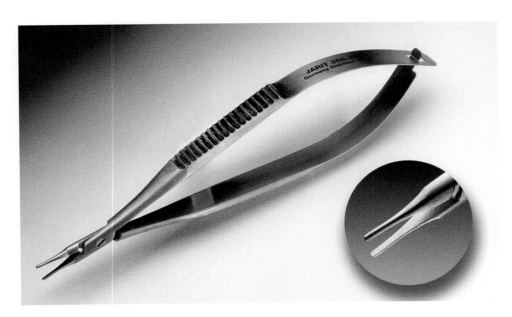

Instrument: McPHERSON NEEDLE HOLDER
Use(s): Used for holding fine suture needles in eye procedures.

Description: Nonlocking needle holder with tapered blunt jaws.

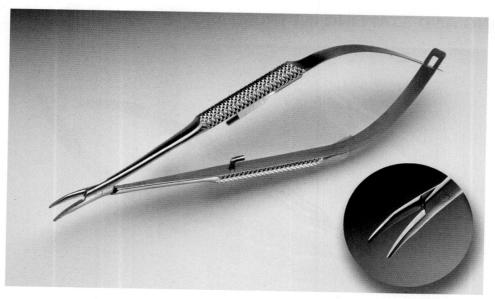

Instrument: BARRAQUER NEEDLE HOLDER

Use(s): Used for holding fine suture needles in eye procedures.

Description: Locking needle holder with curved, narrowed, blunt jaws.

9 Otorhinolaryngology Instruments

ACCESSORY INSTRUMENTS

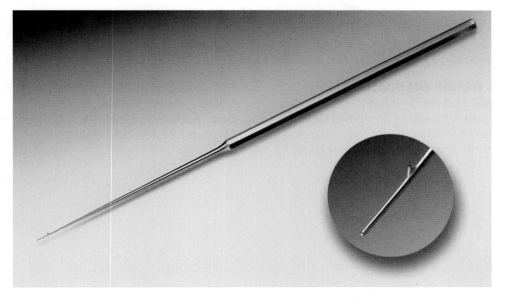

Instrument: HOUSE STRUT CALIPER
Other Names: Measuring tool, strut
Use(s): Used for measuring the ossicles and distances in the middle ear for repair or replacement, especially the stapes.

Description: Sharp instrument with a barb toward the tip for measuring.

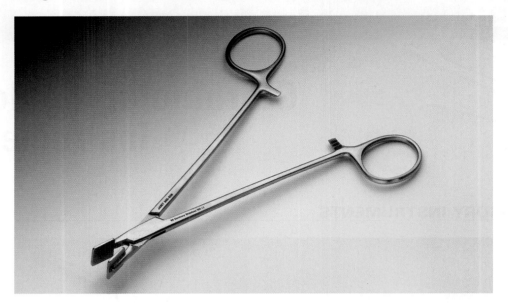

Instrument: HOUSE GELFOAM PRESS
Other Names: Gelfoam masher
Use(s): The press is used to compress Gelfoam into thin sheets that are cut into tiny squares and used for packing after middle ear procedures.

This is done to support and position a graft or to stabilize the prosthesis.
Description: Long shanks with finger rings and flat plates at its working tip.

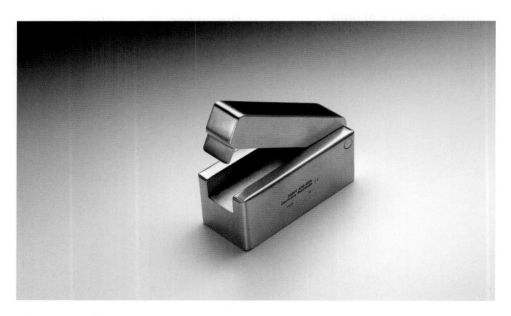

Instrument: COTTLE BONE CRUSHER
Use(s): Used to flattening the septal cartilage before replacing it in the nose.
Description: A rectangular solid box with a channel in the middle and a solid lid that closes

into the channel, compressing the object placed inside.
Instrument Insight: A mallet is used to impact the lid to prepare the cartilage.

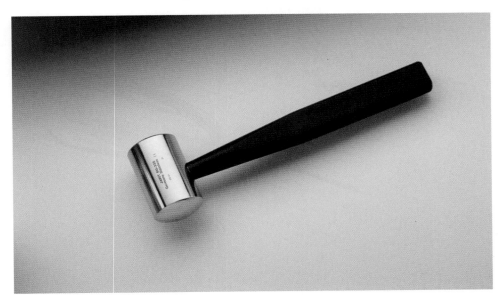

Instrument: COTTLE MALLET
Other Names: Mallet
Use(s): Exerts force on osteotomes, chisels, gouges, tamps, and other specially designed instruments.
Description: Solid stainless-steel head with one flat face and one round face attached to a black aluminum handle. Mallets are hammering-type instruments that weigh between 5 ounces and 2 pounds.
Instrument Insight: The surgeon will use a "tap-tap" rhythm when hitting the osteotome. The second hit is usually slightly harder than the first.

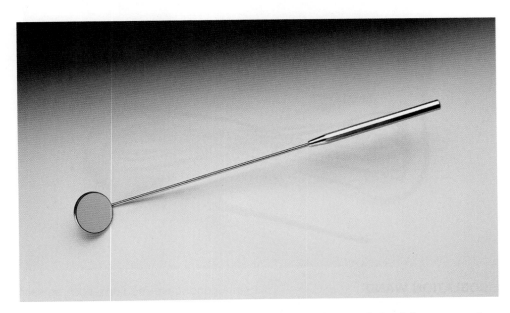

Instrument: LARYNGEAL MIRROR
Use(s): Used for visualization of pharyngeal and laryngeal areas from the back of the throat.
Description: The laryngeal mirror is a round-handled instrument with a small rounded mirror on the end. Mirrors are available in different diameters.
Instrument Insight: Mirrors may fog when inserted into the oral cavity, so the mirrors are dipped into some type of antifog solution or possibly warm water.

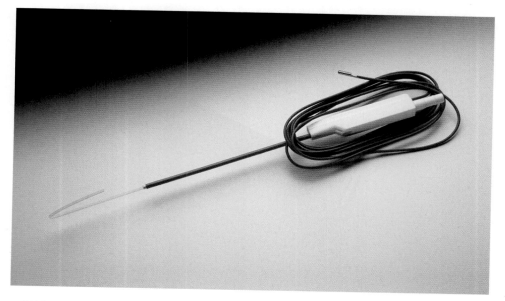

Instrument: SUCTION COAGULATOR TIP
Other Names: Neurocautery suction
Use(s): Used for removing the tonsils and adenoids by cauterizing tissue and at the same time suctioning fluid, debris, and plume from the operative site.
Description: A single-use insulated monopolar suction tip with a relief hole on the handgrip and also with a monopolar cord and stylet.

Instrument Insight: During use the tip may become plugged with charred debris. This can be remedied by inserting the stylet and wiping the tip with a moistened sponge. A dispersive pad must be placed on the patient before use.

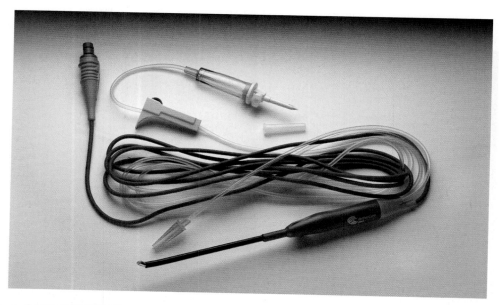

Instrument: COBLATION WAND
Use(s): Used for removing tonsils and adenoids.
Description: A single-use wand with an attached Coblation cord, suction connector, and irrigation tubing.
Instrument Insight: Coblation technology is a controlled, non–heat-driven process that uses radiofrequency energy to excite the electrolytes in a conductive medium, such as saline solution, creating precisely focused plasma. The plasma's energized particles have sufficient energy to break molecular bonds within tissue, causing tissue to dissolve at relatively low temperatures. The result is removal of targeted tissue with minimal damage to surrounding tissue.

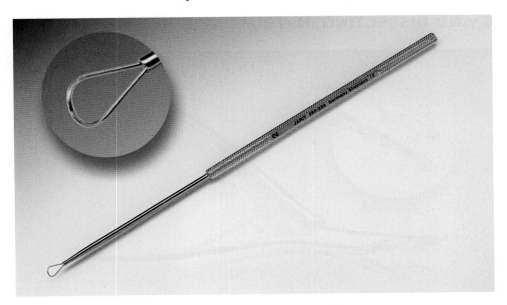

Instrument: BILLEAU EAR LOOP
Other Names: Ear curette
Use(s): Used for removing cerumen from the ear canal.
Description: Long handle with a loop of wire at its working end.

Instrument Insight: Have a sponge ready to clean the tip of the instrument as the surgeon removes debris from the ear canal.

CLAMPING AND OCCLUDING INSTRUMENTS

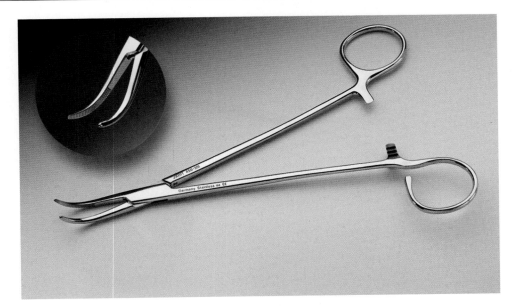

Instrument: ADSON TONSIL/SCHNIDT FORCEPS
Other Names: Adson, Schnidt, fancy clamp
Use(s): Used for clamping small vessels in a deep wound, also for holding tonsil sponges.

Description: The jaws may be curved or straight; they have horizontal serrations running half of their length, ending in fine, blunt tips. The shanks are longer than those of a Crile or a Kelly.

CUTTING AND DISSECTING INSTRUMENTS

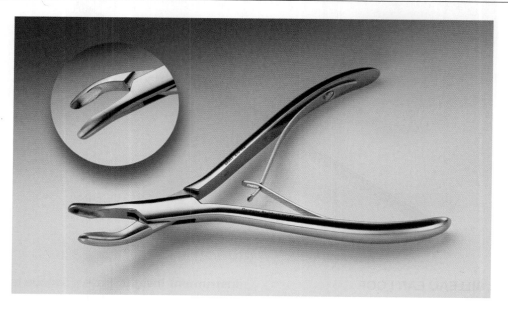

Instrument: DEAN RONGEUR
Use(s): Removes bone.
Description: Single-action instrument with a curved, sharp, cupped tip.

Instrument Insight: Tissues should be removed between uses with a moistened sponge.

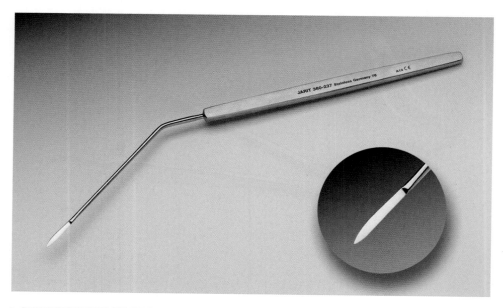

Instrument: MYRINGOTOMY KNIFE
Other Names: Tympanostomy knife, ear knife
Use(s): Used for incising the tympanic membrane for removal of fluid and insertion of aeration tubes.

Description: A long, narrow, angled knife with a lancet blade tip.
Instrument Insight: May also use a Beaver knife handle with #377110 blades.

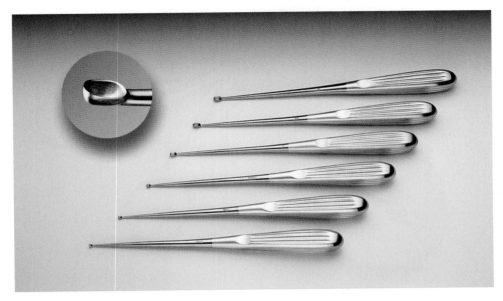

Instrument: SPRATT MASTOID CURETTES
Other Names: Ear curettes
Use(s): Remove diseased bone and tissue during a mastoidectomy.

Description: Small, oval cup shaped curettes.

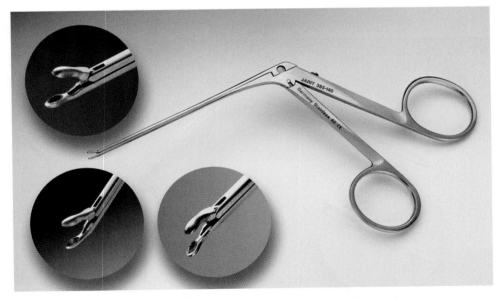

Instrument: OVAL CUP FORCEPS, STRAIGHT, RIGHT, LEFT
Other Names: Micro cups, ear cup forceps
Use(s): Used for removing tissue and ossicles from the middle ear.
Description: Small instrument with finger rings and an oval cupped working tip. The cup tips can be straight, left, right, up, or down-biting for accessing the middle ear.
Instrument Insight: These instruments should be cleaned with an instrument wipe between uses.

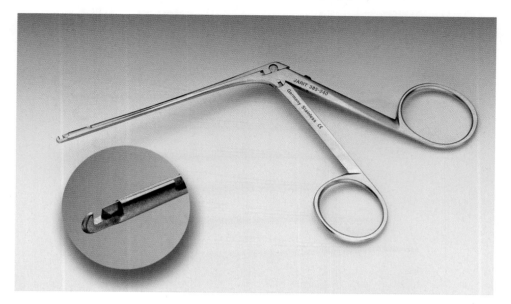

Instrument: HOUSE-DIETER MALLEUS NIPPER
Other Names: Nipper
Use(s): Used for reshaping of the ossicles, especially the malleus, for ossicular reconstruction.

Description: Small instrument with finger rings and a guillotine-type cutting tip.

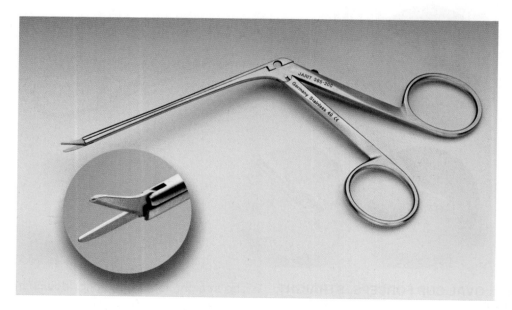

Instrument: BELLUCCI SCISSORS
Other Names: Middle ear scissors
Use(s): Used for cutting tissue in the middle ear.
Description: Small instrument with finger rings and delicate scissors on the working tip.

Instrument Insight: These are very delicate instruments; do not use them to cut packing or suture of any kind, as this will dull the blades.

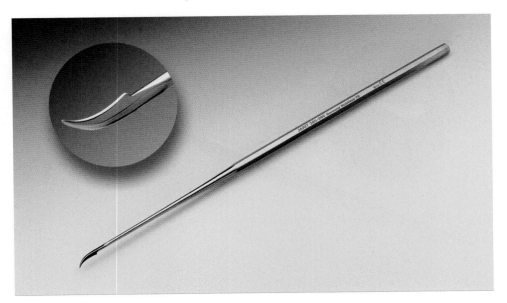

Instrument: HOUSE SICKLE KNIFE
Other Names: Ear knife
Use(s): Used to cut tissue in the ear canal and middle ear; often used to create a tympanic flap when performing middle ear surgery.

Description: Long handle with a sickle-type cutting edge at its working tip.
Instrument Insight: Commonly included in a rack with other delicate instruments for their protection.

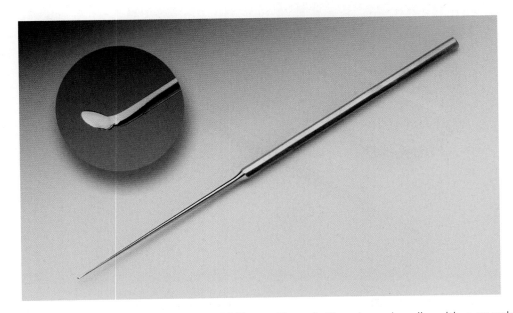

Instrument: HOUSE-SHEEHY KNIFE CURETTE
Other Names: Rosen knife, canal knife
Use(s): Used for removing tissue and bone from the ear canal and middle ear.

Description: Long handle with a rounded, angled, sharp tip.
Instrument Insight: Commonly included in a rack with other delicate instruments for their protection.

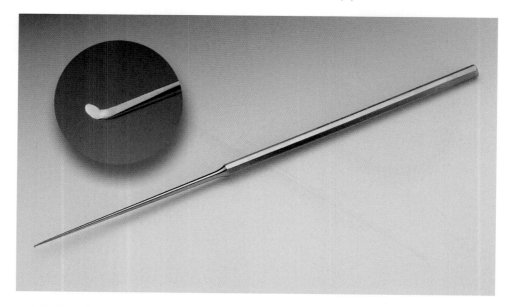

Instrument: HOUSE JOINT KNIFE
Other Names: Canal knife, flap knife
Use(s): Used for incising and dissecting tissue in the ear canal and middle ear, such as creating a tympanic flap, incising the canal during a tympanoplasty, or separating the incus from the stapes during a stapedectomy.

Description: Long handle with a rounded, angled, sharp tip.
Instrument Insight: Commonly included in a rack with other delicate instruments for their protection.

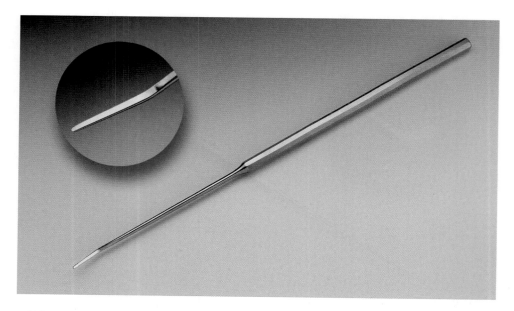

Instrument: HOUSE ELEVATOR
Other Names: Canal elevator, gimmick
Use(s): Used for manipulating and dissecting tissue in the middle ear and ear canal, such as elevating the annulus of the tympanic membrane.

Description: Long handle with an angled, elongated, oval, blunt tip.
Instrument Insight: Commonly included in a rack with other delicate instruments for protection.

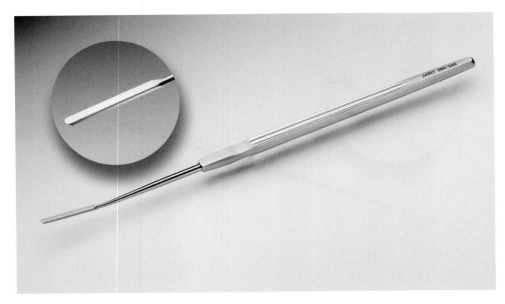

Instrument: LEMPERT ELEVATOR
Use(s): Used to cut and dissect tissue in the middle ear and ear canal.
Description: Long handle with a slightly angled, elongated, oval, blunt tip.

Instrument Insight: Commonly included in a rack with other delicate instruments for protection.

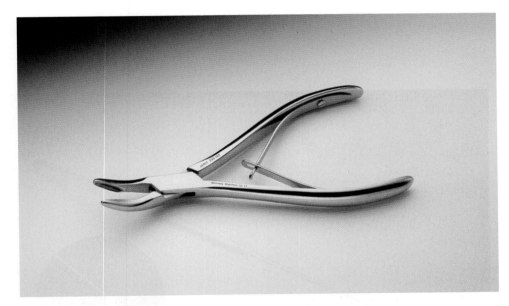

Instrument: CICHERELLI MASTOID RONGEUR
Other Names: Mastoid rongeur
Use(s): Used to cut and remove bone and air cells from the mastoid area.
Description: Small, single-action rongeur, which comes straight or angled.
Instrument Insight: This rongeur is often used in other specialties involving bone or tough tissue removal. Always have a moistened sponge ready when handing the surgeon a rongeur. As the surgeon works to remove tissue and/or bone, the rongeur should be cleaned between uses. While focusing on the wound, the surgeon will point the tip of the rongeur toward the surgical technologist. Using a moistened sponge, the surgical technologist should remove the tissue from the jaws of the rongeur.

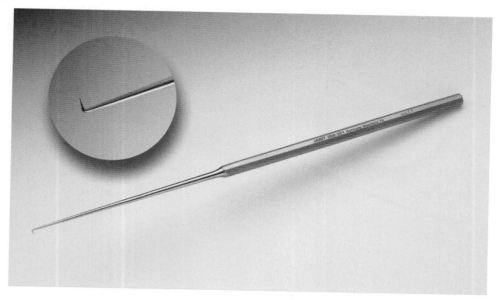

Instrument: HOUSE PICKS
Use(s): Manipulate tissue in the middle ear.
Description: Long handles with, 90° angle sharp tips.

Instrument Insight: Commonly included in a rack with other delicate instruments for protection.

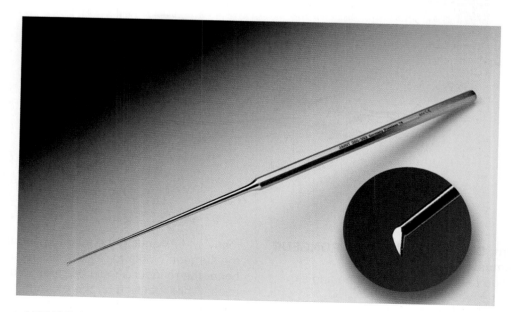

Instrument: HOUSE OVAL WINDOW PICK
Other Names: House pick
Use(s): Used for manipulating the soft tissue graft over the oval window during a stapedectomy.

Description: Long handle with an angled, sharp, triangular tip.
Instrument Insight: Commonly included in a rack with other delicate instruments for protection.

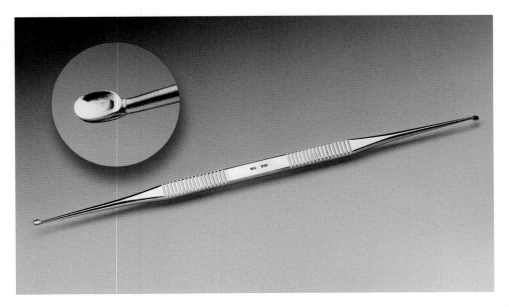

Instrument: HOUSE DOUBLE-ENDED CURETTES
Other Names: Ear curettes, small bone curettes
Use(s): Remove bone from the ear canal and middle ear.

Description: A double-ended curette with cutting cups of different sizes at the ends.
Instrument Insight: Commonly included in a rack with other delicate instruments for protection.

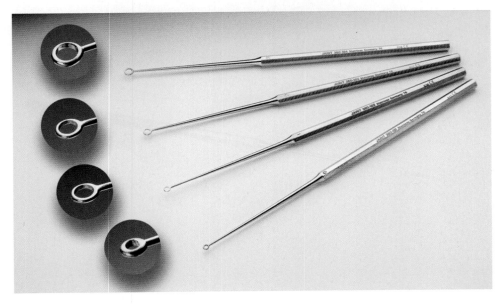

Instrument: BUCK EAR CURETTE
Other Names: Ring curette
Use(s): Removes bone and tissue from the ear canal and middle ear.

Description: Long handle with a blunt or sharp open-ringed tip.

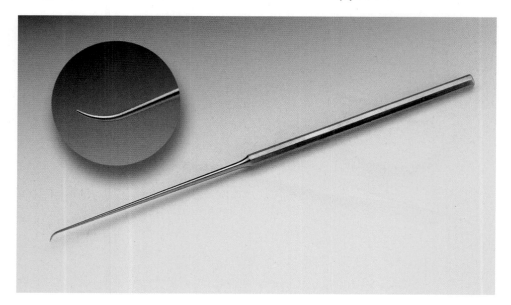

Instrument: ROSEN NEEDLE

Use(s): Used for manipulating tissue in the middle ear.

Description: Long handle with a curved tip that tapers to a blunt point.

Instrument Insight: The Rosen needle is not as sharp as the Barbara needle but is used for the same purposes.

Instrument Insight: Commonly included in a rack with other delicate instruments for protection.

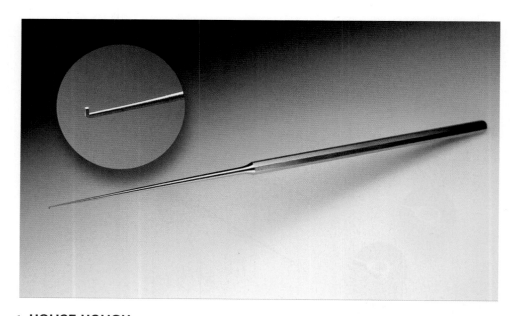

Instrument: HOUSE HOUGH

Use(s): Used for manipulating the ossicles and tissues in the middle ear.

Description: Long handle with a 90° blunt hooked tip.

Instrument Insight: Commonly included in a rack with other delicate instruments for protection.

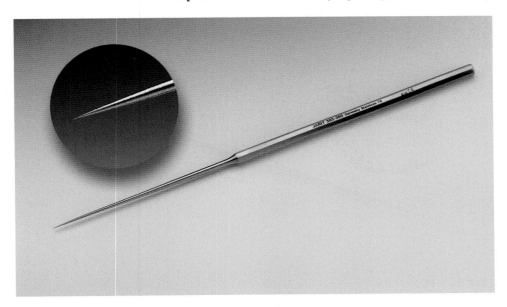

Instrument: HOUSE-BARBARA SHATTERING NEEDLE
Other Names: Barbara needle, shattering needle
Use(s): Used for manipulating tissue and ossicles in the middle ear. It also is used to fracture the superior portion of the stapes from the footplate during a stapedectomy.

Description: Long handle with a straight tip that tapers to a sharp point.
Instrument Insight: This instrument is sharper than a Rosen needle, but used for the same purpose. It is commonly included in a rack with other delicate instruments for protection.

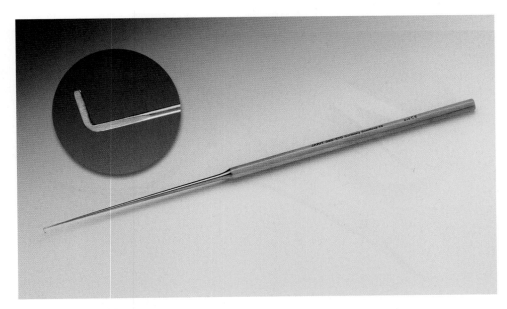

Instrument: CRABTREE DISSECTOR
Other Names: Jimmy
Use(s): Used for manipulating ossicles and tissue in the middle ear.

Description: Long handles with a 90° blunt working tip.
Instrument Insight: Commonly included in a rack with other delicate instruments for protection.

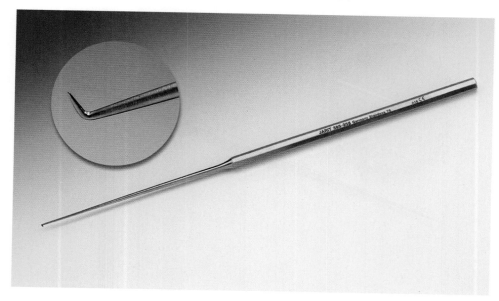

Instrument: HOUSE STRUT HOOK
Other Names: Ditto
Use(s): Used for dissecting and removing ossicles from the middle ear.

Description: Long handles with 90° sharp tips.
Instrument Insight: Commonly included in a rack with other delicate instruments for protection.

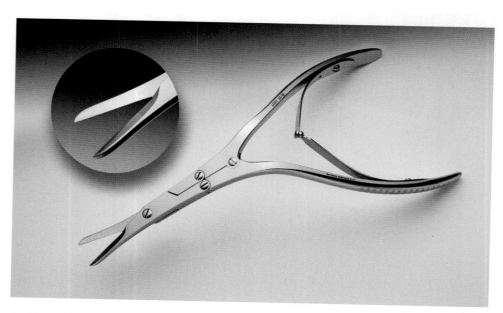

Instrument: CAPLAN SCISSORS
Use(s): Used for cutting tissue within the nasal cavity.

Description: Double-action instrument with angled scissor blades and blunt tips.

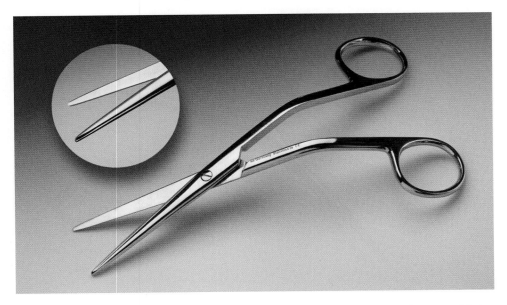

Instrument: COTTLE ANGULAR SCISSORS
Other Names: Turbinate scissors, posterior scissors
Use(s): Used for trimming the turbinate (mucosal) tissue in the nose.

Description: Angled scissors with long, narrow, blunt blades.
Instrument Insight: These scissors come in small and medium sizes.

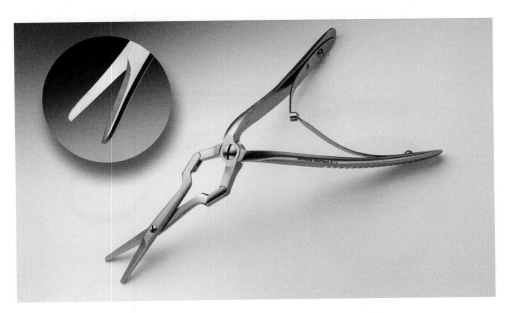

Instrument: BECKER SEPTUM SCISSORS
Use(s): Used for cutting tissue within the nasal cavity.

Description: Angled double-action scissors with straight, blunt-tip blades.

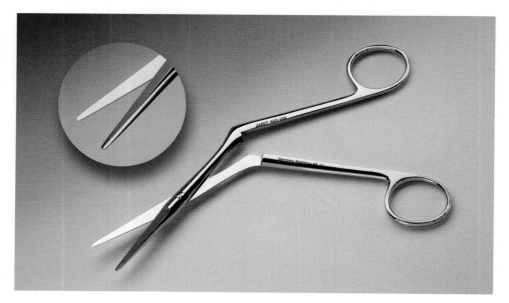

Instrument: KNIGHT ANGULAR SCISSORS
Other Names: Heymann-Knight angular scissors
Use(s): Used for cutting tissue within the nasal cavity.

Description: Angled scissors with narrow, blunt blades.

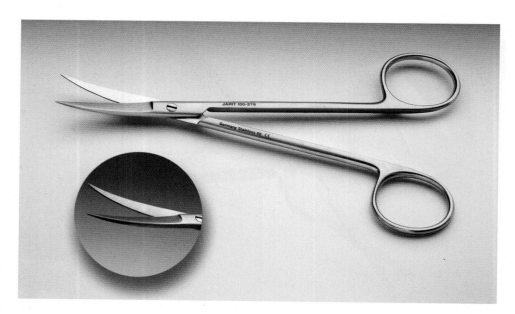

Instrument: JOSEPH SCISSORS
Use(s): Used for cutting fine tissue.
Description: Small, delicate, curved scissors with very sharp points.

Instrument Insight: Because of the sharp points, handle and pass with care.

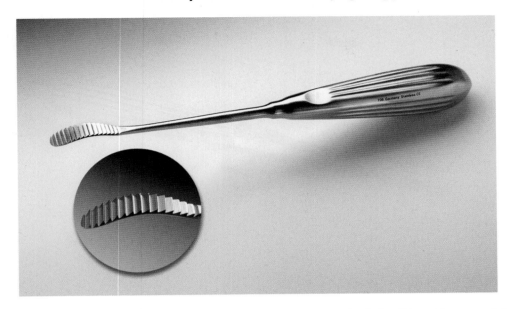

Instrument: AUFRICHT NASAL RASPS
Use(s): Used for filing hard tissue and bone.
Description: This rasp is a round-handled instrument that has a rounded, slightly curved working end with sharp horizontal ridges.

Instrument Insight: Bits of bone and tissue will accumulate in the ridges; clean the rasp by rinsing it in a small basin of water between uses.

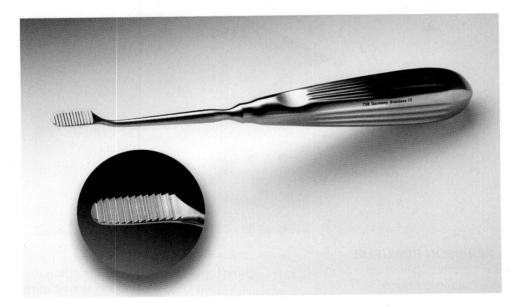

Instrument: LEWIS RASP
Use(s): Used for filing hard tissue and bone.
Description: This rasp is a round-handled instrument that has a rounded, straight working end with sharp horizontal ridges.

Instrument Insight: Bits of bone and tissue will accumulate in the ridges; clean the rasp by rinsing it in a small basin of water between uses.

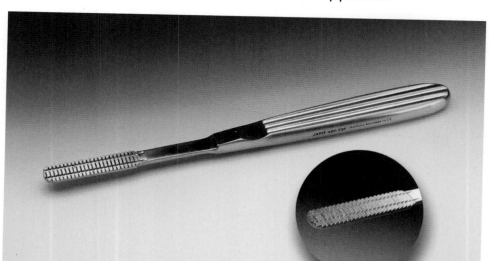

Instrument: MALTZ RASP
Other Names: Maltz-Lipsett
Use(s): Used for filing hard tissue and bone.
Description: Has rectangular sanding edge with horizontal and vertical ridges.

Instrument Insight: Bits of bone and tissue will accumulate in the ridges; clean the rasp by rinsing it in a small basin of water between uses.

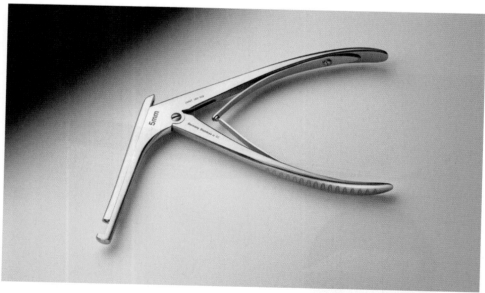

Instrument: KERRISON RONGEUR
Other Names: Up-biter
Use(s): Used for biting off bone.
Description: Gripped handles with a 4-inch shaft and chisel-edge punch at the working tip. The punch tip is available in 3-, 4-, 5-, and 6-mm bites.
Instrument Insight: This rongeur can also have the biting edge positioned downward, called a down-biter or back biter. Always have a moistened sponge ready when handing the surgeon a rongeur. As the surgeon works to remove tissue and/or bone, the rongeur has to be cleaned between uses. While focusing on the wound, the surgeon will point the tip of the rongeur toward the surgical technologist. Using a moistened sponge, the surgical technologist will clean the tissue from the jaws.

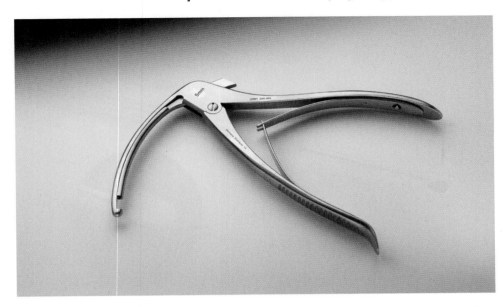

Instrument: KERRISON-COSTEN RONGEUR
Use(s): Used for biting off bone.
Description: This instrument is a variation of the Kerrison rongeur, but this rongeur has an angled arm and the cutting end is facing downward.
Instrument Insight: Always have a moistened sponge ready when handing the surgeon a rongeur.

As the surgeon works to remove tissue and/or bone, the rongeur has to be cleaned between uses. While focusing on the wound, the surgeon will point the tip of the rongeur toward the surgical technologist. Using a moistened sponge, the surgical technologist will clean the tissue from the jaws.

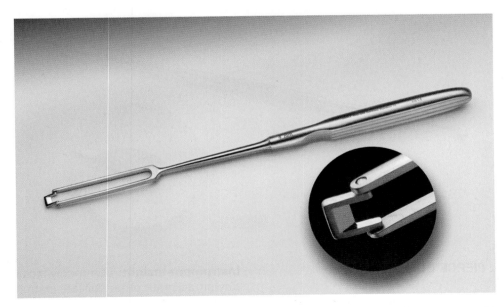

Instrument: BALLENGER SWIVEL KNIFE
Other Names: Swivel knife
Use(s): Used to cut and dissect nasal mucosa.

Description: Handled instrument with a hinged cutting tip for ease of application through nasal tissue.

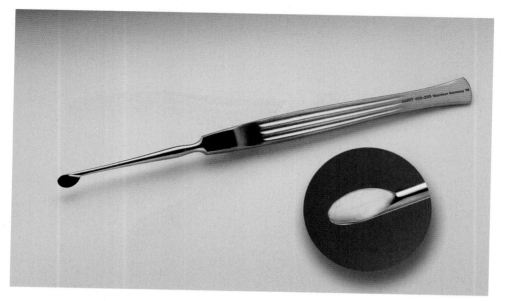

Instrument: FREER SEPTUM KNIFE
Other Names: Septal knife
Use(s): Used to cut and dissect septal mucosa.
Description: Flat-handled instrument with a rounded, sharp cutting end.

Instrument Insight: Commonly included in a tray or rack with other delicate instruments for protection.

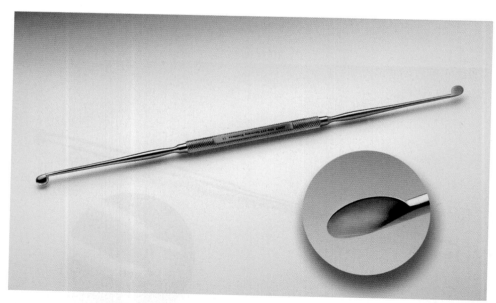

Instrument: PIERCE DOUBLE ENDED ELEVATOR
Use(s): Cuts and dissects septal mucosa.
Description: A double-ended elevator with two rounded sharp blades at each end with one blade larger than the other.

Instrument Insight: Commonly included in a tray or rack with other delicate instruments for protection.

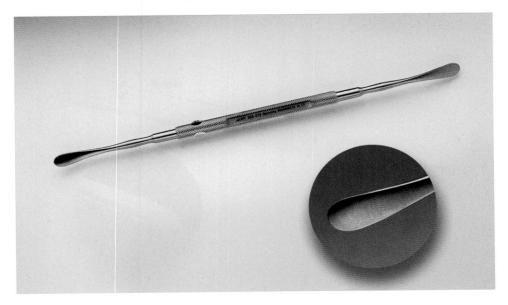

Instrument: FREER SEPTUM ELEVATOR
Other Names: Freer elevator
Use(s): The Freer used to dissect nasal mucosa from the septum.

Description: Round handle with tear-shaped sharp tips at both ends.

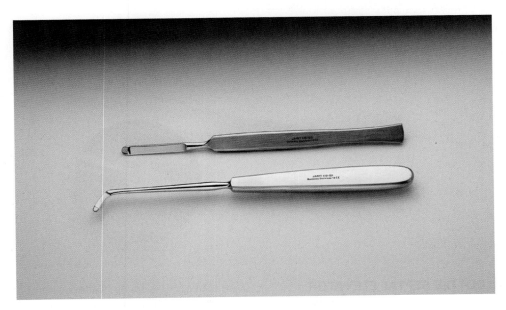

Instrument: JOSEPH BUTTON-END KNIFE
Use(s): Used for dissecting nasal mucosa from the septum.

Description: Solid handled instrument with either an angled or a straight blade.

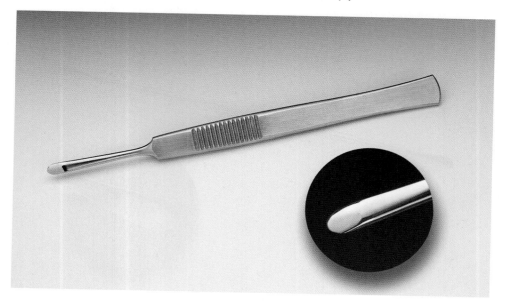

Instrument: COTTLE NASAL KNIFE

Use(s): Used for dissecting nasal mucosa from the septum.

Description: Flat-handled instrument with a smaller, flattened, sharp tip.

Instrument Insight: Commonly included in a tray or rack with other delicate instruments for protection.

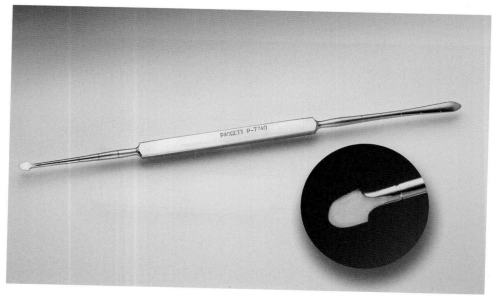

Instrument: COTTLE SEPTAL ELEVATOR

Use(s): Used for cutting and dissecting nasal mucosa.

Description: Double-ended elevator with a flattened handle; one end is sharp and rounded while the other end is sharp, flattened, and tear-shaped. The instrument has calibrations on both arms.

Instrument Insight: Commonly included in a tray or rack with other delicate instruments for protection.

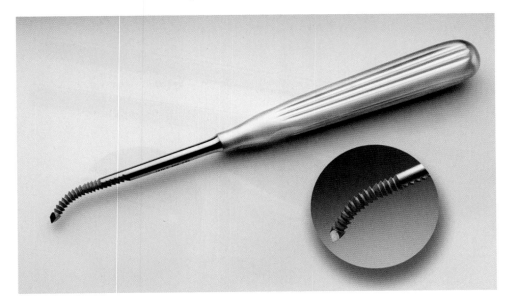

Instrument: WIENER ANTRUM RASP
Other Names: Antrum rasp
Use(s): Used for creating an opening through the nasal wall to the maxillary sinus.

Description: Straight handle and shaft with a curved working end that has a sharp, encircling, raised serration and a trocar tip.

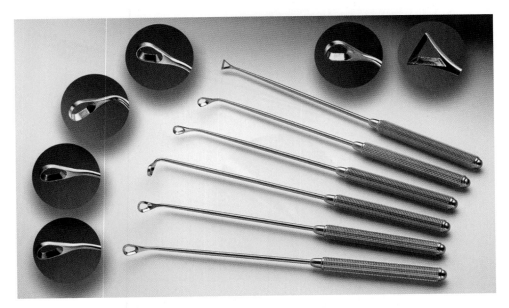

Instrument: COAKLEY ANTRUM CURETTES
Other Names: Nasal curettes
Use(s): Used for removing polyps and diseased sinus tissue.

Description: Round-handled instrument with a circular cutting tip that is available in different sizes and different angles.

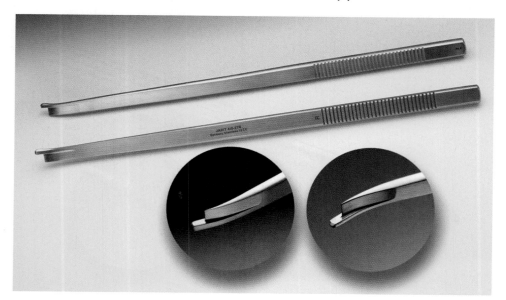

Instrument: NEIVERT-ANDERSON GUARDED OSTEOTOME

Use(s): Used for cutting bone.

Description: Flat-handled instrument with a tip beveled to a point for cutting. One side of the tip extends out and is blunt, which acts as a guard. These osteotomes vary in width.

Instrument Insight: Always hand to the surgeon with a mallet.

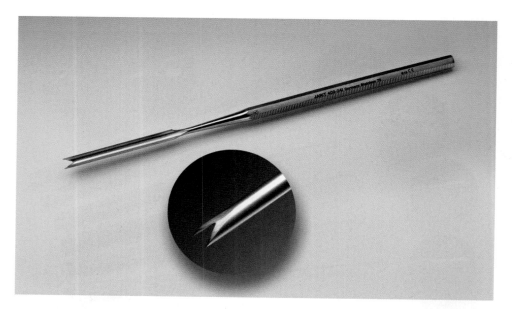

Instrument: BALLENGER V-SHAPED OSTEOTOME

Use(s): Used for removing bone.

Description: Rounded handle with a V-shaped cutting edge.

Instrument Insight: This instrument is finer than other osteotomes but still requires a mallet for use.

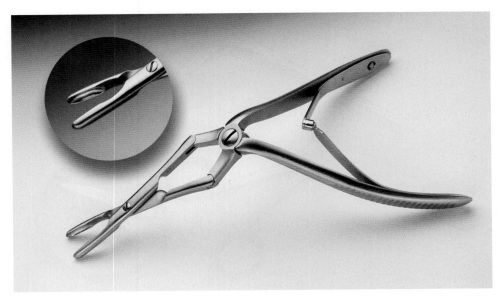

Instrument: JANSEN-MIDDLETON SEPTUM FORCEPS
Use(s): Dissects and removes nasal tissues.
Description: Double-action angled instrument with oval cup jaws.

Instrument Insight: Tissues should be removed between uses with a moistened sponge.

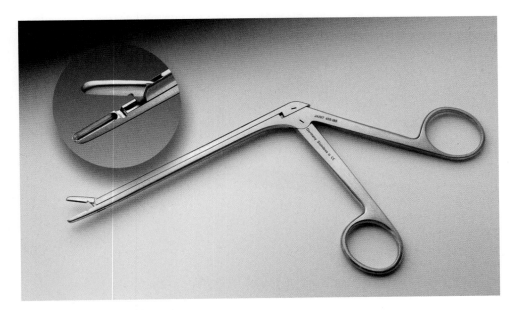

Instrument: TAKAHASHI NASAL FORCEPS
Use(s): Used to grasp and remove nasal tissue and polyps.
Description: Handle with finger rings and a long shaft with an oval cup-shaped tip.

Instrument Insight: Tissues should be removed between uses with a moistened sponge.

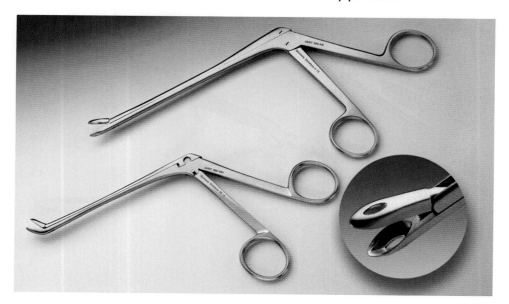

Instrument: WILDE ETHMOID FORCEPS

Use(s): Used to remove infected or inflamed tissue that lines the nasal sinuses or to remove nasal polyps, especially in the ethmoid sinuses.

Description: Handle with finger rings, a long shaft, and an oval cup-shaped tip with fenestrations.

Instrument Insight: Instrument is available in straight and up-biting tips. Tissues should be removed between uses with a moistened sponge.

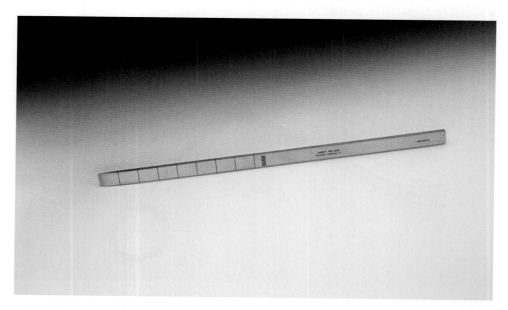

Instrument: COTTLE OSTEOTOMES

Use(s): Used for dissecting and sculpting bone.

Description: Solid stainless-steel strip with a smooth, inclining, sharp blade tip.

Instrument Insight: Always hand to the surgeon with a mallet.

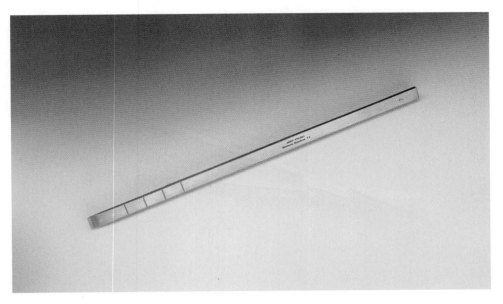

Instrument: COTTLE CHISELS
Other Names: Nasal chisels
Use(s): Used for cutting bone.
Description: Solid stainless-steel strip that ends in a beveled, sharp tip.

Instrument Insight: Always hand to the surgeon with a mallet.

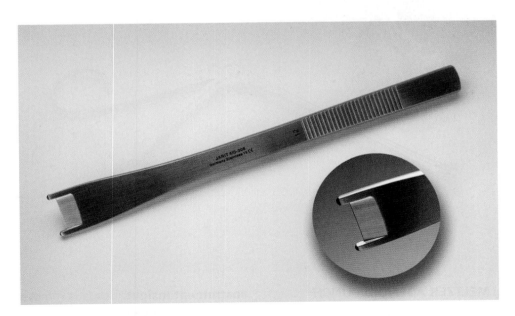

Instrument: CINELLI GUARDED OSTEOTOME
Use(s): Cuts bone.
Description: Solid stainless-steel strip with a widened blade that has a guard on each side.

Instrument Insight: Always hand to the surgeon with a mallet.

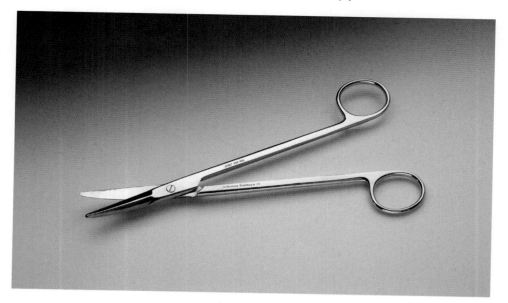

Instrument: BOETTCHER TONSIL SCISSORS
Other Names: Tonsil scissors
Use(s): Used for cutting tissue, especially in the oral pharynx for a tonsillectomy.

Description: Long, narrow, curved scissors with beveled outer blades.
Instrument Insight: These scissors are placed on the surgeon's fingers with the tips pointing downward.

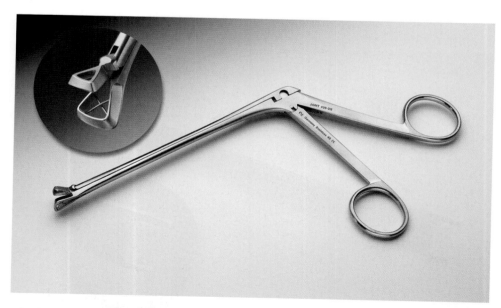

Instrument: MELTZER ADENOID PUNCH
Other Names: Punch
Use(s): Used for dissecting adenoids.
Description: Finger-ringed instrument with a long shaft and triangular sharp jaws that fit inside one another.

Instrument Insight: Tissue is removed with a moistened sponge between uses.

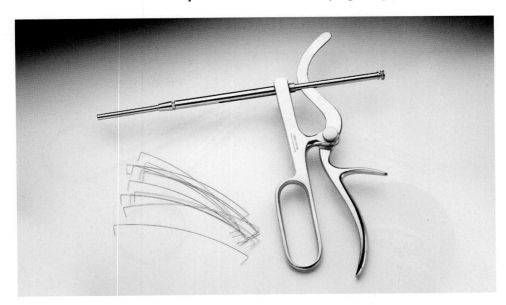

Instrument: TONSIL SNARE

Use(s): Snare wire is placed around the base of each tonsil, the handle is squeezed, and the wire is withdrawn into the cannula, severing the tonsil tissue through a guillotine action.

Description: A handle grip that attaches to a metal cannula and an inner sliding rod. The inner rod has two small holes at the tip in which the snare wires are loaded.

Instrument Insight: When loading the snare wires, expose the rod tip by opening the handles. The bent ends of the snare wire are then threaded into the holes. A slight compression of the handle then pulls the rough ends of the wire into the cannula, creating a loop. Wires become twisted and compressed after use; therefore they should be discarded and replaced with new ones.

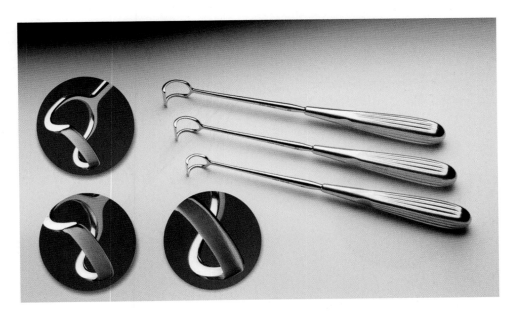

Instrument: BARNHILL ADENOID CURETTES

Use(s): Used for removing adenoid tissue via a scraping action.

Description: Rounded handles with a curved, open frame that contains a cutting edge.

Instrument Insight: Instruments come in sets with various sizes.

GRASPING AND HOLDING INSTRUMENTS

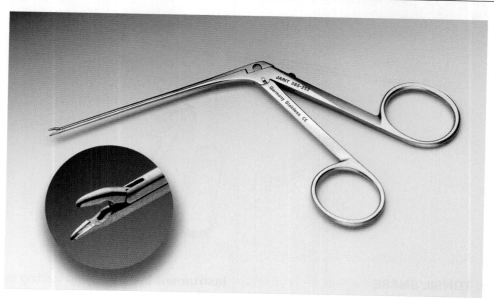

Instrument: McGEE WIRE CRIMPING FORCEPS

Other Names: Crimper

Use(s): Used for ossicular reconstruction to clip or bend the wire on the stapes prosthesis.

Description: Small instrument with finger rings and delicate working tip for use through the ear canal and into the middle ear.

Instrument Insight: Instrument is delicate; do not drop or place heavier instruments on top of it. Keep its tip clean with an instrument wipe or dampened sponge.

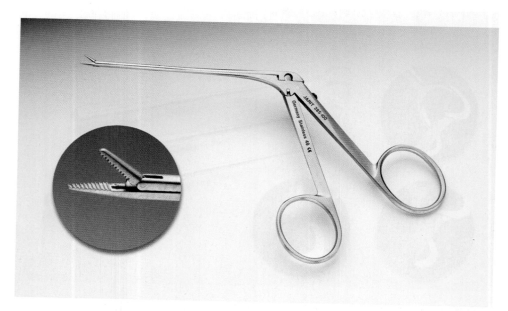

Instrument: WULLSTEIN EAR FORCEPS

Other Names: Alligator forceps

Use(s): Used for manipulating and removing tissue from the ear canal and middle ear, inserting aeration tubes, and placing Gelfoam packing when grafting.

Description: Small instrument with finger rings with tapered, serrated jaws.

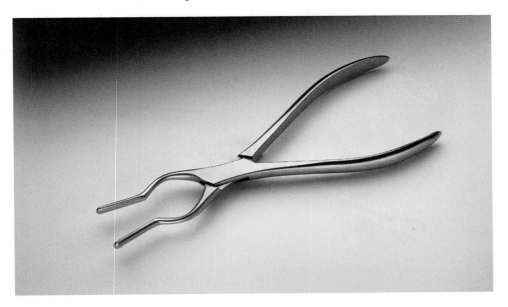

Instrument: WALSHAM SEPTUM STRAIGHTENER

Use(s): This instrument is placed inside the nose, on both sides of the septum, to straighten a displaced nasal fracture.

Description: A single-action handle with a rounded jaw that extends to a flattened end approximately 1 inch on each side of the jaw.

Instrument Insight: The ends are rounded at the tip to prevent injury to the septum during insertion.

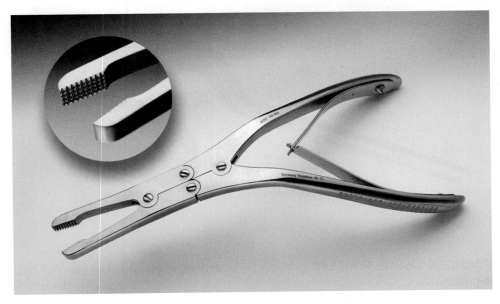

Instrument: RUBIN MORSELIZER

Use(s): Used to grasp and soften nasal cartilage for reinsertion into the septum.

Description: Double-action instrument with a rectangular tip and cross-hatch serrations.

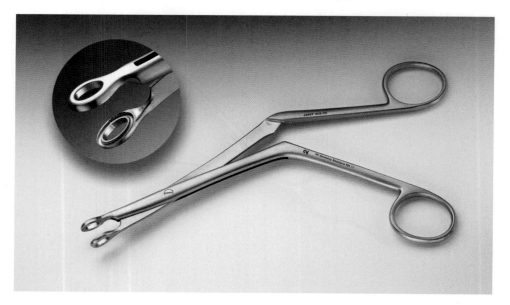

Instrument: BRUENING SEPTUM FORCEPS
Use(s): Used to grasp and hold nasal tissue.

Description: Instrument with finger rings and a cupped, perforated tip.

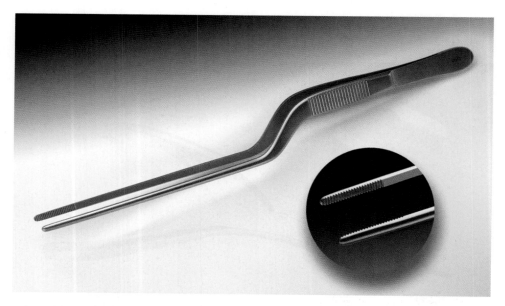

Instrument: JANSEN TISSUE FORCEPS
Other Names: Bayonet
Use(s): Used for grasping and manipulating tissue and placing packing or nasal splints.
Description: Long bayonet-shaped tissue forceps with serrated, round tips.

Instrument Insight: The bayonet has its curved shape to keep the instrument from getting in the surgeon's eyesight when in use.

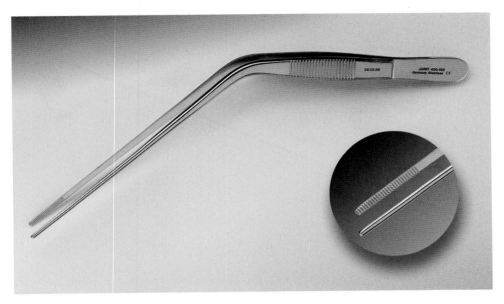

Instrument: WILDE TISSUE FORCEPS
Other Names: Wilde dressing forcep
Use(s): Used for grasping and manipulating tissue and placing packing or nasal splints.

Description: Long, angled tissue forceps with serrated, round tips.

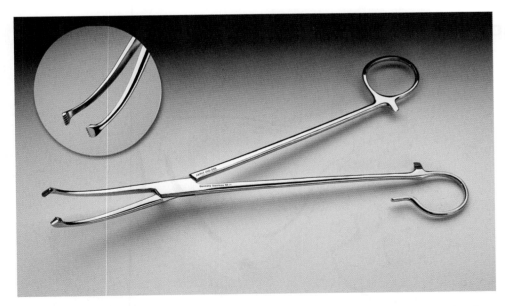

Instrument: CURVED ALLIS FORCEPS
Other Names: Tonsil grasper, tonsil forceps
Use(s): Used to grasp and hold tonsil tissue for removal.
Description: Finger-ringed instrument with one open ring, long shanks with curved jaws, and intertwining fine teeth at the tip.

Instrument Insight: The one ring is open so that, after the tissue is grasped, a suture may slide down the instrument and secure the tissue.

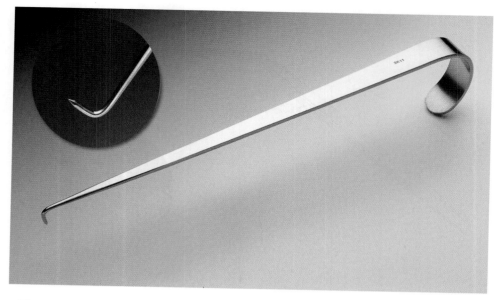

Instrument: HUPP TRACHEAL HOOK
Other Names: Trach hook
Use(s): Used to penetrate the trachea and pull it upwards during a tracheotomy.

Description: Retracting instrument with a curved handle for easy holding and a hooked, sharp end.
Instrument Insight: Use caution when handling to prevent puncture wounds on gloves or drapes.

RETRACTING AND EXPOSING INSTRUMENTS

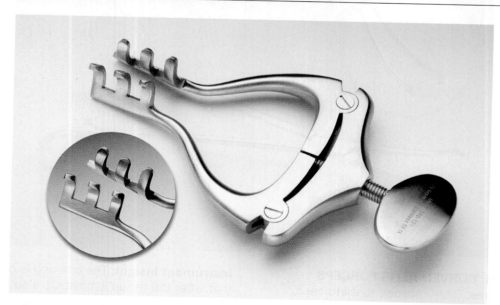

Instrument: JANSEN MASTOID RETRACTOR
Use(s): Used for retracting a postauricular incision.
Description: A small self-retaining retractor with a screw-locking device at the proximal end that holds it open and two small arms that have three sharp or blunt outward-curving prongs on the working end.

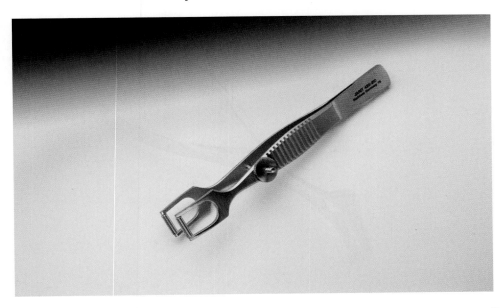

Instrument: COTTLE COLUMELLA FORCEPS
Other Names: Columella retractor
Use(s): Used for manipulating and retracts the nasal columella.
Description: Two-bladed, self-retaining instrument with a screw-down mechanism to hold arms in place.

Instrument Insight: This instrument fits onto the anterior part of the septum (columella), one blade positioned on each side, and screws down to lock.

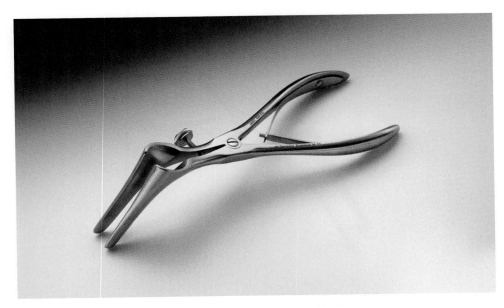

Instrument: COTTLE NASAL SPECULUM
Use(s): Used for retracting the nares for visualization.

Description: A self-retaining instrument with double-bladed tips and a screw opening device. The speculum blades vary in length.

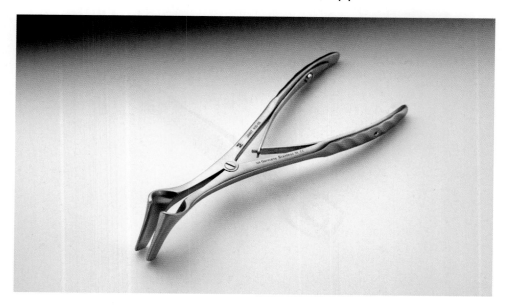

Instrument: VIENNA NASAL SPECULUM
Use(s): Used for retracting the nares for visualization.

Description: A manually held double-bladed instrument with concave tips. The speculum blades vary in length.

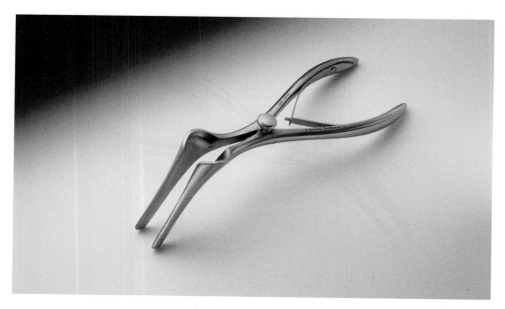

Instrument: KILLIAN NASAL SPECULUM
Use(s): Used for retracting the nares for visualization.

Description: A self-retaining instrument with double-bladed tips and a screw opening device. The speculum blades vary in length.

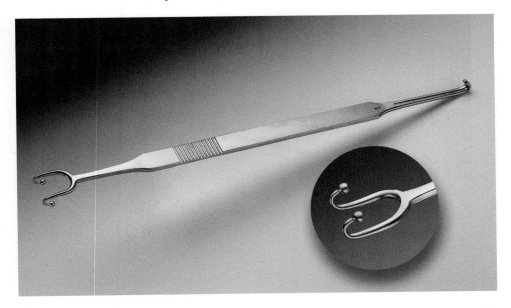

Instrument: COTTLE KNIFE GUIDE AND RETRACTOR

Use(s): Used for retracting the nares for visualization.

Description: Double-ended retractor with a small, blunt hook on one end and two, curved, ball-tip prongs on the other end.

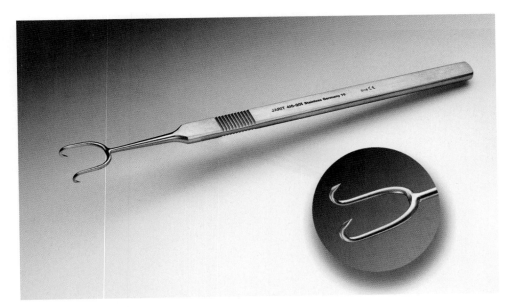

Instrument: COTTLE DOUBLE HOOK RETRACTOR

Use(s): Used for retracting the nares for visualization.

Description: Instrument with a flat handle and two sharp hooks.

Instrument Insight: Use caution not to perforate gloves or drapes with the sharp ends.

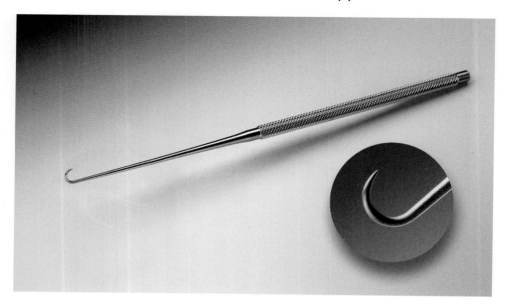

Instrument: JOSEPH SKIN HOOKS
Other Names: Single skin hook
Use(s): Used for retracting tissues.

Description: Round-handled instrument with a single, sharp, hooked end.

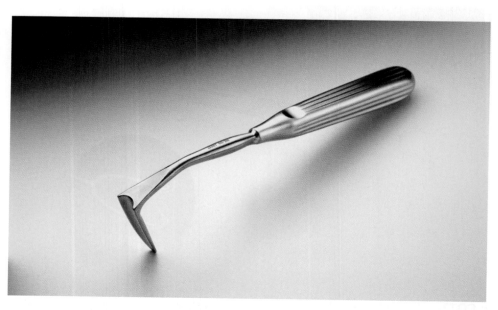

Instrument: AUFRICHT NASAL RETRACTOR
Use(s): Used for retracting the nares for visualization.

Description: Round-handled instrument with a right-angled, slightly concave, blunt blade at its end.

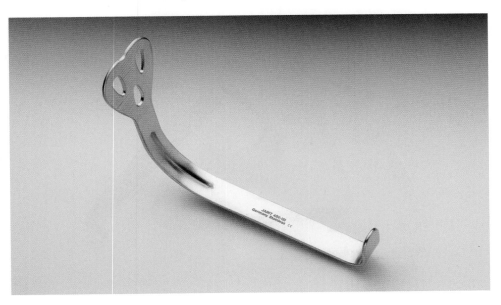

Instrument: WIEDER TONGUE BLADE
Other Names: Tongue depressor
Use(s): Used to depress and thus retract the tongue away from the operative site.

Description: Flat-handled instrument with a heart-shaped tip and three oval-shaped holes.

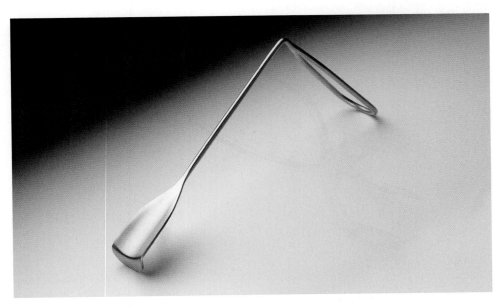

Instrument: LOTHROP UVULA RETRACTOR
Use(s): Used for retracting the uvula and soft palate.

Description: Angled retractor with a looped handle and a flattened end with a lip at the distal end for retracting the soft palate.

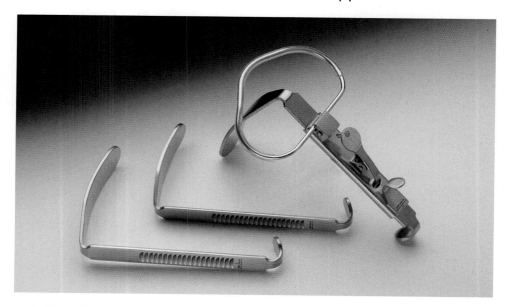

Instrument: McIVOR MOUTH GAG

Use(s): Used for retracting the mouth open and the tongue down for exposure of the oral cavity and the back of the throat.

Description: Self-retaining loop-shaped frame retractor with an attachable tongue blade that slides onto the handle and has a ratchet for adjustment.

Instrument Insight: The mouth gag is available with three different-sized tongue blades. The hook end of the tongue blade slips over the edge of the Mayo stand to hold the patient in proper alignment for maximum exposure.

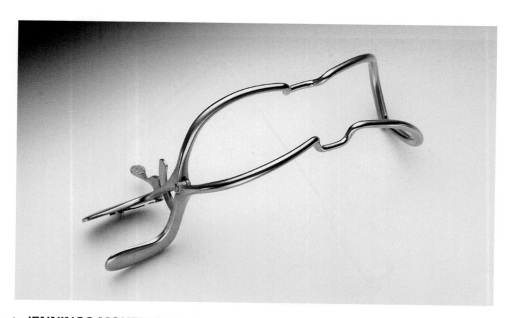

Instrument: JENNINGS MOUTH GAG

Use(s): Used for retracting the mouth open for exposure of the oral cavity and the back of the throat.

Description: A self-retaining eye-shaped retractor with ratchets.

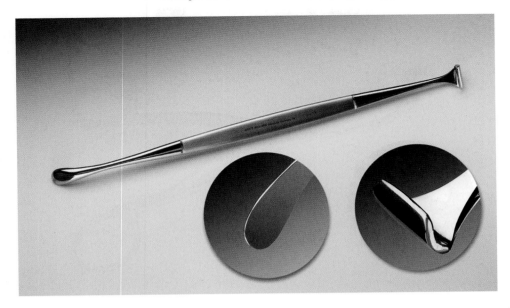

Instrument: HURD DISSECTOR
Other Names: Herd elevator, pillar retractor
Use(s): Retracts the soft palate for oral proce-
dures and dissects tonsil tissue.

Description: Flat-handled instrument with different ends: one is a rounded and slightly sharp
end; the other curves into a lip.

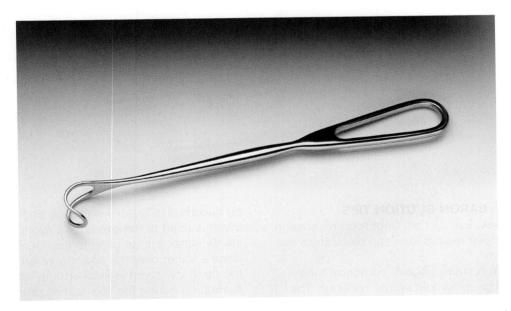

Instrument: GREEN RETRACTOR
Other Names: Thyroid retractor
Use(s): Used for retracting tissue, particularly in
the neck area.

Description: Loop-handled retractor with a
curved, oval, blunt-looped end.

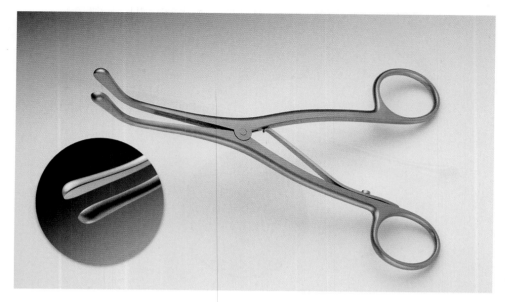

Instrument: TROUSSEAU TRACHEAL DILATOR

Other Names: Tracheal spreader

Use(s): Used for retracting the tracheal edges. This allows for placement of a tracheotomy tube.

Description: Finger-ringed handle with two blunt-angled ends that spread apart when the handle is compressed.

SUCTIONING AND ASPIRATING INSTRUMENTS

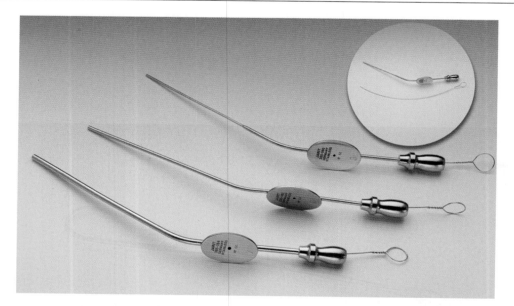

Instrument: BARON SUCTION TIPS

Other Names: Ear suction, finger-control suction

Use(s): Remove excess fluid and blood from the operative site.

Description: A small, angled, cylindrical tube with a relief opening/hole on the handgrip. The diameters are 3F, 5F, and 7F, and they are usually packaged with a metal stylet that fits inside the cylinder.

Instrument Insight: Suction can be increased by covering the relief opening. When the suction tip becomes clogged with tissue and debris, the stylet is used to remove it, or a syringe with sterile water can be used to flush it. Be sure to place a finger over the opening when irrigating the tip. If the stylet is inadvertently left in the suction tip during the sterilization process, do not just remove the stylet and hand it off the field. The inside of the Baron tip and the stylet are considered unsterile, and both should be removed from the field.

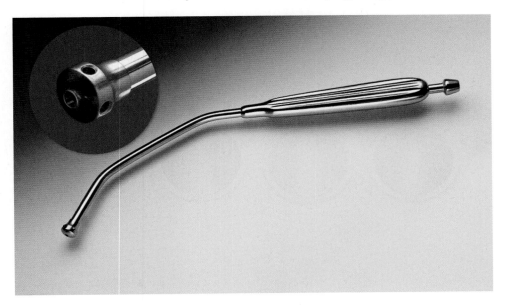

Instrument: NONDISPOSABLE YANKAUER SUCTION TIP
Other Names: Oral tip, oral suction
Use(s): Used for evacuating of tissue, blood, and debris from the surgical site.

Description: A hollow, curved, stainless-steel tube with a ball tip and a grip handle.
Instrument Insight: Note the tip of the suction is removable for cleaning. Make sure the tip is securely tightened before and after the procedure.

VIEWING INSTRUMENTS

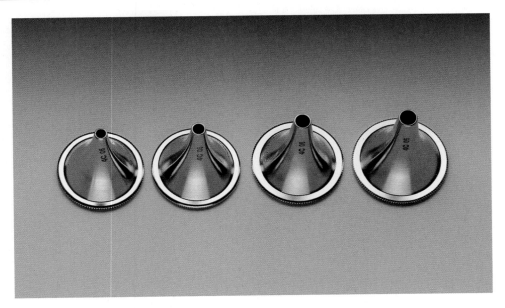

Instrument: BOUCHERON EAR SPECULUM
Use(s): Used for opening the ear canal for exposure of the tympanic membrane and portions of the middle ear.

Description: A bell-shaped speculum with a round opening; available in a set of varying sizes.
Instrument Insight: The size of the speculum is determined by the size of the patient's ear canal.

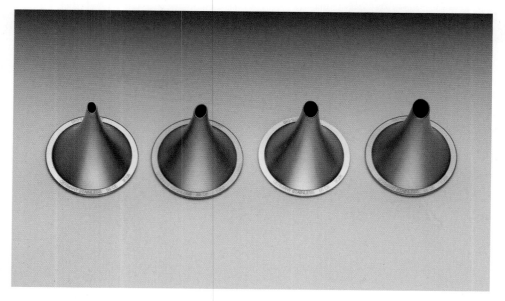

Instrument: FARRIOR EAR SPECULUM
Use(s): Used for opening the ear canal for exposure of the tympanic membrane and portions of the middle ear.

Description: A bell-shaped speculum with an oval opening; available in a set of varying sizes.
Instrument Insight: The size of the speculum is determined by the size of the patient's ear canal.

10

Oral Instruments

ACCESSORY INSTRUMENTS

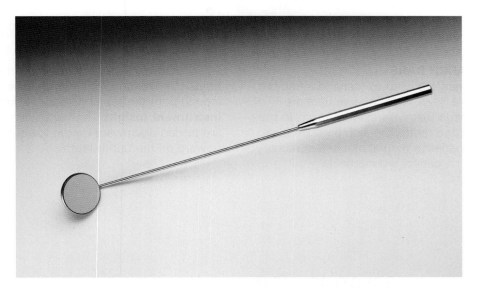

Instrument: MOUTH MIRROR
Other Names: Dental mirror, Laryngeal mirror
Use(s): Used for visualization of the mouth, including the teeth, gums, tongue, palate, and cheeks.
Description: The mouth mirror is a round-handled instrument with a small rounded mirror on the end. Mirrors are available in different diameters.

Instrument Insight: Mirror may fog when inserted into the oral cavity; the mirrors are dipped into some type of antifog solution or possibly warm water. Some oral surgeons will use the patient's saliva to prevent fogging of the mirrors.

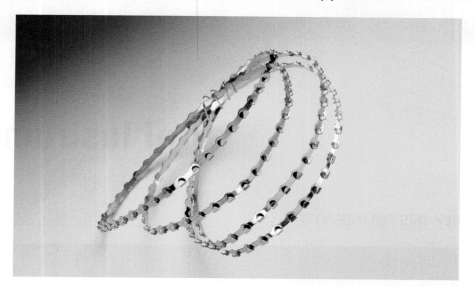

Instrument: ARCH BARS

Use(s): Arch bars are used to manage a fracture of the mandible (jaw). A set of arch bars are placed with wires that will easily conform to the natural arch of the teeth. The arch bars are ideal to maintain a patient's natural bite in a stationary position until the patient's bone heals.

Description: These appliances are rigid metal strips that have hooks in which wire is applied around both the top and bottom and twisted.

Instrument Insight: The hooks on the arch bars are placed downward on the lower teeth and upward on the upper teeth.

CUTTING AND DISSECTING INSTRUMENTS

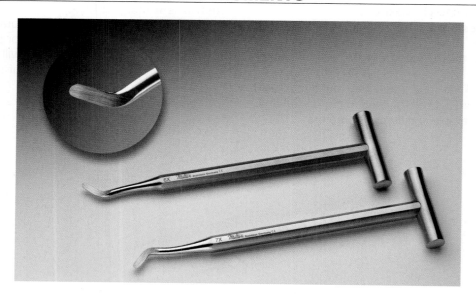

Instrument: POTTS ELEVATOR

Other Names: T-bar Potts elevators

Use(s): To loosen tooth or root from bony socket before use of the extraction forceps.

Description: The working end is right or left curve with a rounded tip in a range of sizes.

Handles may be either T-bar style or a design of heavy tapering to the working end.

Instrument Insight: These are in the set as right and left pairs.

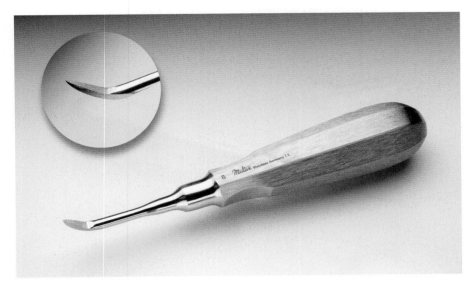

Instrument: CRANE ELEVATOR
Other Names: Angular elevator, root tip pick
Use(s): To loosen tooth or root from bony socket
before use of the extraction forceps.

Description: The working end has an upward
angle with a pointed tip. Handles may be either
T-bar style or a design with heavy tapering to the
working end.

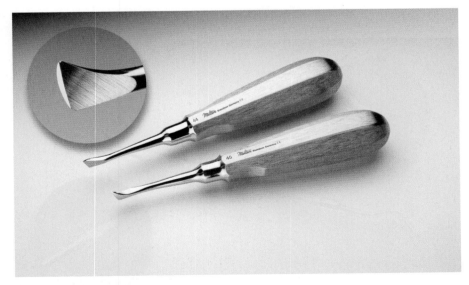

Instrument: CRYER ELEVATOR
Other Names: Flag elevators, root elevators
Use(s): To loosen tooth or root from bony socket
before use of the extraction forceps.
Description: The working end is right or left
with a triangular pointed tip in a range of sizes.

Handles may be either T-bar style or a design
with heavy tapering to the working end.
Instrument Insight: These are in the set as right
and left pairs.

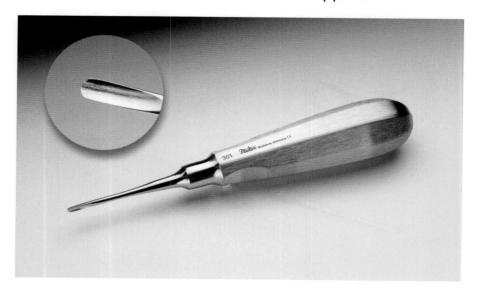

Instrument: APICAL ELEVATOR
Other Names: Straight elevator, luxating elevator
Use(s): To loosen tooth or root from bony socket before use of the extraction forceps.
Description: A round trough-like tip in a range of sizes with a heavy rounded tapering handle.

Instrument Insight: Common sizes are number 1, 34, and 301; these are often referred to by number.

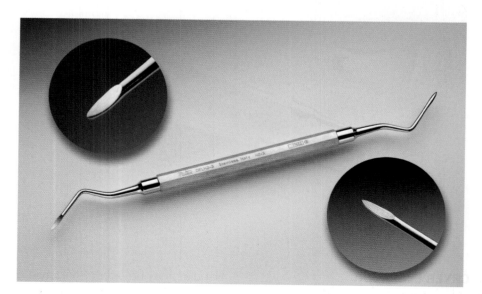

Instrument: ROOT TIP PICK
Other Names: Angle pick, dental pick
Use(s): Used to retrieve loose root fragments from the socket after an extraction.

Description: Double-ended small elevator with thin, angled pointed tip on one end and a blunt tip on the other.

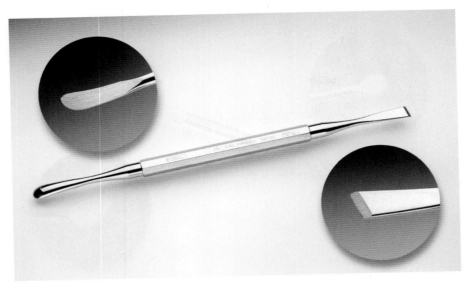

Instrument: WEST PERIOSTEAL
Other Names: Periosteal elevator
Use(s): Primarily are used to retract gingival tissue; also used during an incisional extraction to remove soft tissues from the tooth.

Description: Double-ended straight instrument with one curved, round end and one chisel-like end.

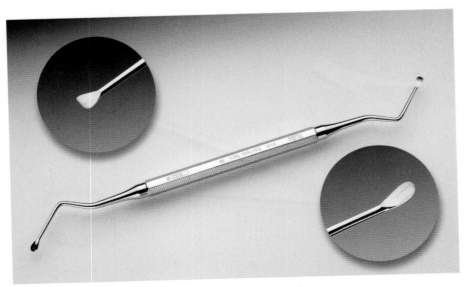

Instrument: LUCAS BONE CURETTE
Other Names: Angled curette
Use(s): Often used after tooth extractions to make sure debris and tissue are removed from the socket.

Description: Angular double-ended, angled, spoon-shaped scraping instrument in a range of sizes.

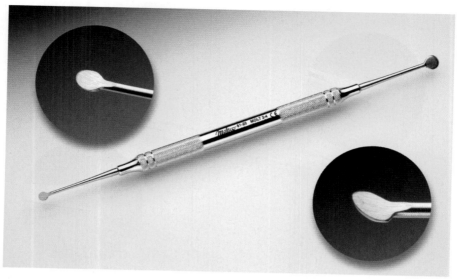

Instrument: MOLT BONE CURETTE
Other Names: Surgical curette, straight curette
Use(s): Often used to remove tissue or debris from bony sockets.

Description: Double-ended, straight instrument with round working ends that are graduated in size. These come in a range of sizes.

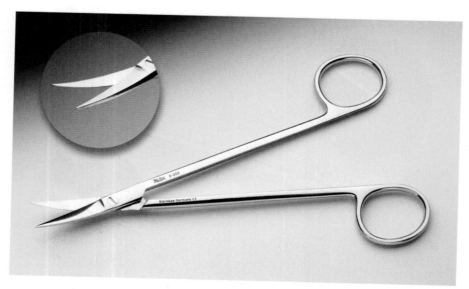

Instrument: KELLY SCISSORS
Other Names: Tissue scissors
Use(s): Used for cutting and excising excess or diseased soft tissue.
Description: Fine curved tip blades.

Instrument Insight: These are tissue scissors and should not be used to cut other items, which will dull the blades and make them unsafe for patient use.

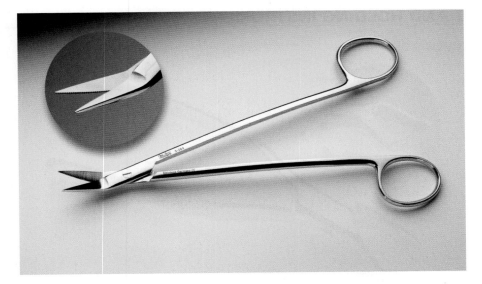

Instrument: DEAN SCISSORS
Other Names: Right-angle scissors
Use(s): Used for cutting and excising excess or diseased soft tissue.
Description: Fine right-angle blades with a sharp tip.

Instrument Insight: These are tissue scissors and should not be used to cut other items, which will dull the blades and make them unsafe for patient use.

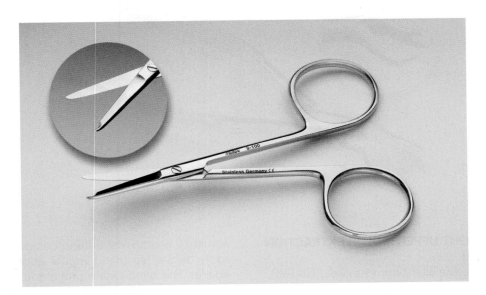

Instrument: SPENCER SUTURE SCISSORS
Other Names: Suture scissors
Use(s): These scissors are used to cut suture intraoperatively and to remove suture post-operatively.

Description: Fine scissors with straight blades.
Instrument Insight: One blade has a hook-like tip to slip under suture to hold suture away from tissue while cutting.

GRASPING AND HOLDING INSTRUMENTS

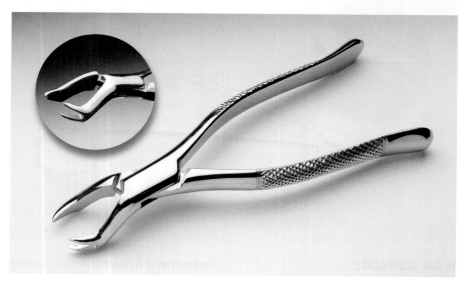

Instrument: LEFT UPPER MOLAR EXTRACTION FORCEPS (88L)

Other Names: Maxillary left forceps, No. 88L, 88L

Use(s): Used for extracting the left first and second maxillary molars.

Description: The tip has a bayonet design with one sharp projection on one jaw and two projections on the other. Each tip is designed to adjust to anatomical differences of the molar roots on the facial and lingual sides of the socket. The handles are straight and have nonslip diamond-cut grips.

Instrument Insight: The two prongs are placed on the palate side of the tooth, and the one prong is placed on the cheek side. Extraction forceps are often asked for by number instead of by proper name.

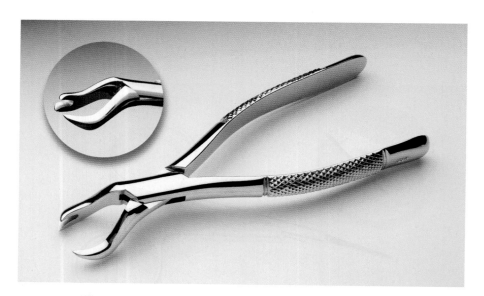

Instrument: RIGHT UPPER MOLAR EXTRACTION FORCEPS (88R)

Other Names: Maxillary right forceps, No.88R, 88R

Use(s): Used for extracting the right first and second maxillary molars.

Description: The tip has a bayonet design with one sharp projection on one jaw and two projections on the other. Each tip is designed to adjust to anatomical differences of the molar roots on the facial and lingual sides of the socket. The handles are straight and have nonslip diamond-cut grips.

Instrument Insight: The two prongs are placed on the palate side of the tooth, and the one prong is placed on the cheek side. Extraction forceps are often asked for by number instead of by proper name.

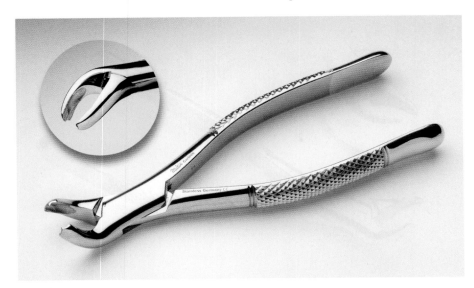

Instrument: LOWER MOLAR EXTRACTION FORCEPS (17)
Other Names: Mandibular forceps (17), #17
Use(s): Used for extracting the first and second maxillary molars of the right and left quadrants.
Description: The jaws are curved with an oval cup-shaped trough on the inner aspect and one sharp projection in the middle of the tip. The tips are universal in design to conform to facial and lingual roots for both the right and left sides. The handles are straight and have nonslip diamond-cut grips.
Instrument Insight: The #17 is handed with the tip curved downward. Extraction forceps are often asked for by number instead of by proper name.

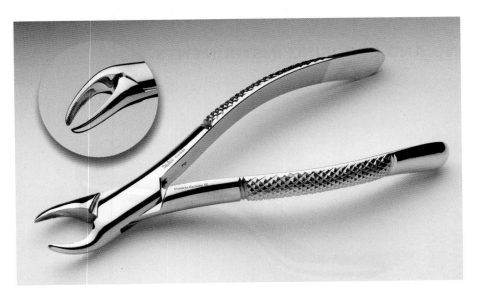

Instrument: UPPER ANTERIOR EXTRACTION FORCEPS (150)
Other Names: Maxillary universal forceps, Cryer forceps, 150
Use(s): Used for extracting the maxillary centrals, laterals, cuspids, premolars, and roots of the right and left quadrants.
Description: The jaws are curved with an oval cup-shaped trough on the inner aspect. The tips are universal in design to conform to facial and lingual roots for both the right and left sides. The handles are curved and have nonslip diamond-cut grips.
Instrument Insight: Maxillary counterpart to the #151 mandibular Cryer forceps; these should be placed on the Mayo together. Extraction forceps are often asked for by number instead of by proper name.

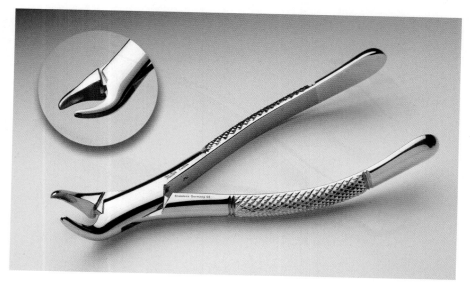

Instrument: LOWER ANTERIOR EXTRACTION FORCEPS (151)

Other Names: Mandibular universal forceps, Cryer forceps, 151

Use(s): Used for extracting the mandibular centrals, laterals, cuspids, premolars, and roots of the right and left quadrants.

Description: The jaws are curved with an oval cup-shaped trough on the inner aspect. The tips are universal in design to conform to facial and lingual roots for both the right and left sides. The handles are curved and have nonslip diamond-cut grips.

Instrument Insight: Mandibular counterpart to the maxillary #150 Cryer forceps; these should be placed on the Mayo together. Extraction forceps are often asked for by number instead of by proper name.

RETRACTING AND EXPOSING INSTRUMENTS

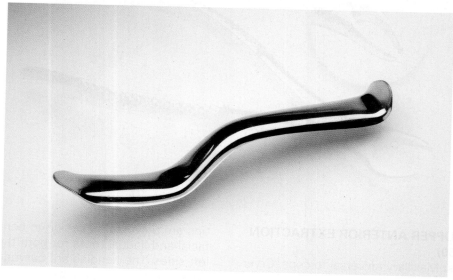

Instrument: MINNESOTA CHEEK RETRACTOR

Other Names: Cheek retractor, University of Minnesota retractor, Cawood retractor

Use(s): To retract the tongue and cheek away from surgical site.

Description: A curved bent and angled ribbon of stainless steel.

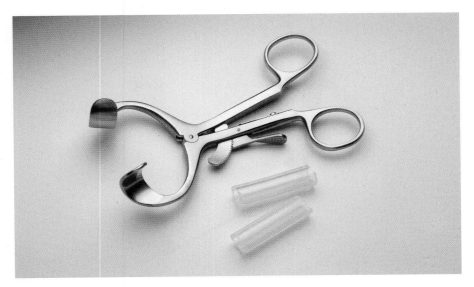

Instrument: MOLT MOUTH GAG
Other Names: Mouth gag, prop
Use(s): To retract the mouth open during procedures.
Description: Self-retaining C-shaped retractor with blades that curve inward and ratcheted finger rings to hold it in place. The rubber tubing slides onto the blades to protect the teeth and soft tissue.

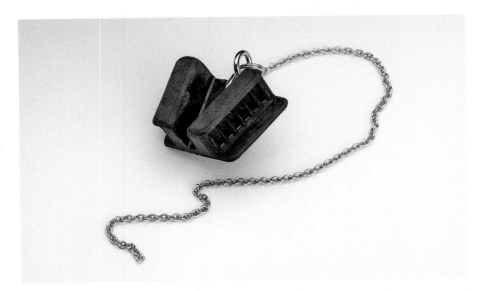

Instrument: MOUTH PROP
Other Names: Bit block, bit wedge
Use(s): To keep mouth propped open during procedures.
Description: A rubber wedge that has a rim on both sides into which the upper and lower teeth fit. The mouth prop comes in four sizes for children and adults. The attached chain is for removal of the wedge.
Instrument Insight: The narrow end of the wedge is placed into the mouth first.

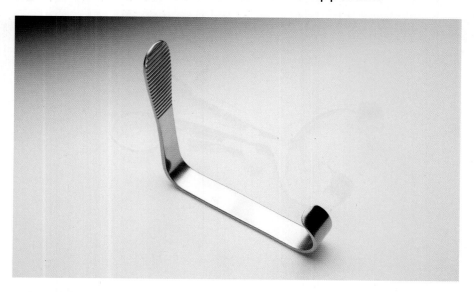

Instrument: ANDREWS'S TONGUE DEPRESSOR

Category: Retracting and exposing

Other Names: Tongue blade

Use(s): Used for retracting the mouth open and the tongue down for exposure of the oral cavity and the back of the throat.

Description: Flat-handled right-angle retractor with a round horizontal serrated blade.

11

Plastic and Reconstructive Instruments

ACCESSORY INSTRUMENTS

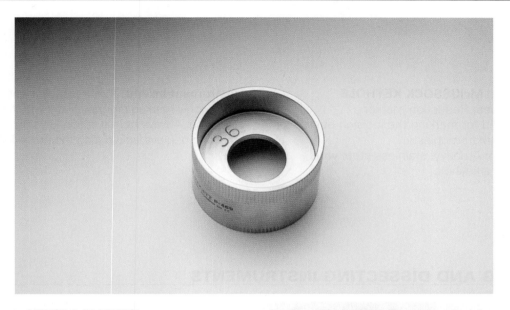

Instrument: AREOLA MARKER

Other Names: Cookie cutter, nipple washer

Use(s): Used for marking an incision line around the areola for a reduction mammoplasty and for marking tissue to become the new areola during reconstruction mammoplasty.

Description: The areola marker is a circular tube with a flat metal ring in the center. These range in size from 24 to 50 mm in diameter.

Instrument Insight: The breast incisions are commonly marked preoperatively with the patient standing. Always have sterile areola markers and marking pen available for marking the new areola site during the procedure.

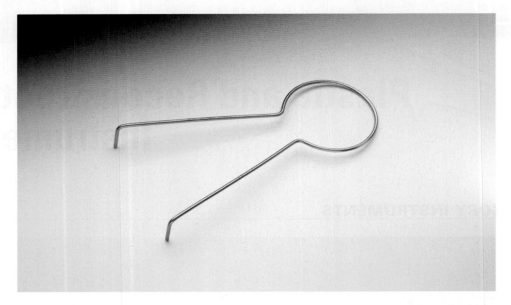

Instrument: McKISSOCK KEYHOLE
Other Names: Reduction marker
Use(s): Used for marking the incision outline for a reduction mammoplasty.
Description: A heavy, stainless-steel wire shaped like a keyhole.

Instrument Insight: The breast incisions are commonly marked preoperatively with the patient standing. Always have a sterile keyhole and marking pen available during the procedure.

CUTTING AND DISSECTING INSTRUMENTS

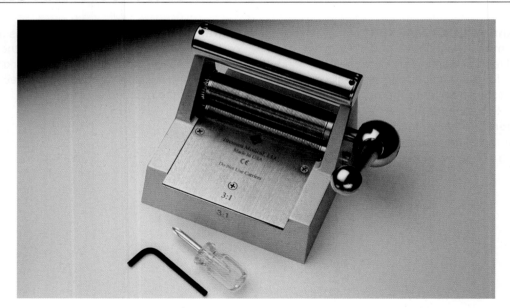

Instrument: DERMAMESHER
Other Names: Skin mesher
Use(s): Used for expansion of a split-thickness skin graft.
Description: A hand-cranked roller-cutting device that creates numerous identical perforations in the skin graft, giving it a mesh appearance. Meshing facilitates fluid drainage and allows the graft to be stretched over a larger surface area.
Instrument Insight: Depending on the type and manufacturer, some meshers use a skin carrier and others take only skin.

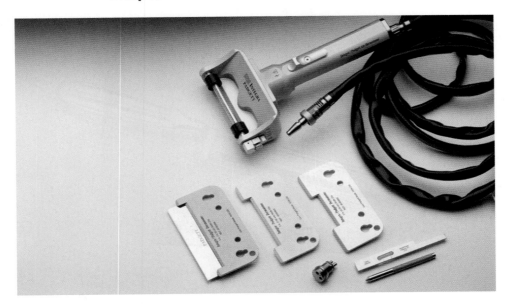

Instrument: DERMATOME

Other Names: Paget dermatome

Use(s): Used for harvesting a split-thickness skin graft.

Description: A power-driven dermatome that uses electricity or compressed gas to move the blade side to side to attain a skin graft. This set includes the dermatome hand piece; power cord; 1-, 2-, and 3-inch width plates; calibration guide; and screwdriver. The dermatome blades are manufacturer packaged for one-time use. There are several manufacturers of mechanical dermatomes.

Instrument Insight: Attaching the blade onto the back of the hand piece assembles the dermatome. The width plate is then placed over the blade by lining up the outer holes with the screws on the hand piece. After this is completed, the plate is slid forward and locked in place by tightening the screws.

⚠ **CAUTION:** Before handing this instrument to the surgeon, the dermatome should always be connected to power and tested to ensure the blade is moving freely. Always have sterile mineral oil and tongue blades available for lubrication and tension at the donor site. The skin should be held taut while the dermatome is cutting.

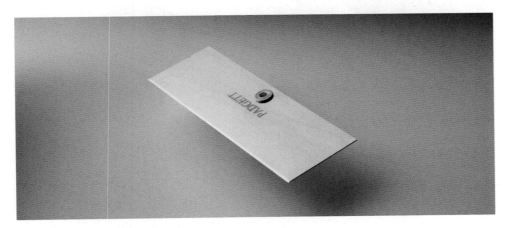

Instrument: DERMATOME BLADE

Other Names: Paget blade

Use(s): Used for harvesting a split-thickness skin graft.

Description: Disposable rectangular-shaped razor blade.

Instrument Insight: The blade attaches onto the back of the hand piece with the bevel down. The dermatome blades are manufacturer packaged for one-time use.

⚠ **CAUTION:** The hand piece should always be tested after being assembled to verify the blade is moving properly.

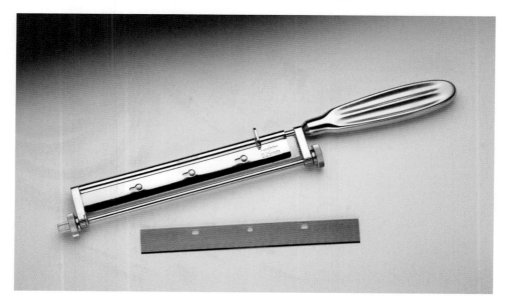

Instrument: WATSON SKIN GRAFT KNIFE
Other Names: Humby
Use(s): Used for harvesting a split-thickness skin graft or for wound debridement.
Description: A handheld dermatome with adjustable roller, which determines the depth of the graft. The blade is manufacturer packaged for one-time use.
Instrument Insight: The blade is attached with the bevel up.

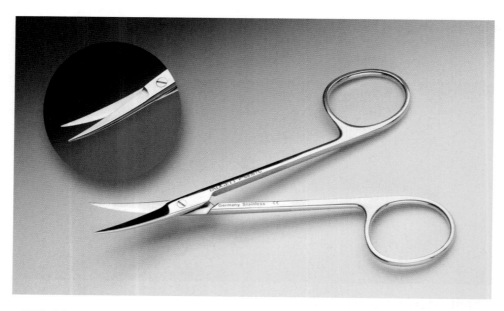

Instrument: IRIS SCISSORS
Use(s): Cut tissues during fine dissection.
Description: Small curved or straight scissors with fine blades and sharp tips.
Instrument Insight: Straight iris scissors are sometimes used to cut very delicate sutures. Curved scissors are for tissue dissection only.

⚠ **CAUTION:** Never place heavy instruments on top of delicate scissors. Never use curved delicate scissors for anything other than delicate tissue dissection because they will dull quickly.

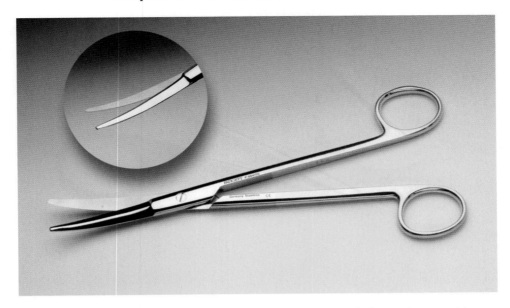

Instrument: KAYE FACELIFT SCISSORS
Other Names: Lift scissors
Use(s): Used for cutting and dissecting tissue during a rhytidectomy.

Description: A fine scissors with curved, beveled blades and blunt tips.

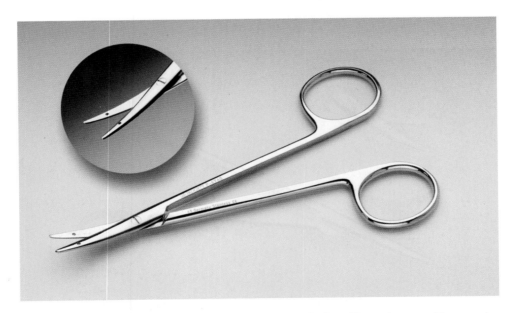

Instrument: LITTLER PLASTIC SURGERY SCISSORS
Other Names: Litler's
Use(s): To cut tissues during fine dissection.

Description: Fine scissors with curved, smooth blades and a single small hole close to the blunt tip.
Instrument Insight: Holes on blades serve as suture carrier.

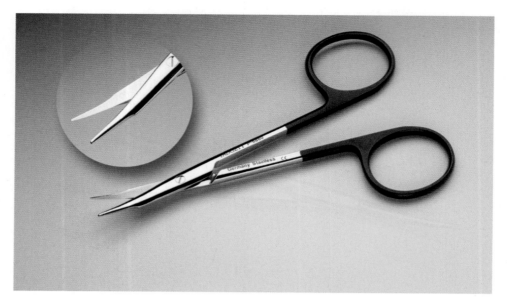

Instrument: STEVENS TENOTOMY SCISSORS
Use(s): To cut tissues during fine dissection.

Description: Small scissors with straight or slightly curved fine blades that narrow to blunt tips.

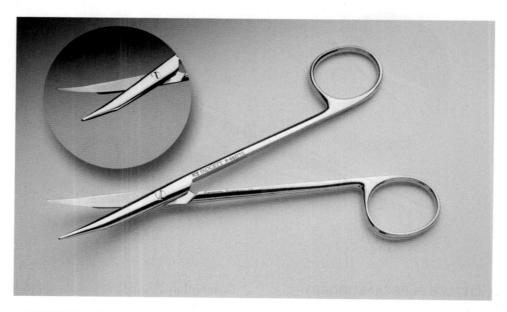

Instrument: JAMISON SCISSORS
Use(s): Cut tissues during fine dissection.

Description: Small scissors with curved elongated blades that narrow to blunt tips.

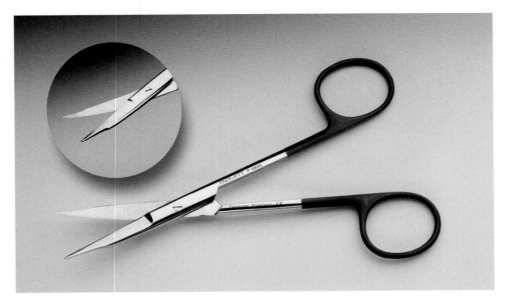

Instrument: REYNOLDS SCISSORS
Use(s): To cut tissues during fine dissection.

Description: Small scissors with curved, widened blades that narrow to blunt tips.

RETRACTING AND EXPOSING INSTRUMENTS

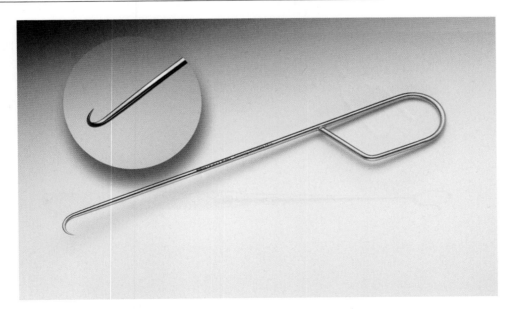

Instrument: MAMMOPLASTY HOOK
Other Names: Breast hook
Use(s): Used for retracting breast tissue during mastectomy or mammoplasty.
Description: A heavy, sharp hook retractor with a wire handle.

Instrument Insight: Always hand to the surgeon with the hook pointed downward.

⚠ **CAUTION:** Care must be taken not to puncture gloves on the sharp point of the hook.

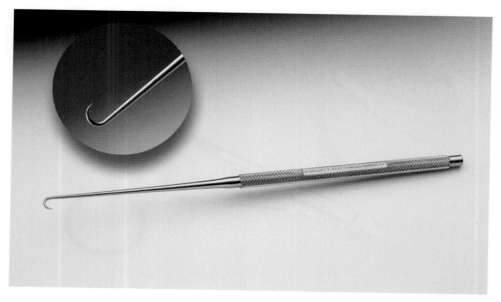

Instrument: JOSEPH SINGLE SKIN HOOK
Use(s): Used for retracting skin edges of small wounds.
Description: A small, sharp hook retractor with a round grip handle.

Instrument Insight: Hand to surgeon with hook pointing downward.

⚠ **CAUTION:** Care must be taken not to puncture gloves on the sharp point of the hook.

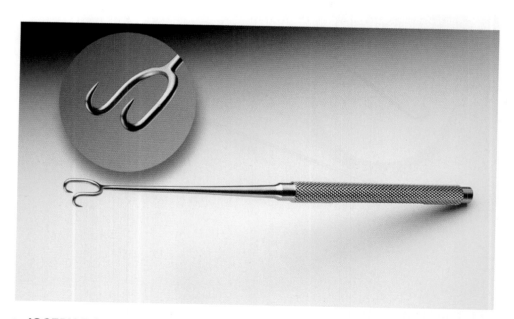

Instrument: JOSEPH DOUBLE SKIN HOOK
Use(s): Used for retracting skin edges of small wounds.
Description: A small, sharp double hook retractor with a round grip handle.

Instrument Insight: Hand to surgeon with hooks pointing downward.

⚠ **CAUTION:** Care must be taken not to puncture gloves on the sharp point of the hooks.

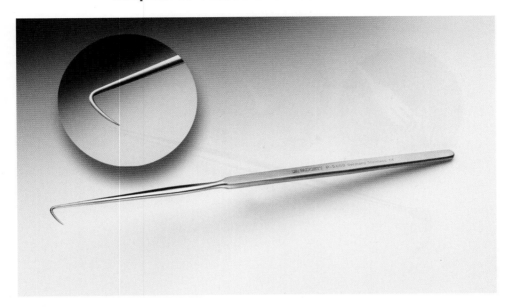

Instrument: SINGLE COTTLE TENACULUM
Use(s): Used for retracting skin edges and deeper tissues of small incisions.
Description: A small, sharp, L-shaped hook retractor with a flattened handle.

Instrument Insight: Hand hook downward.

⚠ **CAUTION:** Care must be taken not to puncture gloves on the sharp point of the hook.

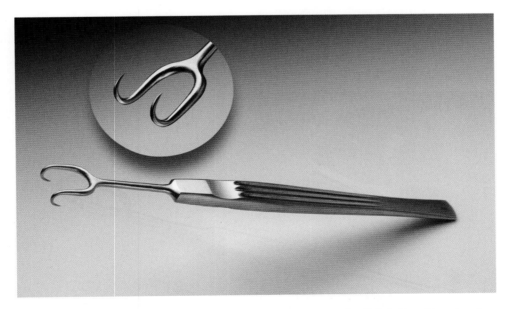

Instrument: DOUBLE COTTLE TENACULUM
Other Names: Tenaculums, hooks
Use(s): Used for retracting skin edges and deeper tissues of small incisions. Often used during nasal procedures.
Description: Sharp, double hook retractor with a flattened, ridged handle.

Instrument Insight: Hand hooks downward.

⚠ **CAUTION:** Care must be taken not to puncture gloves on the sharp point of the hooks.

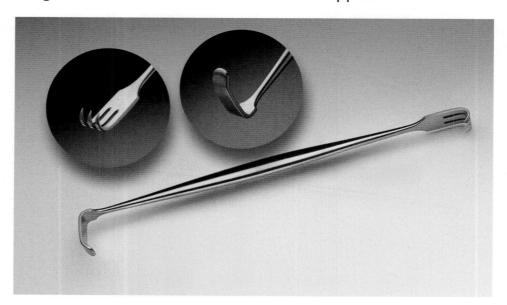

Instrument: MATHIEU RETRACTOR
Other Names: Cat paw
Use(s): Used for retracting skin edges and shallow wound edges.
Description: The Mathieu is a double-ended handheld retractor. One end has three sharp or blunt curved prongs, and the other end is a flat, laterally bent narrow strip.

Instrument Insight: The Mathieu is often confused with the Senn retractor, but it is actually finer than the Senn. Hand with the prongs downward.

⚠ **CAUTION:** Care must be taken not to puncture gloves on the sharp point of the prongs.

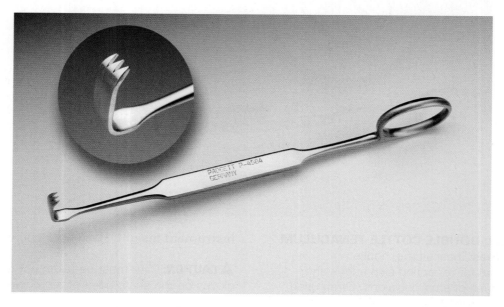

Instrument: MEYERDING FINGER RETRACTOR
Use(s): Used for retracting small wounds.

Description: Laterally bent narrow, flat end with a curved lip and a finger ring handle.

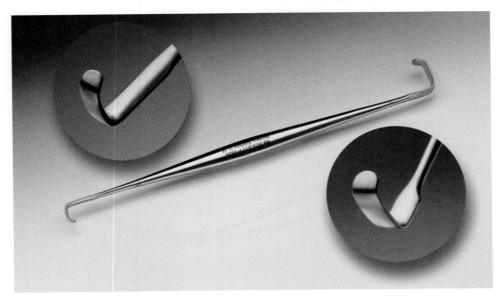

Instrument: RAGNELL RETRACTOR
Use(s): Used to retract superficially and then deeper in a small wound.

Description: Flattened, laterally curved, double-ended retractor with one end larger than the other.

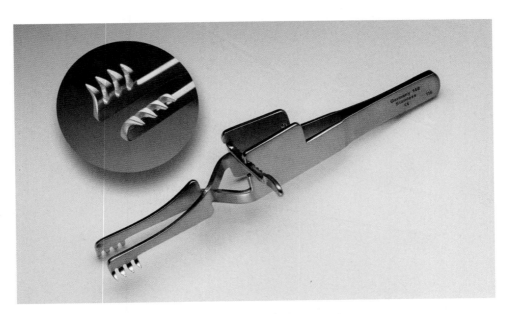

Instrument: JARIT CROSS ACTION RETRACTOR
Other Names: Holzheimer retractor, Cricket retractor, finger retractor, Heiss retractor
Use(s): Used for retracting a small, shallow wound edge.

Description: Self-retaining retractor with four outward-curved claws.

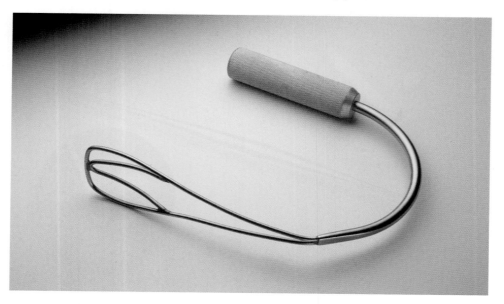

Instrument: BRIGGS MAMMOPLASTY RETRACTOR

Use(s): Used for retracting breast tissues during a mammoplasty.

Description: A large, curved retractor with a teardrop-shaped wire blade and a round grip handle.

SUCTIONING AND ASPIRATING INSTRUMENTS

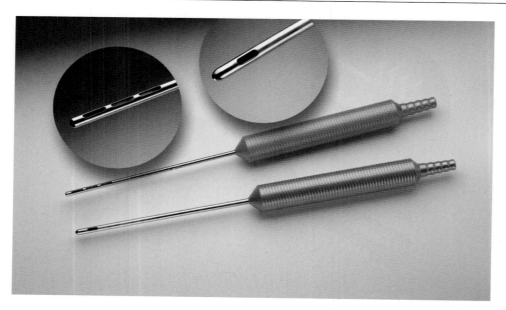

Instrument: LIPOSUCTION CANNULA

Use(s): Used for aspirating adipose tissue during a liposuction procedure.
Description: Rigid suction cannulas with various lengths, sizes, and tips.

Instrument Insight: The cannulas attach to firm, large-bore suction tubing, which is then attached to a high-pressure suction unit.

SUTURING AND STAPLING INSTRUMENTS

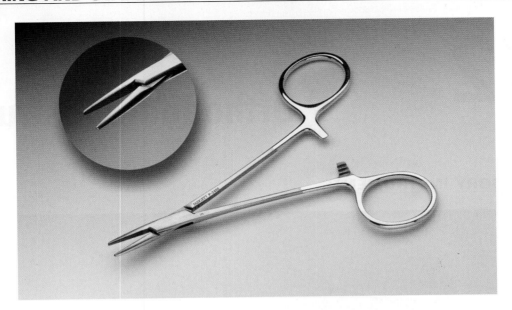

Instrument: WEBSTER NEEDLE HOLDER
Use(s): Used for holding small suture needles during delicate procedures.

Description: A small, fine needle holder with carbide cross-hatch pattern serrations on the inner jaws.

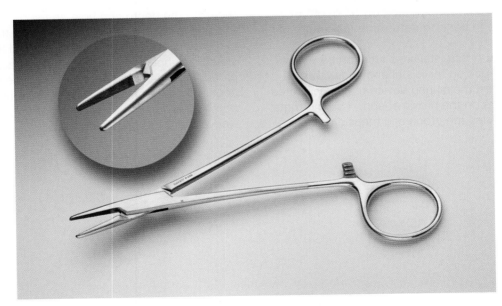

Instrument: HALSEY NEEDLE HOLDER
Use(s): Used for holding small suture needles during delicate procedures.

Description: A small, fine needle holder with carbide cross-hatch pattern serrations on the inner jaws.

12

Orthopedic Instruments

ACCESSORY INSTRUMENTS

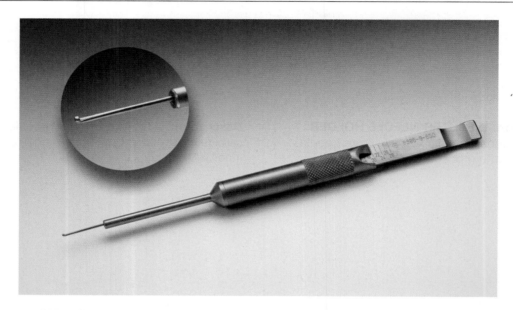

Instrument: DEPTH GAUGE

Other Names: Screw depth gauge

Use(s): Used for confirmation of the depth of the drill hole in bone to determine the length of the screw.

Description: A thin, stainless steel probe with a right-angle hook on the distal end and with a solid, flattened measuring device that is calibrated in millimeters on the proximal end. A sliding metal sleeve encircles the probe and measuring device.

Instrument Insight: Always have the depth gauge available when placing bone screws. To measure the depth of a hole, the surgeon pushes the sleeve against the proximal side of the hole and extends the probe into and beyond the distal side of the hole; the surgeon then retracts the probe, finding the distal side of the hole with the hook. The surgeon reads the measurement of depth by examining the position of the proximal sleeve along the graduated scale.

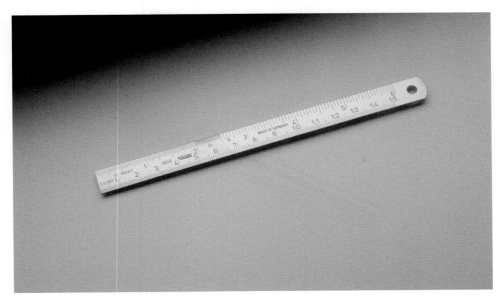

Instrument: RULER
Other Names: Measuring stick
Use(s): Used for measuring structure and distances.

Description: A stainless steel ruler that is calibrated in millimeters and inches.
Instrument Insight: Rulers may also be made of plastic.

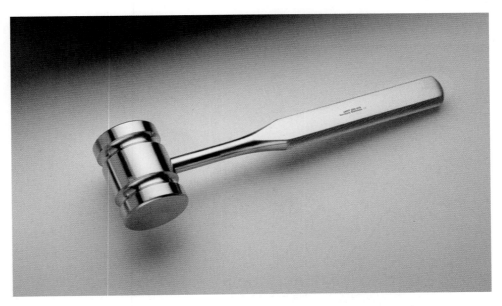

Instrument: MALLET
Other Names: Hammer
Use(s): Used to impact and extract implants or exert force on osteotomes, chisels, gouges, tamps, and other specially designed instruments.

Description: A solid stainless steel hammer-like instrument or may also be brass-filled stainless steel. Weight is usually 1 to 3 pounds. Mallets are used in other specialties that involve bone work.
Instrument Insight: Make available after passing any osteotomes, chisel, tamp, etc.

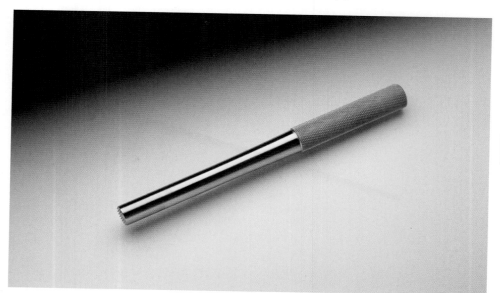

Instrument: BONE TAMP
Other Names: Tamp
Use(s): Used to compact or wedge a structure into place (e.g., a bone wedge).

Description: Solid stainless steel dowel with a grip handle and round, flattened working end.
Instrument Insight: Hand to surgeon with a mallet.

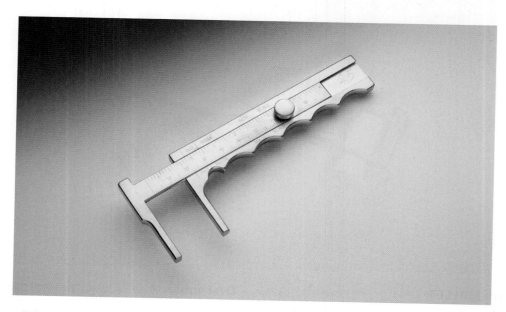

Instrument: TOWNLEY CALIPER
Other Names: Caliper
Use(s): Used for measuring structures and distances. Commonly used for measuring the

thickness of patella before cutting its undersurface during a total knee arthroplasty.
Description: A slide ruler that measures in millimeters and inches between the tips.

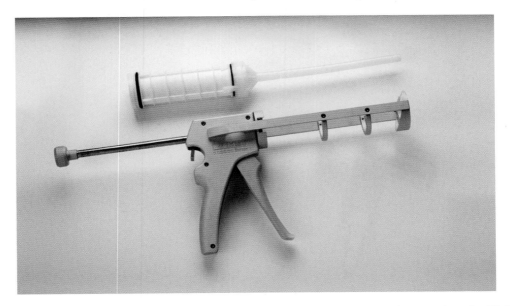

Instrument: BONE CEMENT GUN
Other Names: Cement gun
Use(s): Used for injecting polymethyl methacrylate (PMMA) bone cement during total joint procedures.
Description: The proximal end has a plunger-type disk that moves forward when the handles are compressed. This forces the glue through the chamber and out the tip, similar to a caulk gun.

Instrument Insight: Setting time for PMMA is approximately 8 to 16 minutes after the prosthesis is positioned. The surgeon will need to know how the glue is setting; be sure to obtain a small amount of glue to test for heat and hardening and record the time when the glue was placed in the gun.

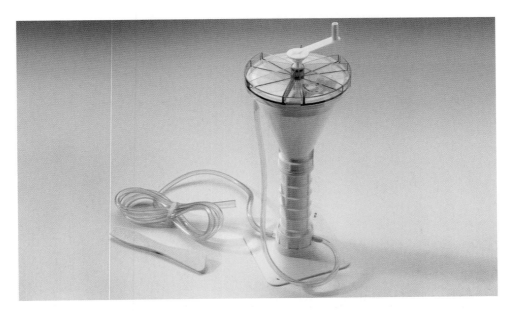

Instrument: BONE CEMENT SYSTEM
Use(s): Used for mixing the liquid (monomer) and powder (polymer) to produce bone cement, also known as polymethyl methacrylate (PMMA).
Instrument Insight: The manufacturer recommends double gloving when mixing

cement. Nonlatex gloves are not recommended because the liquid monomer can be absorbed through gloves.

⚠ **CAUTION:** The liquid monomer is highly flammable; the ESU should never be used near the liquid or the uncured cement.

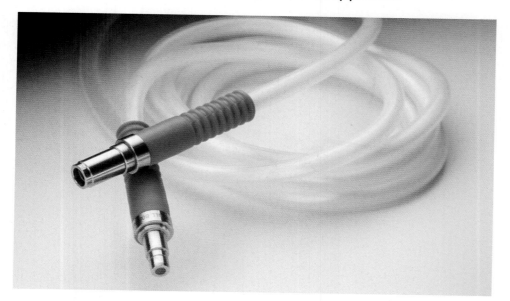

Instrument: FIBEROPTIC LIGHT CORD

Other Names: Light cord

Use(s): Used for delivering high-intensity light to the endoscope for illumination during endoscopic procedures.

Description: A 10-foot-long fiberoptic cable with an endoscope adaptor at the proximal end and a light source adaptor at the distal end.

Instrument Insight: Exercise care when handling a fiberoptic cord; it should never be placed under a heavy object, dropped, twisted, or kinked because the tiny fibers inside can be easily damaged.

⚠ **CAUTION:** When not in use, the light source must be placed on standby or turned off. The intense heat from the beam can cause the patient's drapes or any flammable vapors around the patient to ignite.

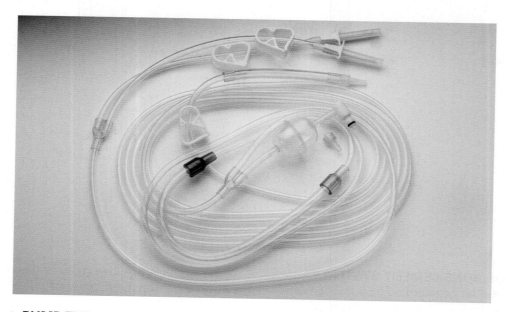

Instrument: PUMP TUBING

Use(s): Attaches irrigation fluid bags to pump at one end with the other end attached to the arthroscopic irrigation cannula.

Description: Hollow tubing with bifurcated spike ports and tubing clamps on one end, and the pump attachment mechanism and a Luer-Lok attachment at the other end.

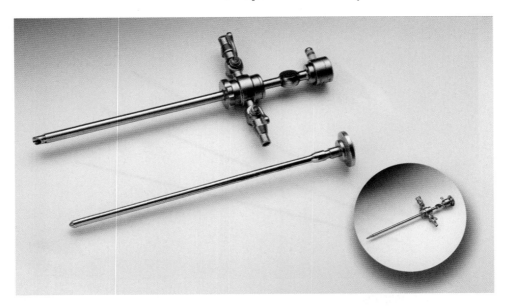

Instrument: 4-MM SHEATH WITH BLUNT OBTURATOR

Use(s): Creates a port in which the endoscope is introduced and exchanged through the sheath or cannula.

Description: A hollow, stainless steel sheath with a blunt tip obturator that fits inside.

Instrument Insight: The blunt tip is less traumatic on the tissues. Tip can be various sizes, depending on the size of the joint.

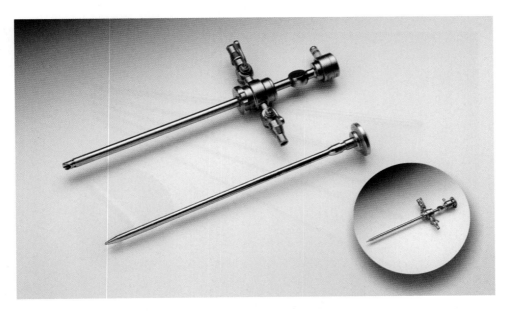

Instrument: 4-MM SHEATH AND SHARP OBTURATOR

Use(s): Creates a port in which the endoscope is introduced and exchanged through the sheath or cannula.

Description: This is a hollow, stainless steel sheath with a sharp tip obturator that fits inside.

Tips are available in various sizes, depending on the size of the joint.

Instrument Insight: The sharp tip is used to pass through tough tissue.

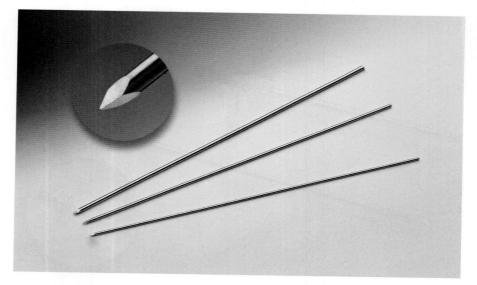

Instrument: KIRSCHNER WIRES

Other Names: K wires, metacarpal pins

Use(s): A steel wire used skeletal fixation of bone fractures and for placing skeletal traction for bone fractures. These are often used on small bones such as phalanges, wrist, and ankle and are often placed percutaneously.

Description: Stainless steel wires are smooth or threaded with trocar and diamond points on one end or on both ends. K wires are available in sizes from 0.7 through 1.6 mm (0.028 through 0.062 inch).

Instrument Insight: Care should be taken when handling because these have very sharp points that can easily puncture skin.

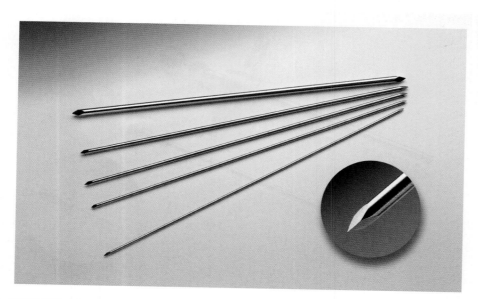

Instrument: SMOOTH STEINMAN PINS

Other Names: Smooth pins

Use(s): These pins can be used for fixation of bone fractures, bone reconstruction, and as a guide pin when placing implants and placing skeletal traction. Often used on larger bones.

Description: Smooth stainless steel pin with a trocar or diamond point. Steinmann pins are available in sizes from 2.0 through 4.8 mm (5/64 through 3/16 inch).

Instrument Insight: Care should be taken when handling; these have very sharp points that can easily puncture skin.

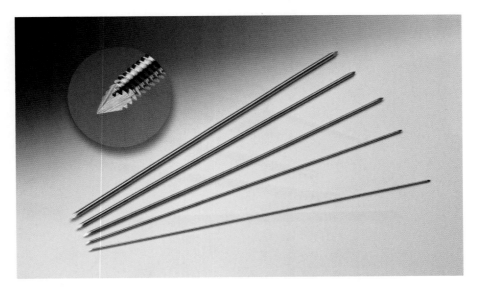

Instrument: THREADED STEINMAN PINS
Other Names: Threaded pins
Use(s): These pins can be used for fixation of bone fractures, bone reconstruction, and as a guide pin when placing implants and placing skeletal traction. Often used on larger bones.
Description: Threaded stainless steel pins with a trocar or diamond point. Steinmann pins are available in sizes from 2.0 through 4.8 mm (5/64 through 3/16 inch).
Instrument Insight: Care should be taken when handling; these have very sharp points that can easily puncture skin.

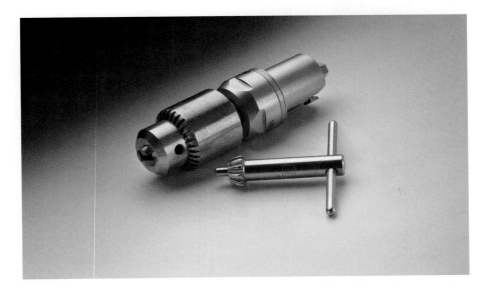

Instrument: CHUCK AND KEY
Other Names: Drill chuck
Use(s): Most commonly used to hold rotating devices, such as the drill bit or a pin in a power tool. Some chucks can also hold irregularly shaped objects and those that lack radial symmetry. Often the jaws will be tightened or loosened with the help of a chuck key, which is a wrench-like device made to tighten or loosen the jaws.
Description: A chuck is a specialized type of clamp in which the jaws, which are arranged in a radially symmetrical pattern like the points of a star, are used to hold a cylindrical object.

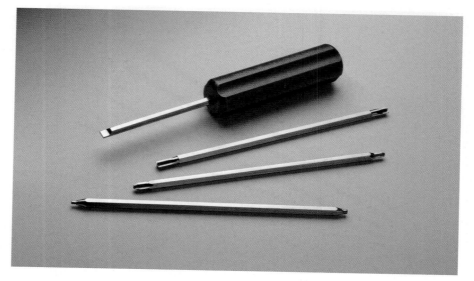

Instrument: UNIVERSAL SCREWDRIVER SET
Other Names: Screwdriver kit
Use(s): Used during revision of total joint surgery in which screws were used, removal of bone plates, fracture fixation screws, or bone graft screws.
Description: Set consists of a handle that accommodates any of the four double-ended screwdriver bits and one each of small and large single slot, cross and cruciate, 3.5-mm and 4.5-mm hex, and small and large Phillips heads.
Instrument Insight: The set helps eliminate the opening of multiple sterile packs when a specific size or style of screwdriver is needed.

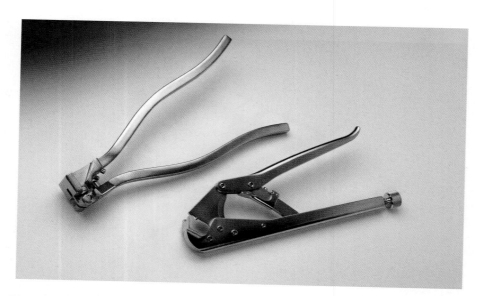

Instrument: PLATE BENDING PLIERS
Other Names: Plate bender
Use(s): Used during open reduction internal fixation (ORIF) to bend the plate to conform to the contour of the bone in which it is being implanted.
Description: Pictured are large forceps. The plate is slid into the jaws and compressed to bend the plate. These come in various sizes and designs depending on the type of plating system that is being used and the size and type of bone that is being fixated.
Instrument Insight: Often plate benders will be found in the fixation set that you are using.

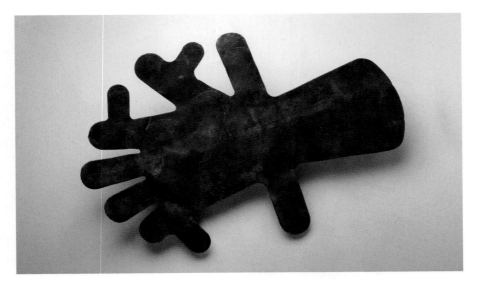

Instrument: LEAD HAND
Use(s): Often used during hand procedures to position the hand open for exposure.
Description: A hand-shaped malleable metal device with tabs.
Instrument Insight: The patient's hand is generally laid onto the lead hand palm up. The metal fingers are bent up over the top of the patient's fingers to hold them down, then the tabs are molded around the wrist, index finger, and little finger to secure the hand open.

CUTTING AND DISSECTING INSTRUMENTS

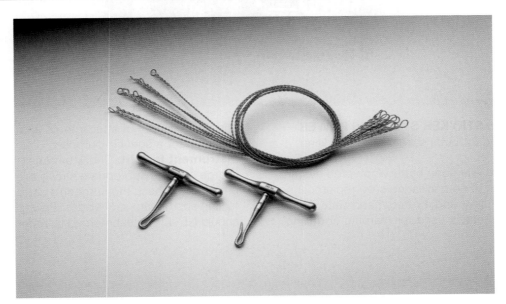

Instrument: GIGLI SAW
Use(s): A type of hand saw used for cutting bone. A back and forth movement of the "T" handle slides the cable over the bone, creating a notch that continues through the bone. Often used for amputations and can be use to open the skull for craniotomies.

Description: A flexible, twisted wire cable with looped ends that affix to the hooks on the two "T" handles. The handles may also be oval or box shaped. The wire cable may be replaced after each use or when it becomes dull.

⚠ **CAUTION:** Do not run fingers and/or hand along the blade; this could tear gloves and skin.

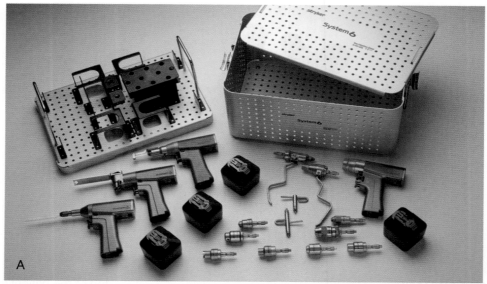

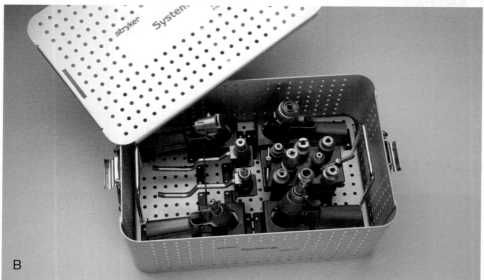

Instrument: STRYKER SYSTEM 6 POWER

Use(s): Used for cutting, reaming, or drilling large bones.

Description: All-in-one battery-powered system that consists of an oscillating saw, reciprocating saw, sternal saw, and a rotary handpiece. The rotary handpiece is used for reaming or drilling and has a variety of attachments and chucks that are used for a specific purpose.

Instrument Insight: Check batteries for a full charge and the appropriate saw blade for the procedure. Check the surgeon's preference card for the appropriate saw blades. Power instruments should NEVER be submerged in water.

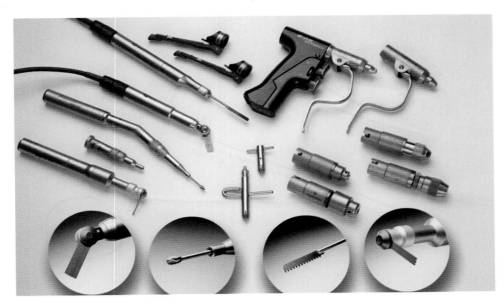

Instrument: STRYKER CORE SYSTEM
Other Names: TPS system
Use(s): Used for cutting, drilling, or burring small bones.
Description: An all-in-one electrical-powered system that consists of sagittal, oscillating, and reciprocating saws, microdrill, and universal driver handpiece. The universal drivers are capable of pin and wire driving, sawing, drilling, tunneling, or reaming and have a variety of attachments, collets, and chucks that are used for a specific purpose.
Instrument Insight: Refer to the surgeon's preference card for type of blades or burrs used. Power instruments should NEVER be submerged in water.

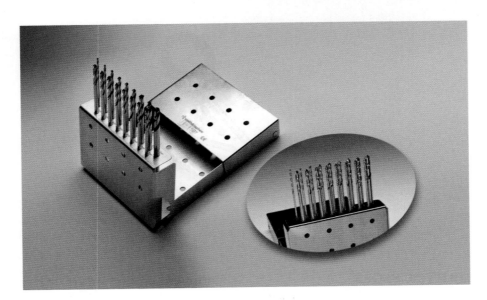

Instrument: DRILL BIT SET
Other Names: Drill box
Use(s): Drill bits are used to drill holes in bone, usually before the placement of a screw.

Description: The drill bits in this case range from 1.6 mm to 4.7 mm.

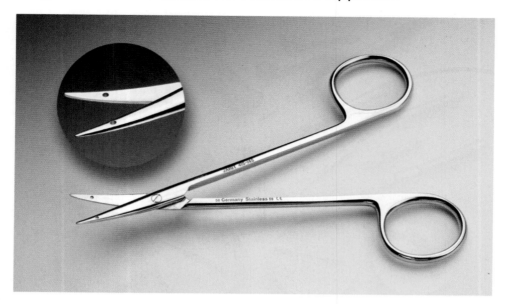

Instrument: LITTLER SCISSORS

Use(s): Used for fine tissue dissection.

Description: Slightly curved, blunt-tip, sharp blades. The holes on the blades serve to draw suture or muscle through a tunnel dissection.

Instrument Insight: Use caution when passing because of sharp edges; only use on tissue—never use to cut drapes or suture.

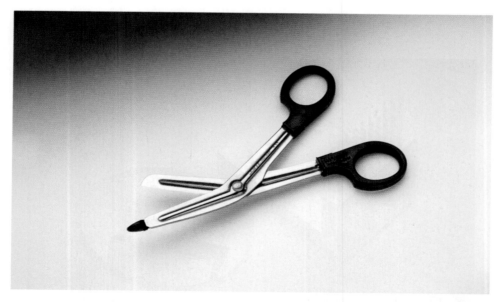

Instrument: UTILITY SCISSORS

Other Names: Bandage scissors

Use(s): Cut bandages, casting material, clothing, and other nonsterile items.

Description: Serrated edge with blunt tip on lower jaw to prevent cutting tissue or skin.

Instrument Insight: Used to cut dressing, drapes, cast material, etc. These scissors should never be used to cut tissues or suture.

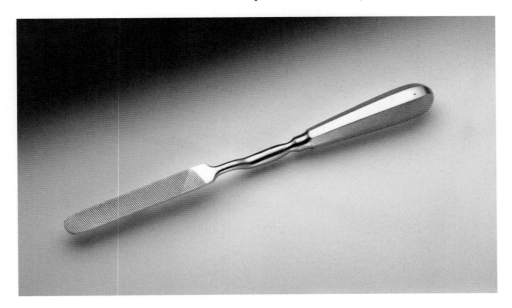

Instrument: BONE FILE
Other Names: Rasp
Use(s): Used for smoothing rough edges or surfaces of large bones.

Description: A single-handle instrument with flat end with serrations in a crisscross pattern.
Instrument Insight: This should always be available during total joint procedures to smooth bone surfaces.

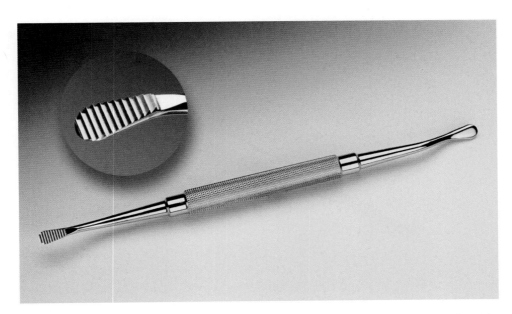

Instrument: MILLER RASP
Other Names: Small rasp
Use(s): Used for smoothing rough edges or surfaces of small bones.
Description: A double-ended instrument with tear-shaped ends. One end has fairly thick ridges

in parallel lines; the ridges on the other end are closer together.
Instrument Insight: Instrument is used to smooth bone surfaces in small areas or when the areas are hard to reach.

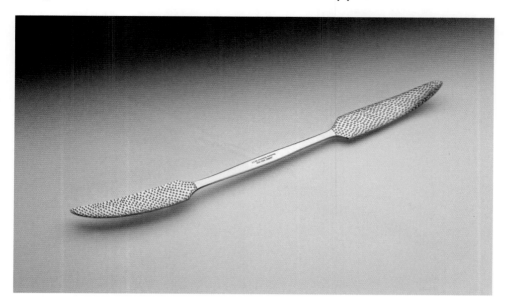

Instrument: PUTTI BONE RASP
Other Names: Putti Platte, rat tail
Use(s): Used for smoothing rough edges or surfaces of large bones.
Description: A flattened, double-ended rasp with a rounded blade on one end and a half-rounded blade on the other end. The blade surfaces are covered with tiny spikes.

Instrument Insight: Immerse and gently stir the rasp in water to keep instrument surface clean between uses.

⚠ **CAUTION:** Do not run fingers and/or hand along the blade; this could tear gloves and skin.

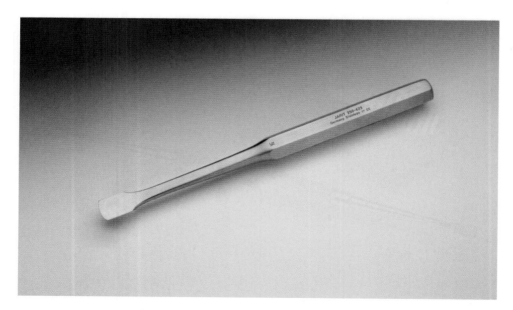

Instrument: KEY ELEVATOR
Use(s): Dissects or separates hard tissue (e.g., periosteum from bone).
Description: A solid, smooth, octagonal handle with a squared, flat, and sharp working end that comes in a variety of sizes.

Instrument Insight: Inspect edge before and after each use for nicks to ensure sharpness.

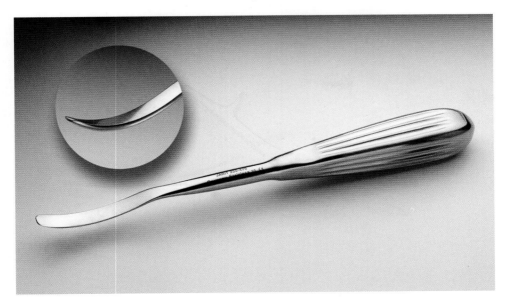

Instrument: CREGO ELEVATOR
Use(s): Dissects or separates tissue; retracts tissue.
Description: Thick handle with long, thin, curved, flat edge.

Instrument Insight: Inspect edge for nicks to ensure sharpness.

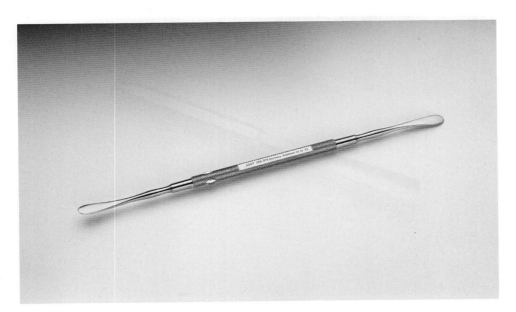

Instrument: FREER ELEVATOR
Use(s): Lifts the periosteum from bone or retracts in confined spaces.
Description: Round handle with flattened, tear-shape tips at both ends; one end is sharper than the other.

Instrument Insight: Small balls of bone wax are pressed onto the tip and then are smeared in bone edges for hemostasis.

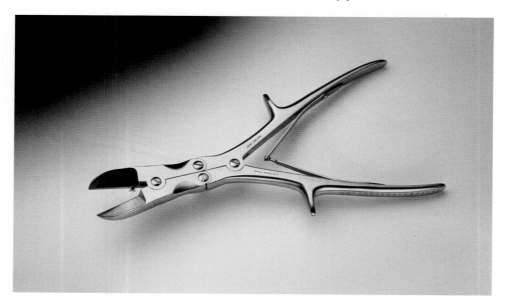

Instrument: LISTON BONE CUTTING FORCEPS
Other Names: Large bone cutters
Use(s): Used for cutting large bones.
Description: Large double-action forceps with curved or straight blades that are rounded to the tip with sharp inner jaw edges.

Instrument Insight: The double action gives the forceps more torque at the tip for better cutting action.

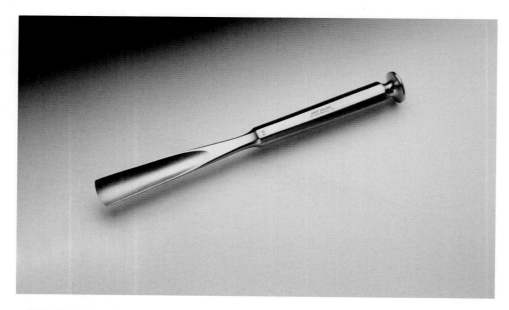

Instrument: STILLE BONE GOUGE
Use(s): Used to cut or scoop out a channel of bone.
Description: A flat, round impaction platform with a solid octagonal handle that extends to a trough-like blade that has a sharp cutting edge.

Gouges are available in cases or in sets with a variety of sizes.
Instrument Insight: Always hand the gouge to the surgeon with a mallet. Inspect edges for breaks or nicks to ensure precision, sharpness, and patient safety.

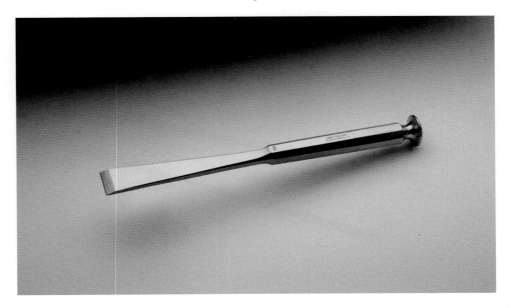

Instrument: STILLE BONE CHISEL

Use(s): Used to cut or shape bone. The chisel is often used when harvesting a bone graft.

Description: A flat, round impaction platform with a solid octagonal handle that extends to a flattened, flared blade with a beveled edge. Chisels are available in cases or in sets with a variety of sizes.

Instrument Insight: Always hand the chisel to the surgeon with a mallet. Inspect edges for breaks or nicks to ensure precision, sharpness, and patient safety.

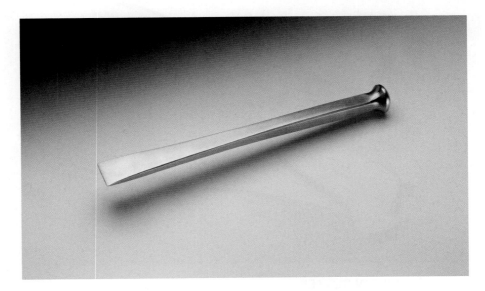

Instrument: STILLE BONE OSTEOTOME

Use(s): Used to cut or shape bone. The osteotome is often used when harvesting a bone graft.

Description: A flat, round impaction platform with a solid octagonal handle that extends to a flattened, flared blade. Osteotomes are available in cases or in sets with a variety of sizes.

Instrument Insight: Always hand the osteotome to the surgeon with a mallet. Inspect edges for breaks or nicks to ensure precision, sharpness, and patient safety.

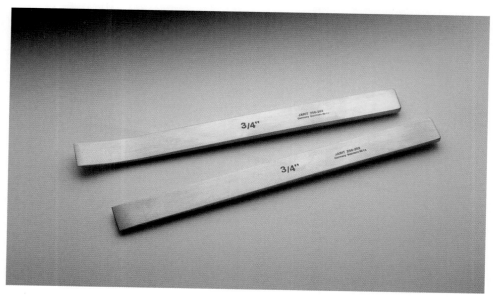

Instrument: LAMBOTTE OSTEOTOME

Use(s): Used to cut or shape bone. An osteotome is often used when harvesting a bone graft.

Description: A flattened, stainless steel ribbon that tapers to a sharp cutting edge; osteotomes are available in various size widths.

Instrument Insight: Osteotomes may come in cases or sets with a variety of sizes and may be straight or curved. Inspect edges for breaks or nicks to ensure precision, sharpness, and patient safety.

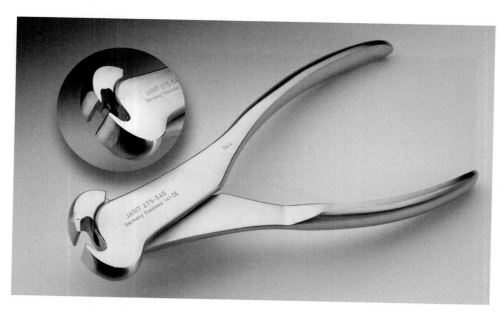

Instrument: CANNULATED PIN CUTTER

Other Names: Pin cutter

Use(s): Used for cutting wire or small pins, such as Kirschner wires (K wires) or Steinmann pins.

Description: Heavy, curved handles with extremely curved jaws that meet flush against one another and have extremely sharp edges. There is a circular pin channel between the jaws that runs through the lock box and between the handles. The channel allows the pin to slide through the jaws so the proper length can be cut.

Instrument Insight: Inspect jaw edges for breaks or nicks to ensure precision and sharpness.

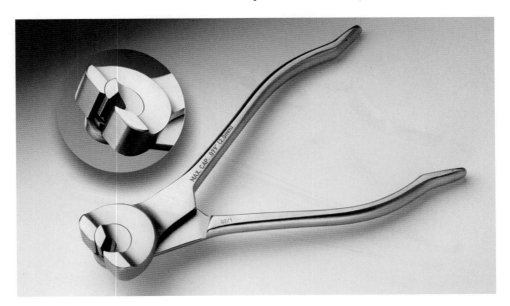

Instrument: DIAMOND PIN CUTTER
Other Names: Pin cutter
Use(s): Used for cutting wire or small pins, such as Kirschner wires (K wires) or Steinmann pins.
Description: Heavy, curved handles with a guillotine-action tip. The working end has an angled channel that allows the pin to be placed into the jaw so the proper length can be cut.
Instrument Insight: Double-action jaws allow for more power when cutting. Inspect for sharpness and smooth action of jaw and cutting surfaces.

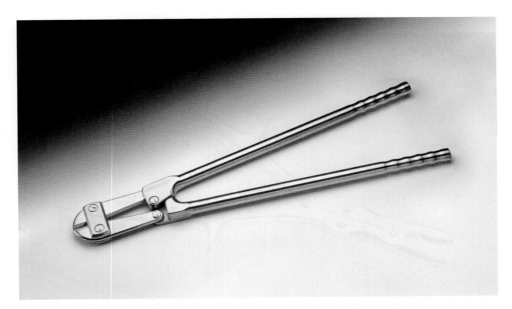

Instrument: LARGE PIN CUTTER
Other Names: Bolt cutter, rod cutter
Use(s): Used for cutting heavy pins and rods.
Description: Very long handles with double-action hinges and a sharp, small cutting surface.
Instrument Insight: A long handle with double action allows a great amount of force to be applied to the jaws.

⚠ **CAUTION:** When setting up, always check the screw to ensure it is tightened down and can not fall out into the wound when in use.

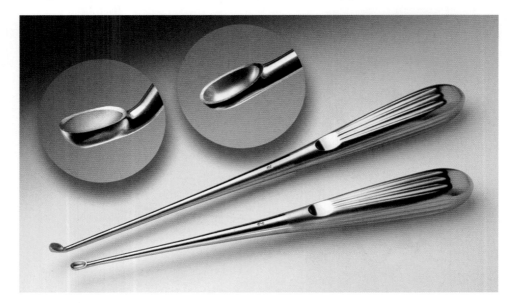

Instrument: BRUNS OVAL BONE CURETTES
Other Names: Curettes
Use(s): Used for scooping out tissue or material from small, tight areas.

Description: Thick handles with a small scoop at one end; scoops have a variety of shapes and angles.

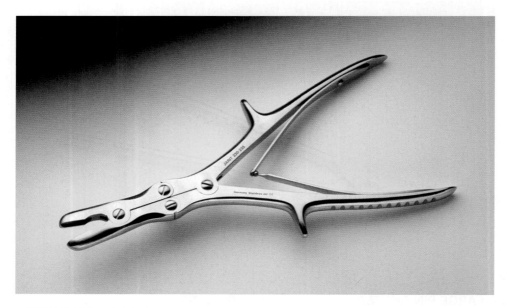

Instrument: STILLE-LUER RONGEUR
Other Names: Straight rongeur, large mouth rongeur
Use(s): Used to grasp, bite, and detach large amounts of tissue.
Description: Large-handled double-action mechanism with large, oval cup shape jaws.

Instrument Insight: Frequently used instrument for large cases that require significant dissection or cleaning of the area.

⚠ **CAUTION:** When setting up, always check the screw to ensure it is tightened down and can not fall out into the wound when in use.

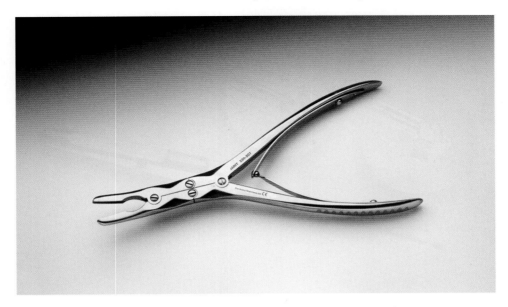

Instrument: ZAUFEL-JANSEN RONGEUR
Other Names: Small-mouthed rongeur
Use(s): Used for removing pieces of bone and the soft tissue surrounding the bone.
Description: Large handle with double-action mechanism and thin, sharp jaws.
Instrument Insight: The double-action mechanism gives the rongeur more torque at the tip for better biting action. Always have a moistened sponge ready when handing the surgeon a rongeur. As the surgeon works to remove tissue and/or bone, the rongeur has to be cleaned between uses. While focusing on the wound, the surgeon will point the tip of the rongeur toward the surgical technologist. Using a moistened sponge, the surgical technologist will clean the tissue from the jaws.

⚠ **CAUTION:** When setting up, always check the screw to ensure it is tightened down and can not fall out into the wound when in use.

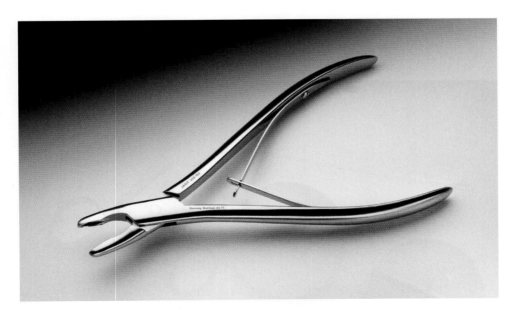

Instrument: CUSHING RONGEUR
Use(s): Used for removing pieces of bone and the soft tissue surrounding the bone.
Description: Medium-sized handle with a single hinge and short, oval, cup-shaped jaws.
Instrument Insight: Always have a moistened sponge ready when handing the surgeon a rongeur. As the surgeon works to remove tissue and/or bone, the rongeur has to be cleaned between uses. While focusing on the wound, the surgeon will point the tip of the rongeur toward the surgical technologist. Using a moistened sponge, the surgical technologist will clean the tissue from the jaws.

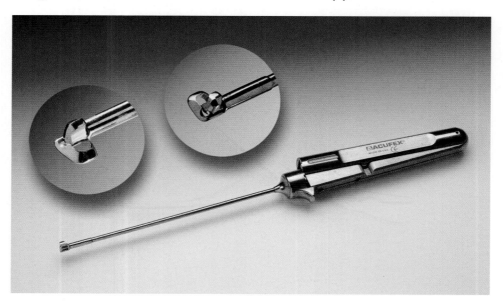

Instrument: DUCKBILL RIGHT AND LEFT BITER

Use(s): Cuts and dissects tissue during arthroscopy procedures.

Description: A thick handle with thumb lever that opens and closes the jaws. Has a square-shaped cutting tool on the right or left side of the instrument.

Instrument Insight: Before handing to the surgeon, hold this instrument by the handle with the cutting end away from you so that you may visualize what side the cutter is facing.

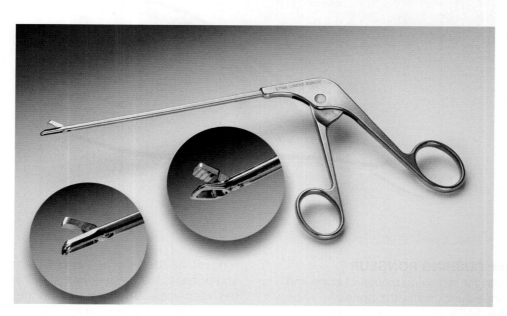

Instrument: DUCKBILL STRAIGHT BITER

Use(s): Cuts and dissects tissue facing the surgeon.

Description: Ringed handles with a thin rod that has a rectangular-shaped cutter attached distally.

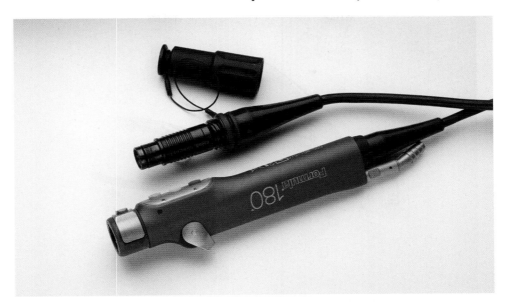

Instrument: SHAVER

Use(s): Houses various shaver attachments to remove, trim, or burr tissue and bone.

Description: Motorized handpiece (pictured in blue) is an attachment for various burrs and blades that move at various speeds and directions. Suction tubing is connected to the adaptor next to the cord attachment. The black cord end is handed off the field and connected to the control panel. The shaver is activated by stepping on the foot pedal or with buttons on the handpiece.

Instrument Insight: Shaver often gets clogged with debris. Remove shaver attachment, separate it into its two parts, and remove tissue. HINT: Strike the two parts together to remove tissue.

GRASPING AND HOLDING INSTRUMENTS

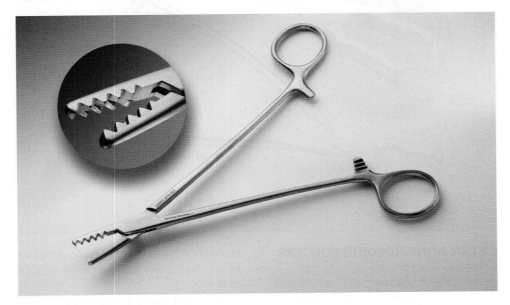

Instrument: MARTIN CARTILAGE CLAMP

Other Names: Meniscus clamp

Use(s): Used for grasping heavy tissues and cartilage. The Martin is often used to grasp the meniscus for dissection during total knee arthroplasty.

Description: Ringed handles with large serrations placed in opposition.

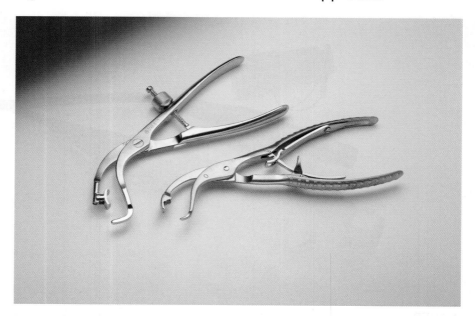

Instrument: PLATE FORCEPS
Other Names: Plate holding forceps, plate holders, plate clamp
Use(s): During an open reduction internal fixation, these are used to hold the plate in alignment while drilling and screw placement takes place.
Description: These come in various sizes and designs depending on the type of plating system that is being used and the size and type of bone that is being fixated. The foot of the forceps fits into the counter of the plate, ensuring a firm grip of the plate and the back side of the bone. The foot often has the ability to swivel for precise positioning of the forceps onto the plate.

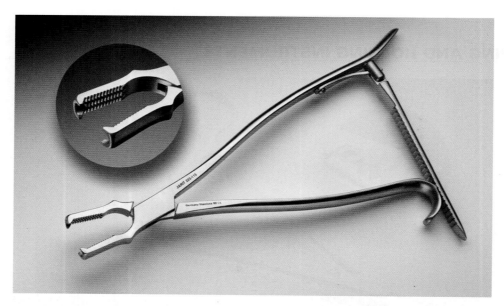

Instrument: KERN BONE-HOLDING FORCEPS
Use(s): Used for manipulating bone fractures into place and for holding the fracture in alignment while plates and screws are placed. Also used during total joint procedures to grasp bone segments.
Description: Long, thin handles with a bar ratchet device between them to lock jaws in place. The inner jaws have four heavy teeth and heavy serrations that allow for secure grasping of the bone.
Instrument Insight: Hands and instruments should be kept away from the ratchet bar during the procedure to prevent inadvertently releasing it.

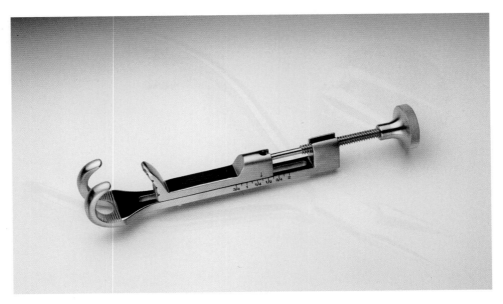

Instrument: LOWMAN BONE CLAMP
Use(s): Used for holding the fractured bone in alignment while plates and screws are placed.
Description: Three curved, grasping, blunt claws at the working end that are tightened into position by turning the screw mechanism at the proximal end.
Instrument Insight: Inspect the screw mechanism before surgery to ensure that it is working properly.

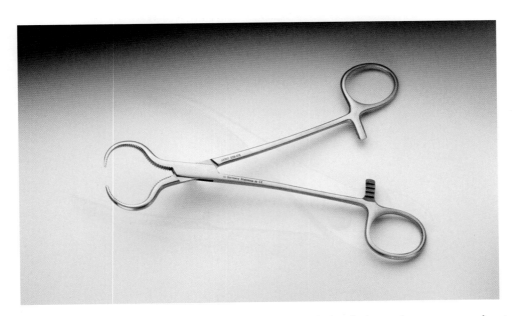

Instrument: LEWIN BONE-HOLDING FORCEPS
Other Names: Joplin
Use(s): Used for manipulating bone fractures into place and to holding the fracture in alignment while plates and screws are placed. The Lewin can also be used during a hip arthroplasty to punch holes in bone for passage of sutures when closing the joint.
Description: Ringed handles with very sharp double-curved graspers.
Instrument Insight: Because of sharp ends, use extreme caution when handling.

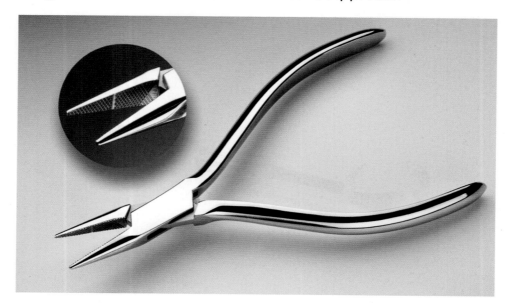

Instrument: NEEDLENOSE PLIERS
Use(s): Remove pins and hardware and twist wires.

Description: Thin, single-action handles with serrated jaws that narrow to a point.

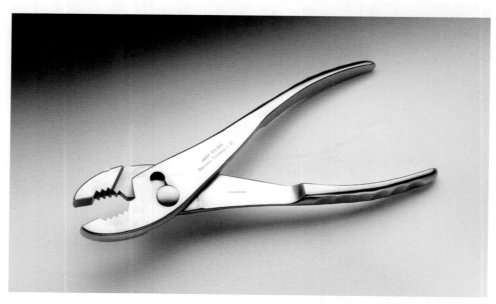

Instrument: PLIERS
Other Names: Channel locks
Use(s): Used to place or remove hardware and to grasp pointed trocar during drain insertion of deep wounds.

Description: Thin, single-action handles with thin and thick serrations and rounded-end jaws. Hinge provides two opening sizes of the jaws.

RETRACTING AND EXPOSING INSTRUMENTS

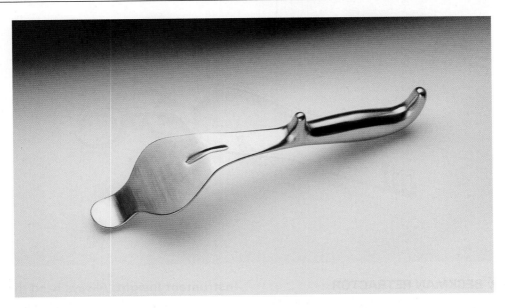

Instrument: BENNETT RETRACTOR

Use(s): Used for retracting tissues during procedures involving large bones (e.g., the proximal or mid-shaft of the femur).

Description: A smooth, solid grip type handle with a downward-curved, rounded, flared blade and a smaller upward-curved round lip.

Instrument Insight: The lip of the Bennett is slid behind and around the bone shaft for leverage when retracting tissues. There is no pulling needed when holding this retractor; once it is placed, simply hold the handle down or back.

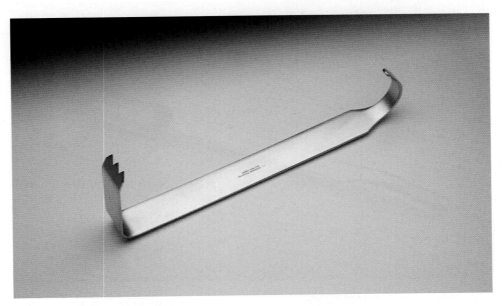

Instrument: HIBBS RETRACTOR

Use(s): This is a tissue retractor for either deep or superficial areas. The Hibbs is often used in large bone cases.

Description: This is a flattened, double-ended retractor that has a laterally bent blade and slightly bent lip with V-shaped teeth on one end and a small, crescent-shaped blade on the other.

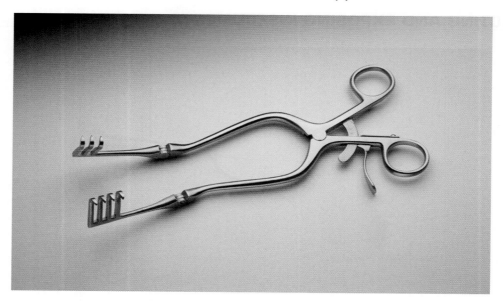

Instrument: BECKMAN RETRACTOR

Use(s): Used for retraction in procedures involving deep tissue, such as the spine, and in proximal femur fractures.

Description: Self-retaining, finger-ringed instrument with a ratcheted/release device on the shanks. Two hinged arms extend from the shank to three outward-curved prongs on one side and four on the other. These prongs can be sharp or dull.

Instrument Insight: Always hand this retractor to the surgeon with the prongs pointing downward.

⚠ **CAUTION:** The prongs may be very sharp. Exercise care when handling sharp instruments to avoid puncture to gloves and/or skin.

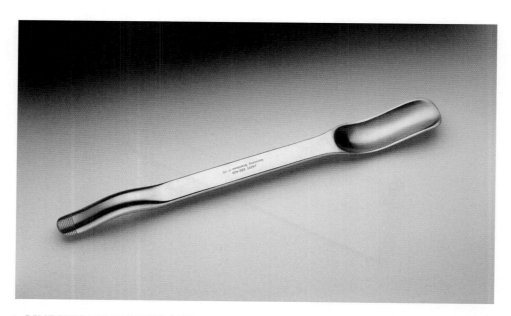

Instrument: MURPHY-LANE BONE SKID

Use(s): Used for removing the femoral head from the joint during total hip arthroplasty.

Description: Double ended with large or small curved spoons at each end.

Instrument Insight: The size of the femoral head and the acetabulum will determine which end of the bone skid to use.

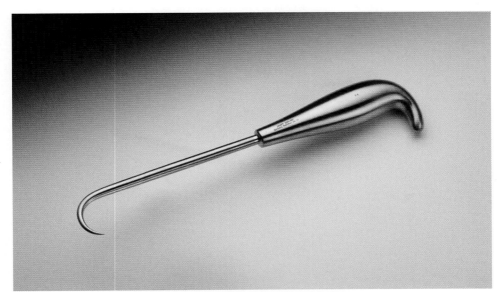

Instrument: BONE HOOK
Use(s): Used for retracting bone or heavy tissue.
Description: Thick handle with an extremely sharp curved hook at the working end.
Instrument Insight: Always hand the bone hook to the surgeon with the prongs pointing downward.

⚠ **CAUTION:** The prongs are very sharp. Exercise care when handling sharp instruments to avoid puncture to gloves and/or skin.

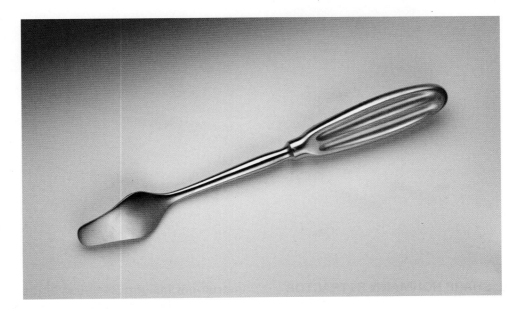

Instrument: CHANDLER RETRACTOR
Other Names: Chandler elevator
Use(s): Used for retracting bone and tissue.
Description: Thick handle with medium-curved, blunt blade.

Instrument Insight: This instrument is used to hold soft tissue away from bone, like a lever, when the surgeon is performing fixation.

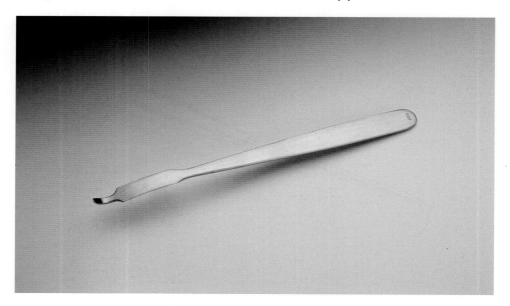

Instrument: MINI HOHMANN RETRACTOR
Use(s): Used for retracting tissue or bone in tight, small areas. The mini Hohmann is often used during open reduction internal fixation (ORIF) of the ankle.
Description: A flattened, smooth handle with thin, slightly curved blades and with a small, upward-curved, pointed tip.

Instrument Insight: The tip of the Hohmann is slid behind and around the bone for leverage when retracting tissues. There is no pulling needed when holding this retractor; after it is placed, simply hold the handle down or back.

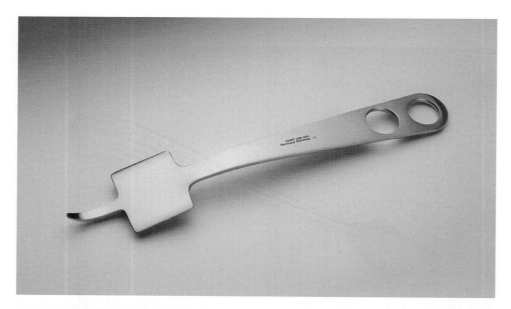

Instrument: SHARP HOHMANN RETRACTOR
Use(s): Used for retracting a large area of tissue, usually close to bone.
Description: Flat handle with two holes placed distally to aid in grasping the handle. The blade is shaped in a square with an upward, slightly curved prong at the end.

Instrument Insight: The prong of the Hohmann is slid behind and around the bone for leverage when retracting tissues. There is no pulling needed when holding this retractor; after it is placed, simply hold the handle down or back.

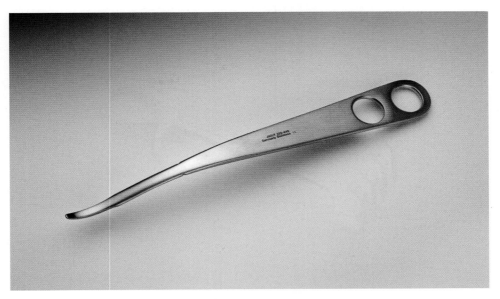

Instrument: BLUNT HOHMANN RETRACTOR
Use(s): Used for retracting a small amount of tissue in a very tight area.
Description: Flat handle with two holes placed distally. The blade is blunt, very thin, and slightly curved. There is no pulling needed when holding this retractor; after it is placed, simply hold the handle down or back.

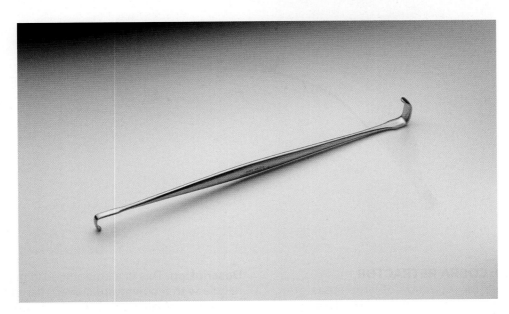

Instrument: RAGNELL RETRACTOR
Use(s): Used for retracting varying amounts of tissue at different depths.
Description: Double ended with right-angle, blunt blades that are available in different sizes.

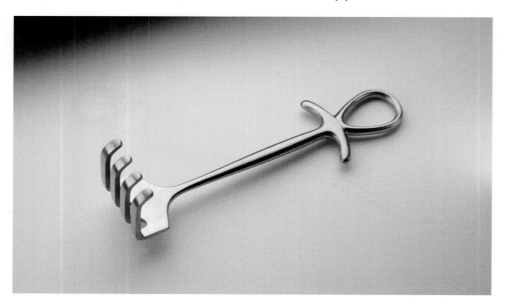

Instrument: ISRAEL RAKE RETRACTOR

Use(s): Used for retracting large amounts of tissue that usually does not involve bone.

Description: The handle has a teardrop opening with two prongs on each side. Has four large claws that may be blunt or sharp.

Instrument Insight: This instrument is also available with sharp prongs.

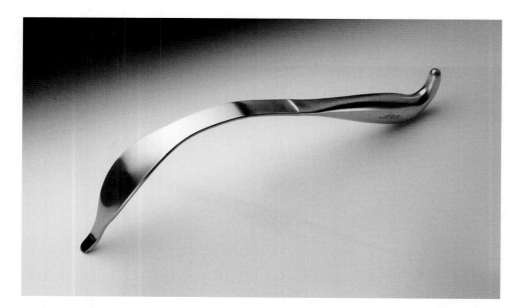

Instrument: COBRA RETRACTOR

Use(s): Used for retraction of large areas of tissue. The large bend in the blade allows tissue to be retracted far away from the field, allowing for better visualization.

Description: This is a smooth, solid grip type handle with a downward-curved, flared blade and with a smaller upward-curved, round tip.

Instrument Insight: There is no pulling needed when holding this retractor; after it is placed, simply hold the handle down or back.

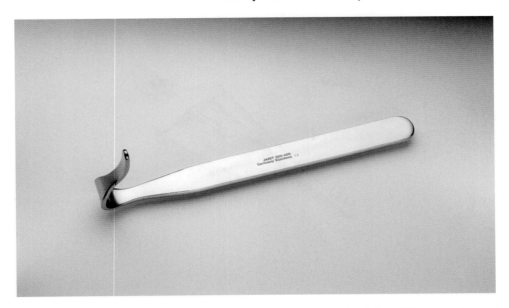

Instrument: BLOUNT KNEE RETRACTOR
Use(s): Used for retracting tissue at a right angle.
Description: Thin, flat handle with a blunt blade at a right angle and slightly curved.

Instrument Insight: Often used as a lever to retract. There is no pulling needed when holding this retractor; after it is placed, simply hold the handle down or back.

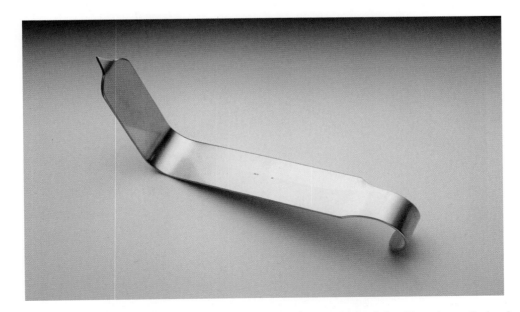

Instrument: TAYLOR HIP RETRACTOR
Use(s): Used for retracting tissue for exposure in total hip arthroplasties.
Description: Thin handle with curved, rounded end and blade at a right angle with a sharp tip.

Instrument Insight: The sharp tip is placed next to or on the bone for leverage. There is no pulling needed when holding this retractor; after it is placed, simply hold the handle down or back.

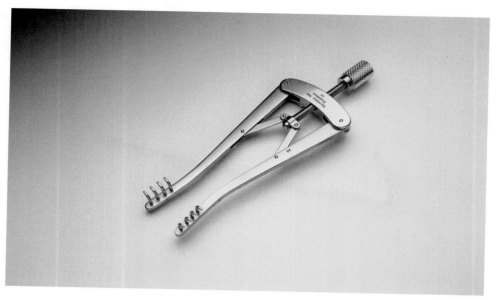

Instrument: ALM RETRACTOR
Use(s): Used for retracting in small areas.

Description: A self-retaining retractor. Thumb screw with flaring wings to open the arms of the retractor. Four sharp prongs on each side.

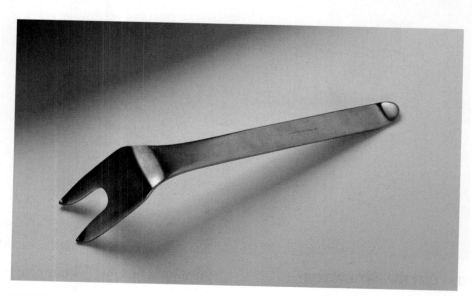

Instrument: HUMERAL HEAD RETRACTOR
Use(s): Placed between the glenoid and the humeral head to obtain exposure.

Description: An angled two-prong blade with a straight flat handle.

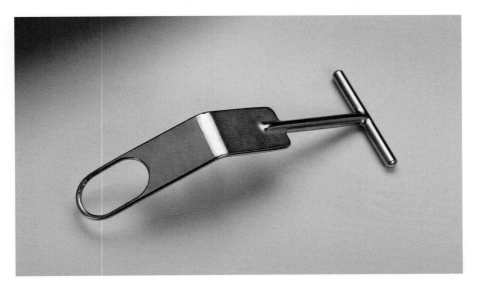

Instrument: FUKUDA HUMERAL HEAD RETRACTOR
Other Names: Humeral head, Fukuda
Use(s): Used to retract the humeral shaft posteriorly and helping to expose the entire glenoid surface.

Description: The Fukuda is available in small and large sizes; it has a T-bar style handle with an angled blade with and oval fenestration at the working end.

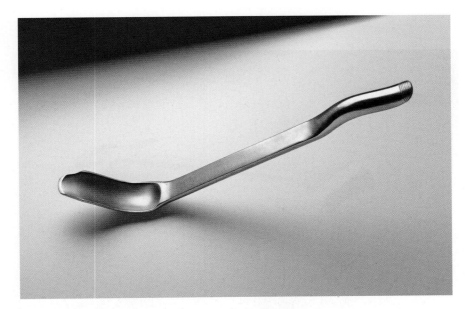

Instrument: LEVER SKID HUMERAL HEAD RETRACTOR
Other Names: Bone skid, shoulder skid
Use(s): Removal of the humeral head from the joint during a total shoulder arthroplasty.

Description: Double ended with large and small curved spoons at each end.

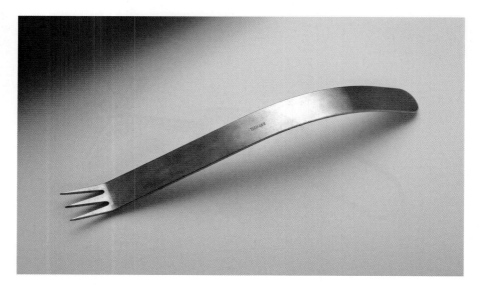

Instrument: CAPSULE RETRACTOR
Other Names: Fork
Use(s): The two- and three-prong retractors are designed to be placed medially along the scapular neck to retract the anterior capsule and labrium. The single prong retractor is commonly used when retracting on the inferior rim of the glenoid.
Description: A curved ribbon of steel with three angled sharp prongs at the working end. These come with one, two, or three prongs, which are design to retract in different areas.

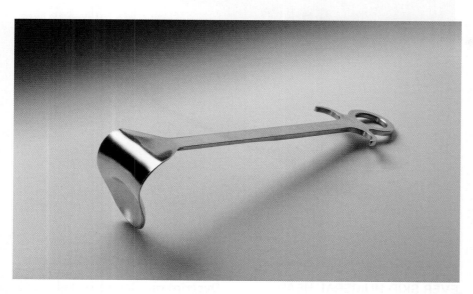

Instrument: BROWNE DELTOID RETRACTOR
Use(s): Placed to contour the humeral head for deltoid retraction to allow for exposure.

Description: The blade is concave and angled with a cup-like indentation at the working end. The handle is flat with a round opening with two curved prongs to each side at the distal end.

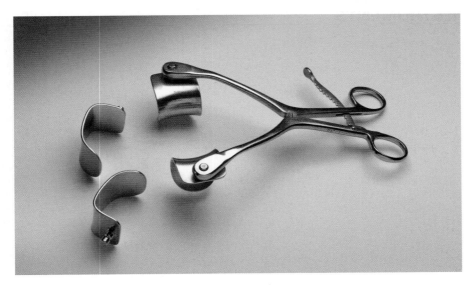

Instrument: KOLBEL SELF-RETAINING GLENOID RETRACTOR
Use(s): For retracting the capsule open during shoulder procedures.

Description: A finger-ring ratcheted self-retaining retractor that has exchangeable shallow to deep blades.

SUCTIONING AND ASPIRATING INSTRUMENTS

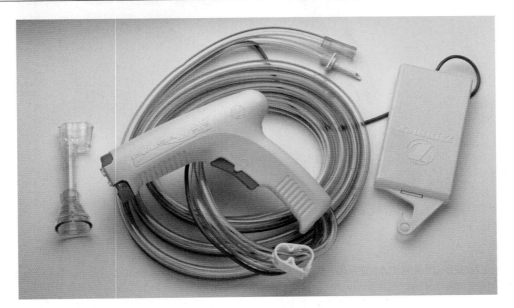

Instrument: PULSAVAC
Other Names: Pulse lavage
Use(s): Used for irrigation and debridement of tissues. The Pulsavac is commonly used for high-pressure irrigation during total joint arthroplasties.

Description: A battery pack provides power. The irrigation spike and the suction connection are handed off the sterile field. Pulsavac gun has two speeds with controls on the handle. A barrel is attached to the gun with a funnel at the distal end of the gun.

VIEWING INSTRUMENTS

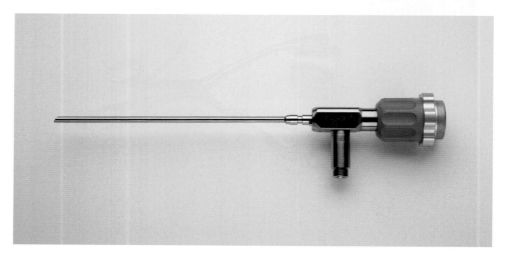

Instrument: 25° 4-MM LENS
Other Names: Arthroscope
Use(s): Used for viewing the inside of a joint.
Description: A rigid, stainless steel tube containing an optical chain of precisely aligned glass lenses and spacers. The objective lens is located at the distal tip of the scope. This determines the viewing angle. The stainless steel cylinder is called the optical element or the telescope, providing both images and light. The light connector allows attachment of the light cord to the telescope. At the proximal end is the eyepiece or ocular lens; this attaches to the camera coupler, or the surgeon may view the surgical field directly.
Instrument Insight: 25° is the angle in which the objective lens views. 25° endoscopes are very expensive and fragile. Care should be exercised when handling an endoscope; it should never be picked up by the distal telescope end, placed under heavy objects, or dropped.

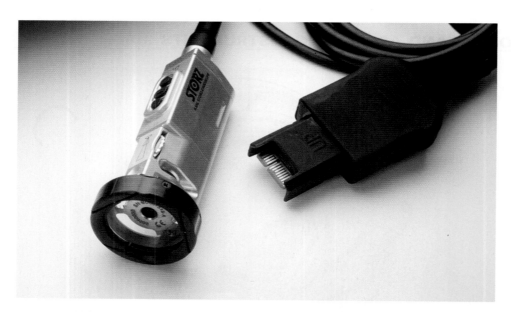

Instrument: ENDOSCOPIC CAMERA
Use(s): Used for the transmission of images from the rigid or flexible endoscope to the video monitor.
Description: At the distal end of the camera is the coupler, which attaches the camera to the eyepiece of the rigid scope. The coupler is attached to the camera head, which provides the image quality. Attached to the camera head is the cord, which relays the images back to the video system.
Instrument Insight: Most camera failures are related to a damaged cord. Care should be exercised when handling the camera and cord. They should never be placed under a heavy object, dropped, twisted, or kinked. Also keep the distal end covered until it is ready to be plugged into the unit.

INSTRUMENT SETS

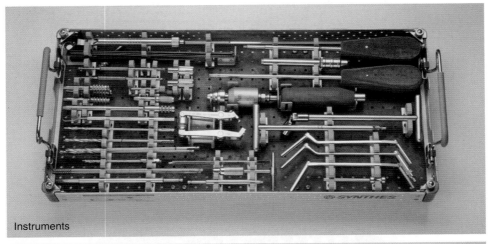

Instruments

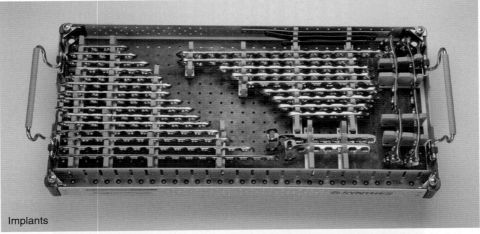

Implants

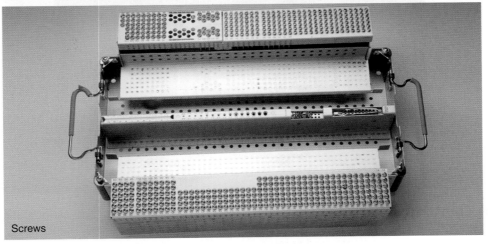

Screws

Instrument: LARGE FRAGMENT SET
Other Names: Large frag set
Use(s): These instruments, plates, and screws are used to secure fractures in large bones.
Description: First tray (instruments): Different types of screwdrivers, depth gauge, variety of drill bits, taps, chuck, drill guides, and plate holders.

Second tray (implants): Narrow plates, broad plates, T-plates, and bending templates.

Third tray (screws): Variety of screws, locking screws, other implants, and screw forceps.
Instrument Insight: Check surgeon's preference card for type of screws, implants, drill bit sizes, and drill guides. Check each tray before use to determine that all instruments and sizes are in each tray. This is especially needed for screws because they are placed in the patient and not reused.

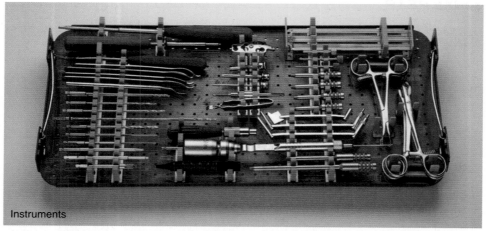

Instruments

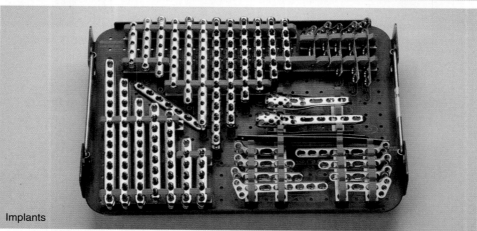

Implants

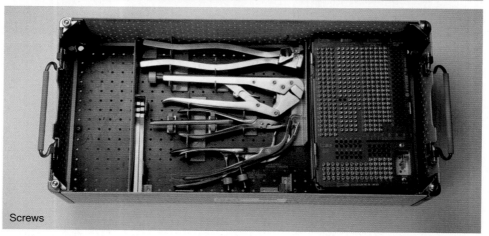

Screws

Instrument: SMALL FRAGMENT SET
Other Names: Small frag
Use(s): These instruments, implants, and screws are used to secure fractures in small bones.
Description: First tray (instruments): Variety of screwdrivers, drill bits, depth gauge, bone holding clamps, and screw retriever.

Second tray (implants and screws): Implants—LCP plates, T-plates, one third tubular, proximal humerus, straight reconstruction plates, curved reconstruction plates, and oblique and right angle plates; Screws—cortex, cancellous, shaft, and self-tapping; Kirschner wires and washers also in this tray.

Instrument Insight: Check surgeon's preference card for type of screws, implants, drill bit sizes, and drill guides. Check each tray before use to determine that all instruments and sizes are in each tray. This is especially needed for screws because they are placed in the patient and not reused.

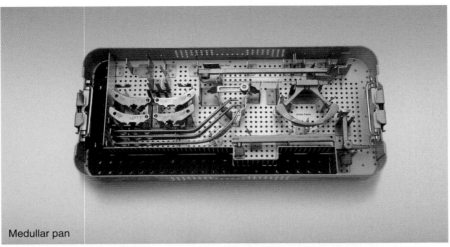

Medullar pan

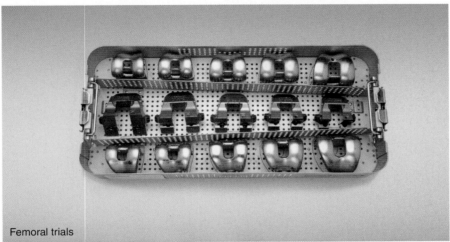

Femoral trials

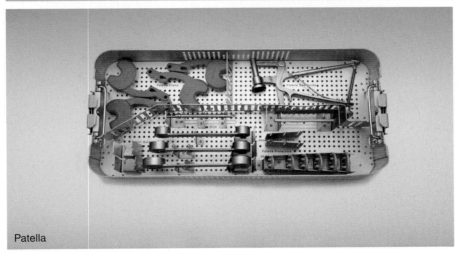

Patella

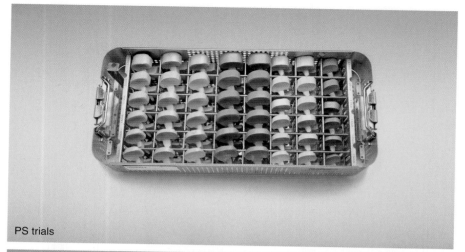

PS trials

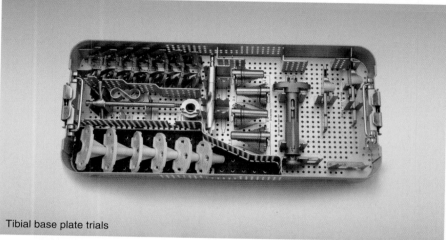

Tibial base plate trials

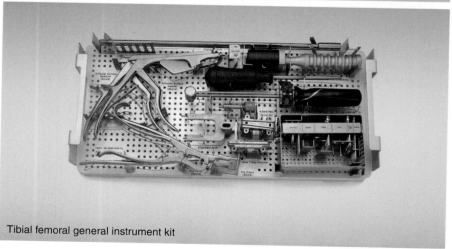

Tibial femoral general instrument kit

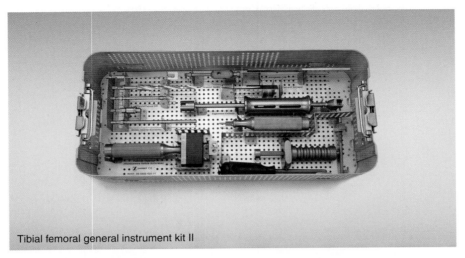

Tibial femoral general instrument kit II

Instrument: TOTAL KNEE INSTRUMENTS
Other Names: Knee arthroplasty set
Use(s): These are used to perform a total knee replacement (arthroplasty).
Description: Several pans are opened to perform the arthroplasty. Shown here:
Medullar pan
Femoral trials
Patella
PS trials
Tibial base plate trials

Tibial femoral general instrument kit
Tibial femoral general instrument kit II
Instrument Insight: There are many different systems and companies that have their own systems. Total knee instrument pans are often set by the company sales representative for a specific surgeon or group of surgeons according to their preference; these systems will differ accordingly. These pictures were set up by a Zimmer representative for a specific surgeon. Sets can vary by facility.

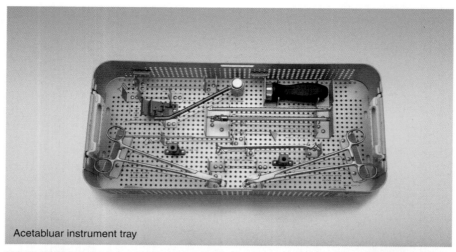

Acetabluar instrument tray

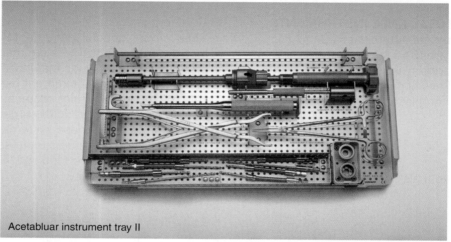

Acetabluar instrument tray II

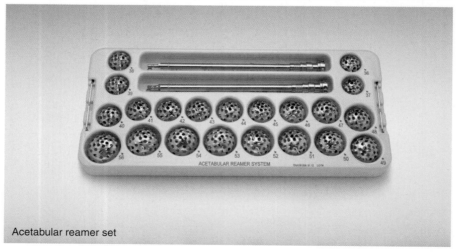

Acetabular reamer set

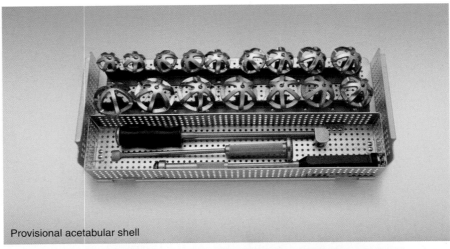

Provisional acetabular shell

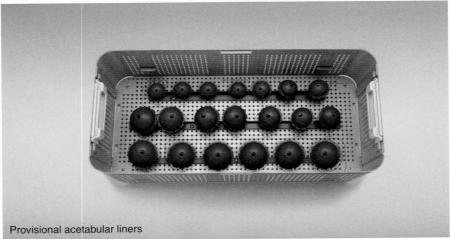

Provisional acetabular liners

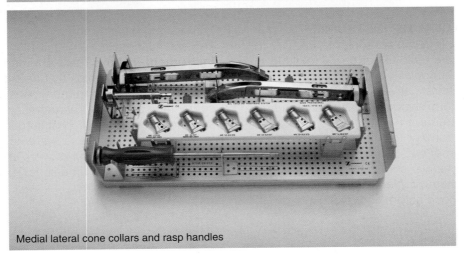

Medial lateral cone collars and rasp handles

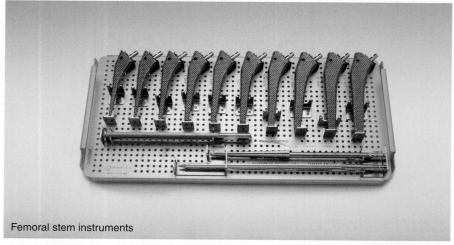

Femoral stem instruments

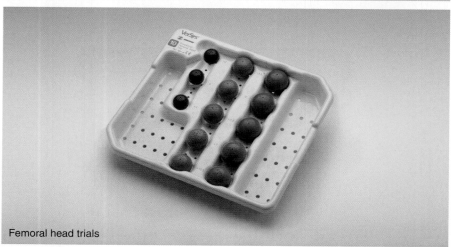

Femoral head trials

Instrument: TOTAL HIP INSTRUMENTS
Other Names: Total hip arthroplasty set
Use(s): These are used to perform a total hip replacement (arthroplasty).
Description: There a several pans that are opened to perform the arthroplasty. Shown here:
Acetabluar instrument tray
Acetabluar instrument tray II
Acetabular reamer set
Provisional acetabular shell
Provisional acetabular liners
Medial lateral cone collars and rasp handles

Femoral stem instruments
Femoral head trials
Instrument Insight: There are many different systems and companies that have their own systems. Total hip instrument pans are often set by the company sales representative for a specific surgeon or group of surgeons according to their preference; these systems will differ accordingly. These pictures were set up by a Zimmer representive for a specific surgeon. Sets can vary by facility.

13

Neurosurgical Instruments

ACCESSORY INSTRUMENTS

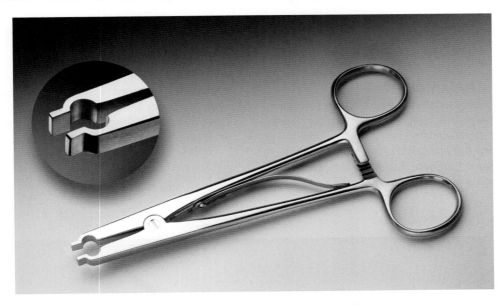

Instrument: RANEY CLIP APPLIERS

Other Names: Scalp clip applier

Use(s): Used for applying Raney clips to scalp flap edges during a craniotomy.

Description: Finger-ringed ratcheted instrument with heavy, smooth jaws that have a crescent-shaped fenestration, which leads to a flattened tip. The jaws of the applier are spread apart when the instrument is ratcheted down and are brought together when the ratchet is released.

Instrument Insight: To load a clip, the flattened tips of the applier are inserted into the opening on the back of the Raney clip. Upon compression of the ratchet, the jaws and clip open and are ready for application. Each clip controls bleeding only at the site on which it is applied. The length of the incision will determine the number required for hemostasis. Clips are placed along the incision edge with no more than a 1-cm gap between clips.

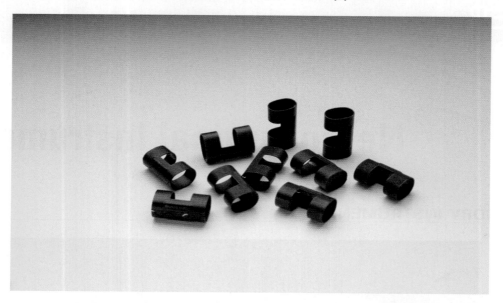

Instrument: **RANEY CLIPS**

Use(s): Provide hemostasis by compressing the tissue layers of the scalp edges when turning a flap during a craniotomy.

Description: A disposable plastic or reusable metal spring-action clip with wavelike jaws on one side and a slot on the other.

Instrument Insight: The disposable clips are typically packaged in sets of 10 or 20. Several clips must be placed on each side of the incision, so multiple packages may be needed.

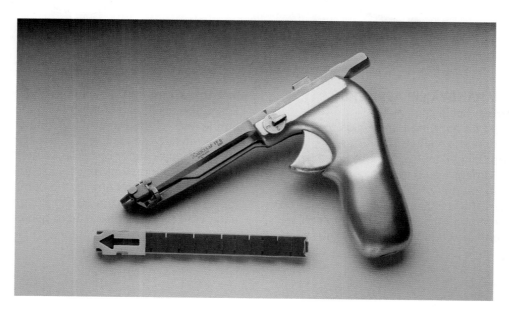

Instrument: **SCALP CLIP GUN**

Use(s): Used for providing hemostasis by compressing the tissue layers of the scalp edges when turning a flap during a craniotomy.

Description: A reusable, gun-shaped device with disposable clip cartridges. The system components are a reusable clip gun, disposable scalp clip cartridges, and clip removal forceps.

Instrument Insight: With activation of the trigger, the clip is opened, closed, and released by the applier. The successive clip automatically slides into position and can be applied in the same manner. The disposable clip cartridge is packaged with 10 clips. Each clip controls bleeding only at the site on which it is applied. The length of the incision will determine the number required for hemostasis. Clips are placed along the incision edge with no more than a 1-cm gap between clips.

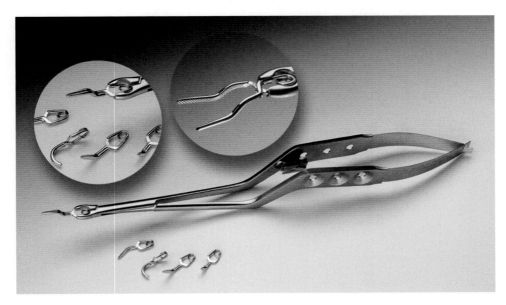

Instrument: ANEURYSM CLIP APPLIER AND CLIPS

Use(s): Used to clip the base or neck of an intracranial aneurysm to isolate it from normal circulation, thus causing it to deflate or obliterate.

Description: A bayoneted spring-action forceps with slotted, inward-curving jaws that grasp around the clip. There are many different manufacturers and a variety of aneurysm clips available for use. Most of the clips are spring-loaded, are made of titanium, and are manufactured in an assortment of types, sizes, shapes, and lengths to accommodate the various needs of the aneurysms (such as location, dimension, and form). Aneurysm clips are classified as permanent or temporary. Temporary clips are used to assure proper position of the permanent clip or to clip the vessels that supply the aneurysm if rupture occurs or if the aneurysm is very large.

Instrument Insight: There are many different aneurysm clip manufacturers (e.g., Sugita, Yasargil, Sundt, McFadder, and Heifetz).

⚠ **CAUTION:** An aneurysm clip should never be compressed between the fingers or with any other device; this should only be done with the clip appliers. A clip that has been compressed open should never be used again. The closing force on a clip that has been opened, closed, and opened again can be become sprung and unstable and endanger the patient.

⚠ **CAUTION:** Always have a temporary clip loaded in case a rupture occurs.

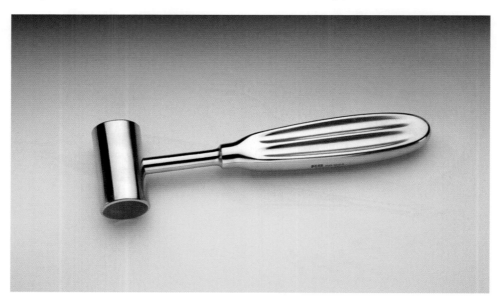

Instrument: MALLET
Use(s): Used to exert force on osteotomes, chisels, gouges, tamps, and other specially designed instruments. Commonly used during spinal surgery to harvest the bone graft.
Description: A solid stainless-steel or brass-filled, stainless steel hammer-like instrument.

Weight is 1 to 3 pounds. Mallets are used in other specialties that involve bone work.
Instrument Insight: Make available after passing any chisel, tamp, etc.

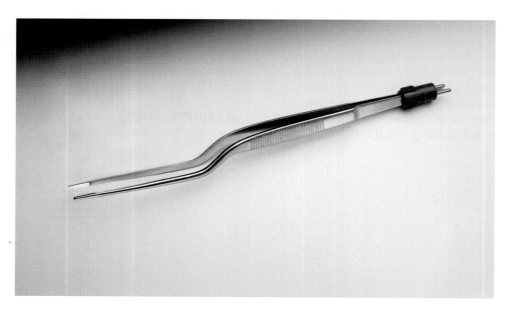

Instrument: CUSHING BIPOLAR FORCEPS
Other Names: B.B. forceps (bipolar bayonet)
Use(s): Used for coagulating tissue that is grasped between the tips.
Description: Bayonet-style forceps with fine, smooth tips and an ESU cord connection post at the proximal end. Bipolar forceps can be either insulated or noninsulated.
Instrument Insight: The bipolar forceps uses a disposable cord that attaches to the post end and is then connected to the ESU generator located

off the field. Stepping on a foot pedal activates the bipolar. The electricity travels from the ESU generator, to one tip of the forceps, through the grasped tissue, into the other tip, and back to the generator. The current does not pass through the patient's body, so a dispersive electrode is not needed. The ESU bipolar uses less energy that travels a shorter pathway, and is much safer than the monopolar. Bayonet-shaped instruments are designed so that the user can see beyond his/her fingers.

CLAMPING AND OCCLUDING INSTRUMENTS

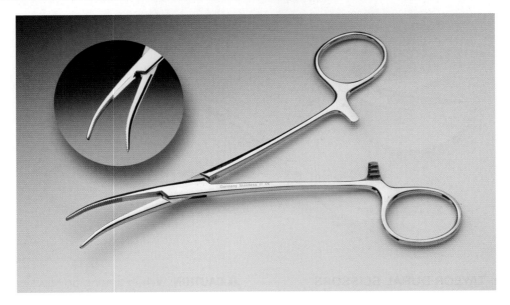

Instrument: DANDY HEMOSTATIC FORCEPS
Other Names: Dandy clamp
Use(s): Used for providing hemostasis on the scalp edges when lifting the flap during a craniotomy.

Description: A sideways-curved forceps with horizontal serrations running halfway down the jaws.

CUTTING AND DISSECTING INSTRUMENTS

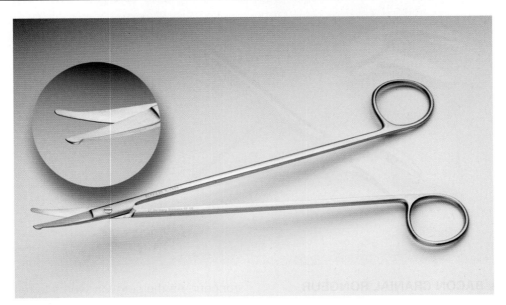

Instrument: STRULLY SCISSORS
Use(s): Used for blunt and sharp dissection of delicate tissues.
Description: A fine scissors with a slightly curved blade and with crescent-shaped probe tips.
Instrument Insight: The crescent-shaped tips are to protect underlying tissue from trauma during cutting (e.g., protecting brain tissue when cutting the dura).

⚠ **CAUTION:** When setting up, always check the screw to ensure it is tightened down and can not fall out into the wound when in use.

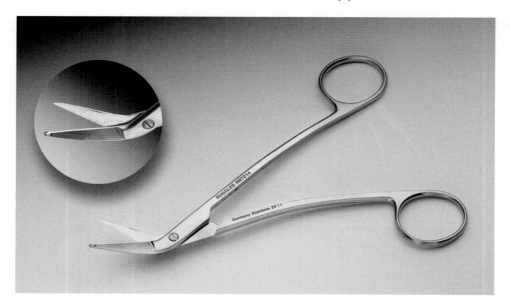

Instrument: TAYLOR DURAL SCISSORS
Other Names: Angled dura scissors
Use(s): Extend the incision into the dura mater during a craniotomy.
Description: An angled bladed scissors with a blunt tip on the lower blade to prevent damage to underlying tissue.

⚠ **CAUTION:** When setting up, always check the screw to ensure it is tightened down and can not fall out into the wound when in use.

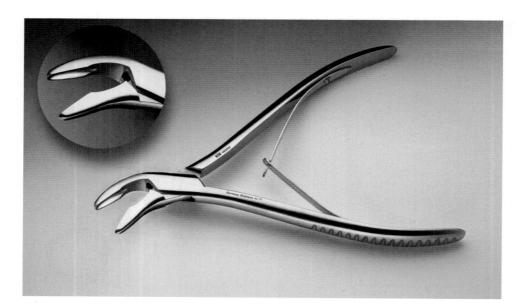

Instrument: BACON CRANIAL RONGEUR
Use(s): Removes pieces of bone and the soft tissue surrounding the bone. The Bacon is often used to remove the jagged skull edges when drilling burr holes or creating a flap.
Description: An angled rongeur with fine, oval-cupped jaws.
Instrument Insight: Always have a moistened sponge ready when handing the surgeon a rongeur. As the surgeon works to remove tissue and/or bone, the rongeur has to be cleaned between uses. While focusing on the wound, the surgeon will point the tip of the rongeur toward the surgical technologist. Using a moistened sponge, the surgical technologist will grasp the tissues from the jaws.

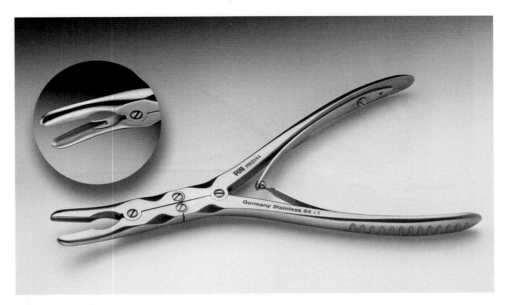

Instrument: BEYER RONGEUR

Use(s): Used for removing pieces of bone and the soft tissue surrounding the bone.

Description: Double-action, slightly angled rongeur with broad, elongated, trough-like jaws.

Instrument Insight: The double action gives the rongeur more torque at the tip for better biting action. Always have a moistened sponge ready when handing the surgeon a rongeur. As the surgeon works to remove tissue and/or bone, the rongeur has to be cleaned between uses.

While focusing on the wound, the surgeon will point the tip of the rongeur toward the surgical technologist. Using a moistened sponge, the surgical technologist will clean the tissue from the jaws. All biting or gripping instruments should be inspected at the cups for chipping and sharpness.

⚠ **CAUTION:** When setting up, always check the screw to ensure it is tightened down and can not fall out into the wound when in use.

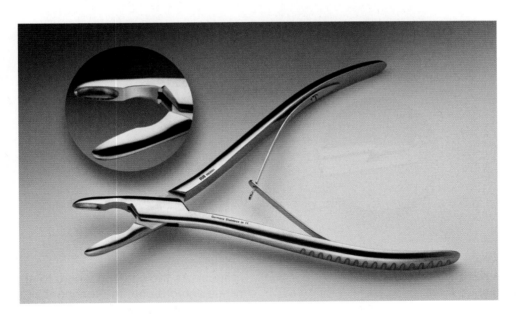

Instrument: ADSON CRANIAL RONGEUR

Use(s): Used for removing pieces of bone and the soft tissue surrounding the bone.

Description: A straight rongeur with oval cup jaws.

Instrument Insight: Always have a moistened sponge ready when handing the surgeon a

rongeur. As the surgeon works to remove tissue and/or bone, the rongeur has to be cleaned between uses. While focusing on the wound, the surgeon will point the tip of the rongeur toward the surgical technologist. Using a moistened sponge, the surgical technologist will grasp the tissue from the jaws.

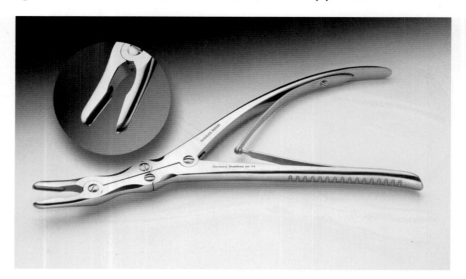

Instrument: **LEKSELL RONGEUR**

Use(s): Used for removing pieces of bone and the soft tissue surrounding the bone. The Leksell is often used in spinal surgery to remove the spinous process.

Description: Double-action, slightly angled rongeur with narrow, trough-like jaws.

Instrument Insight: The double action gives the rongeur more torque at the tip for better biting action. Always have a moistened sponge ready when handing the surgeon a rongeur. As the surgeon works to remove tissue and/or bone, the rongeur has to be cleaned between uses. While focusing on the wound, the surgeon will point the tip of the rongeur toward the surgical technologist. Using a moistened sponge, the surgical technologist will grasp the tissues from the jaws.

⚠ **CAUTION:** When setting up, always check the screw to ensure it is tightened down and can not fall out into the wound when in use.

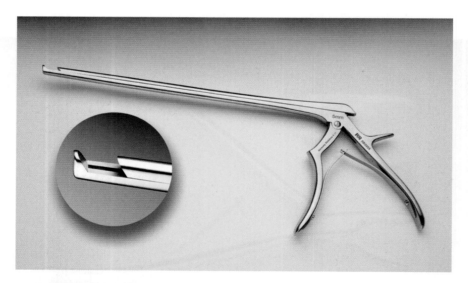

Instrument: **KERRISON RONGEUR**

Other Names: Up-biter

Use(s): Used for removing pieces of bone and lamina during spinal procedures.

Description: Compression handles that are attached to a long shaft with an angled guillotine-style action tip. The tips have a 40° or 90° angle and are either up-biting or down-biting with the dimension of the bite ranging from 1 to 6 mm.

Instrument Insight: Always have a moistened sponge ready when handing the surgeon a rongeur. As the surgeon works to remove tissue and/or bone, the rongeur has to be cleaned between uses. While focusing on the wound, the surgeon will point the tip of the rongeur toward the surgical technologist. Using a moistened sponge, the surgical technologist will grasp the tissues from the jaws.

⚠ **CAUTION:** When setting up, always check the screw to ensure it is tightened down and can not fall out into the wound when in use.

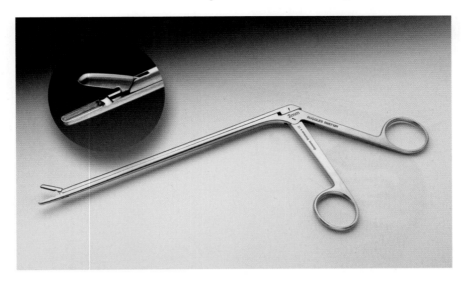

Instrument: CUSHING PITUITARY RONGEUR
Other Names: Pituitary forceps, bean rongeur
Use(s): Used for removing herniated disk fragments when performing a diskectomy.
Description: A finger-ringed instrument with a long shaft that extends to narrow, elongated, oval cup jaws. The jaws may be straight, up-angled, or down-angled.
Instrument Insight: Always have a moistened sponge ready when handing the surgeon a rongeur. As the surgeon works to remove tissue,

the rongeur has to be cleaned between uses. While focusing on the wound, the surgeon will point the tip of the rongeur toward the surgical technologist. Using a moistened sponge, the surgical technologist will grasp the tissues from the jaws.

⚠ **CAUTION:** When setting up, always check the screw to ensure it is tightened down and can not fall out into the wound when in use.

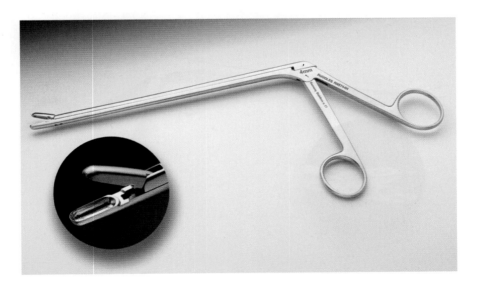

Instrument: SPURLING RONGEUR (STRAIGHT)
Use(s): Used for removing herniated disk fragments when performing a diskectomy.
Description: A finger-ringed instrument with a long shaft that extends to oval cup jaws. The jaws may be straight, up-angled, or down-angled.
Instrument Insight: Always have a moistened sponge ready when handing the surgeon a rongeur. As the surgeon works to remove tissue, the rongeur has to be cleaned between uses.

While focusing on the wound, the surgeon will point the tip of the rongeur toward the surgical technologist. Using a moistened sponge, the surgical technologist will grasp the tissues from the jaws.

⚠ **CAUTION:** When setting up, always check the screw to ensure it is tightened down and can not fall out into the wound when in use.

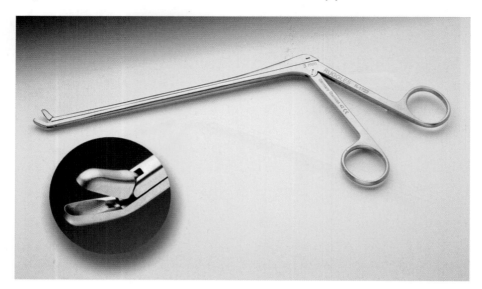

Instrument: PEAPOD RONGEUR

Use(s): Used for removing herniated disk fragments when performing a diskectomy.

Description: A finger-ringed instrument with a long shaft that extends to upward-bent, oval cup jaws.

Instrument Insight: Always have a moistened sponge ready when handing the surgeon a rongeur. As the surgeon works to remove tissue and/or bone, the rongeur has to be cleaned between uses. While focusing on the wound, the surgeon will point the tip of the rongeur toward the surgical technologist. Using a moistened sponge, the surgical technologist will grasp the tissues from the jaws.

⚠ **CAUTION:** When setting up, always check the screw to ensure it is tightened down and can not fall out into the wound when in use.

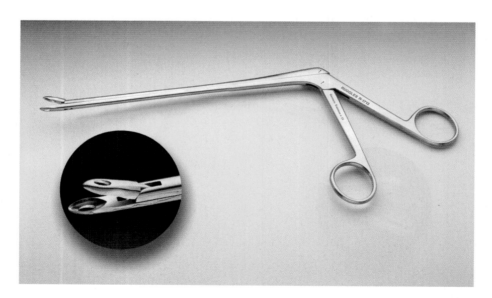

Instrument: WILDE RONGEUR

Other Names: Fenestrated

Use(s): Used for removing herniated disk fragments when performing a diskectomy.

Description: A finger-ringed instrument with a long shaft that extends to eye-shaped, fenestrated-cupped jaws. The jaws can be straight or up-angled.

Instrument Insight: Always have a moistened sponge ready when handing the surgeon a rongeur. As the surgeon works to remove tissue and/or bone, the rongeur has to be cleaned between uses. While focusing on the wound, the surgeon will point the tip of the rongeur toward the surgical technologist. Using a moistened sponge, the surgical technologist will grasp the tissues from the jaws.

⚠ **CAUTION:** When setting up, always check the screw to ensure it is tightened down and can not fall out into the wound when in use.

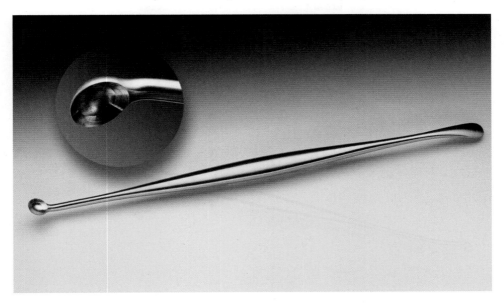

Instrument: #1 PENFIELD DISSECTOR
Use(s): Used for retracting, manipulating, and dissecting of nerves, vessels, bone, and tissues during craniotomies, carotid endarterectomies, and spinal procedures.

Description: A double-ended instrument with a broad, curved dissector at one end and a sharp, round spoon at the other end.

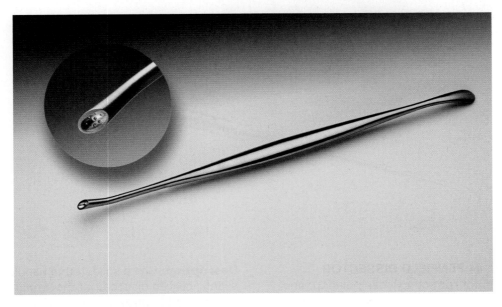

Instrument: #2 PENFIELD DISSECTOR
Use(s): Used for retracting, manipulating, and dissecting of nerves, vessels, bone, and tissues during craniotomies, carotid endarterectomies, and spinal procedures.

Description: Double-ended instrument with a slightly curved dissector at one end and a wax packer at the other end.

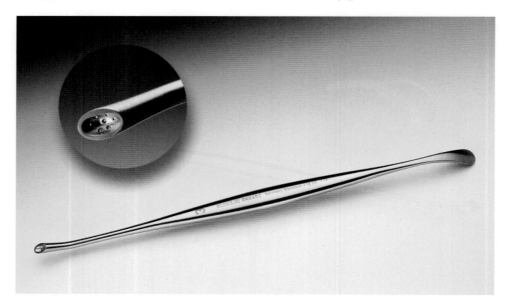

Instrument: #3 PENFIELD DISSECTOR
Use(s): Used for retracting, manipulating, and dissecting nerves, vessels, bone, and tissues during craniotomies, carotid endarterectomies, and spinal procedures.

Description: Double-ended instrument with a full curved dissector at one end and a wax packer at the other end.

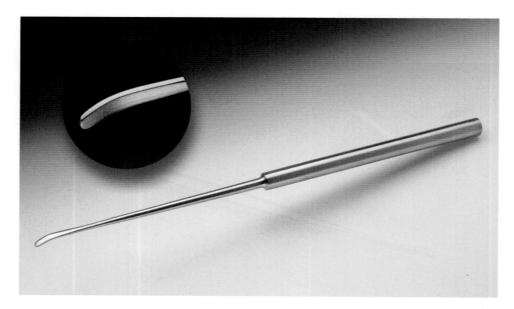

Instrument: #4 PENFIELD DISSECTOR
Use(s): Used for retracting, manipulating, and dissecting nerves, vessels, bone, and tissues during craniotomies, carotid endarterectomies, and spinal procedures. The Penfield #4 is commonly used to remove arterial plaque from the walls of the carotid artery.

Description: Has a solid, round handle with a slightly curved dissector at the working end.
Instrument Insight: Small balls of bone wax are pressed onto the tip and then are smeared on the cranial edges for hemostasis.

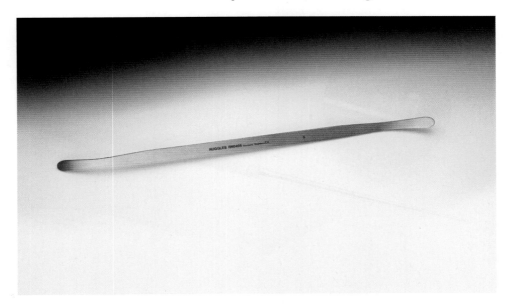

Instrument: #5 PENFIELD DISSECTOR
Use(s): Used for retracting, manipulating, and dissecting nerves, vessels, bone, and tissues during craniotomies, carotid endarterectomies, and spinal procedures.

Description: Double-ended flattened dissector with a full curved dissector at one end and a slightly curved blunt dissector at the other end.

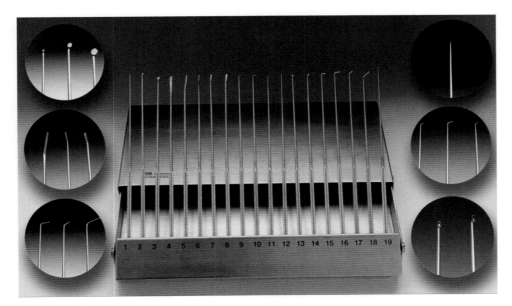

Instrument: RHOTON DISSECTOR EXTENDED SET
Use(s): Used for manipulation and dissection of very fine nerves, tissues, and tumors of the brain when performing a craniotomy.
Description: Extremely precise and delicate micro dissecting instruments. The Rhoton set contains round and spatula micro dissectors, micro hooks, micro curettes, micro needlepoint, and micro elevators.
Instrument Insight: These instruments should be wiped clean after every use with a moistened sponge. They are very delicate and should be handled with extreme care.

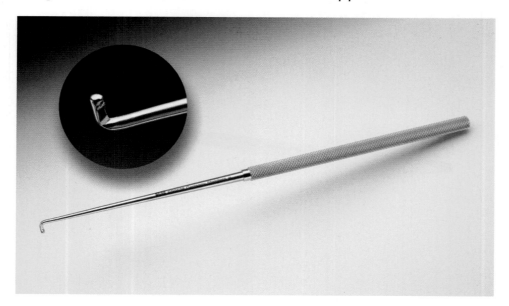

Instrument: MICRO KNIFE

Use(s): Used for dissection of very fine nerves, tissues, and tumors of the brain when performing a craniotomy.

Description: A round grip handle with a right hook at the distal end that has a sharp edge on the inner side.

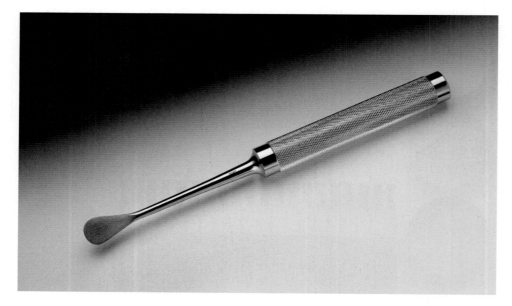

Instrument: COBB ELEVATORS

Use(s): Used for stripping the paraspinous muscles and the periosteum off the laminae. This is done when performing a laminectomy during spinal surgeries.

Description: An elongated, solid, rounded grip handle that extends to a narrowed, smooth shaft that terminates with a flat, broad, tear-shaped, sharp working end.

Instrument Insight: As the area is stripped, Raytex sponges that have been opened are packed along the side of the spine to compress the bleeding.

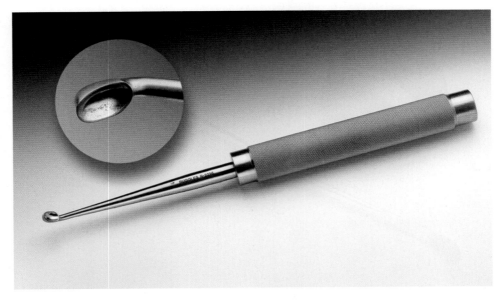

Instrument: COBB CURETTES

Use(s): Used for scraping bone during spinal surgery.

Description: An elongated, solid, round grip handle that extends to a narrowed, smooth shaft that terminates with a sharp-edged, oval-scooped working end. The tips may be straight, angled, or reverse-angled.

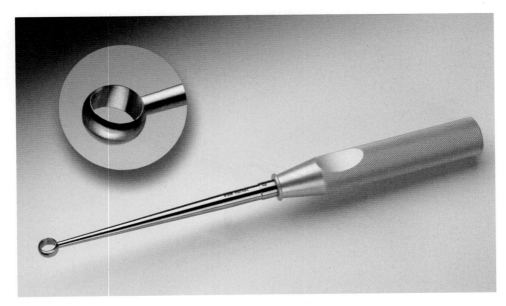

Instrument: COBB RING CURETTES

Use(s): To strip muscle and the periosteum off bone.

Description: An elongated, solid, round grip handle that extends to a narrowed, smooth shaft that terminates with a sharp ring-shaped working end.

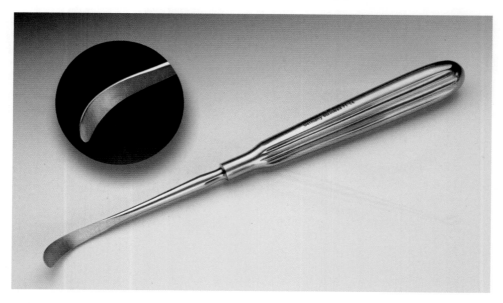

Instrument: ADSON PERIOSTEAL ELEVATOR
Other Names: Joker
Use(s): Used for elevating the skull off the dura when turning a flap or for scraping the periosteum off bone.

Description: A narrowing handle that leads to a flattened, curved, rounded tip.

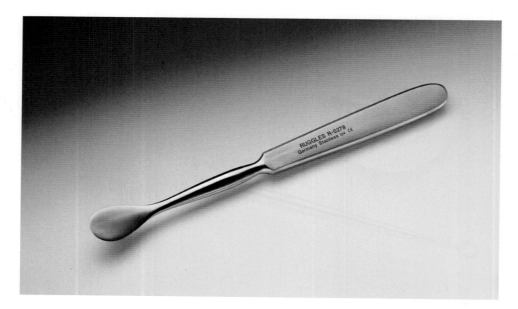

Instrument: HOEN PERIOSTEAL ELEVATOR
Use(s): Used for reflecting the scalp flap off the skull and/or scraping the periosteum off the skull when creating a bone flap during a craniotomy procedure.

Description: A smooth, elongated handle that extends to a narrowed, smooth shaft that terminates with a flattened, broad, rounded, sharp working end.

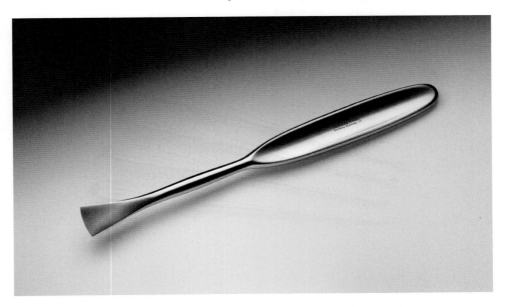

Instrument: LANGENBECK PERIOSTEAL ELEVATOR

Use(s): Used for reflecting the scalp flap off the skull and/or scraping the periosteum off the skull when creating a bone flap during a craniotomy procedure.

Description: A smooth, elongated, concave handle that extends to a narrowed, smooth shaft that terminates with a flattened, fan-shaped, sharp working end.

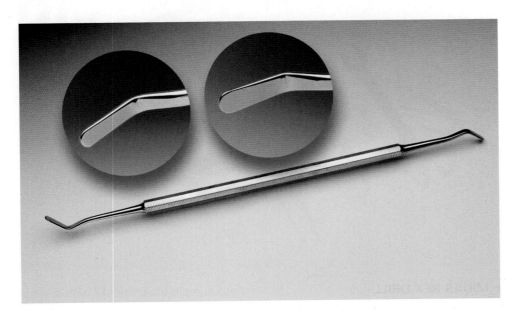

Instrument: WOODSON ELEVATOR

Use(s): Used for separating the dura from the cranium when creating a burr hole or turning a bone flap.

Description: Double-ended instrument with slightly angled, rounded spatula ends, with one end being wider than the other.

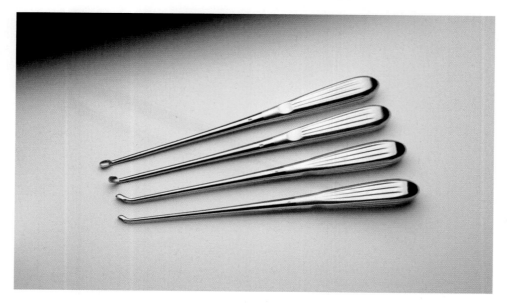

Instrument: SPINAL CURETTES
Other Names: Brun curettes
Use(s): To scrape out bone and tissue.

Description: This is a small spoon-like instrument with sharp edges. The tips can be straight, angled, or reverse-angled. They come in a variety of sizes.

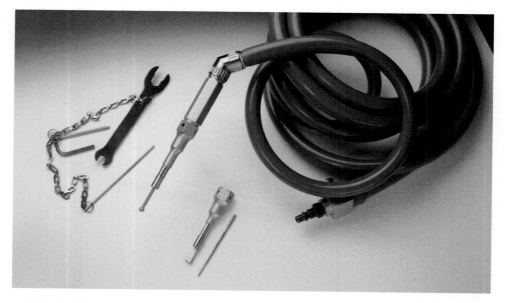

Instrument: MIDAS REX DRILL
Use(s): Used for perforating the skull when creating burr holes or for turning a bone flap during a craniotomy.
Description: This is a high-speed pneumatic drill that is activated by a foot pedal. The hand piece has multiple attachments with disposable burrs and blades.
Instrument Insight: As the burr holes and/or flap are prepared, the bit of the drill should be irrigated with saline to reduce the heat and bone dust that is generated from the friction.

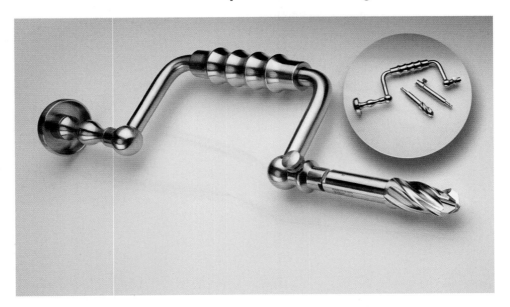

Instrument: HUDSON HANDHELD DRILL
Other Names: Hudson brace
Use(s): Used for perforating the skull when creating burr holes.
Description: A hand-held drill with a stabilizing handle on the proximal end that is in succession with a handle that rotates in a circle. The distal end has a thumbscrew chuck, which locks the bits in place. The bits come in a variety of shapes and sizes.

Instrument Insight: The perforator bit has a sharp cutting point that is designed to penetrate the skull. The burr bits are rounded and are used to enlarge the hole made by the perforator.

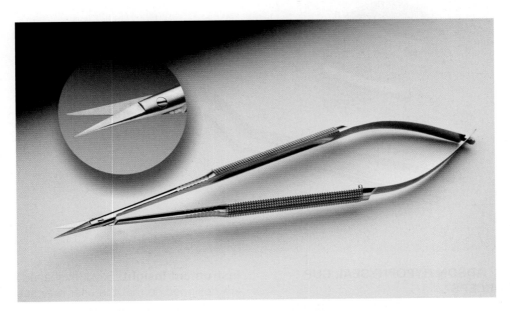

Instrument: RHOTON MICRO SCISSORS
Other Names: Micro scissors
Use(s): Used for micro dissection of delicate tissues.

Description: Fine spring-operated scissors that may be curved or straight.

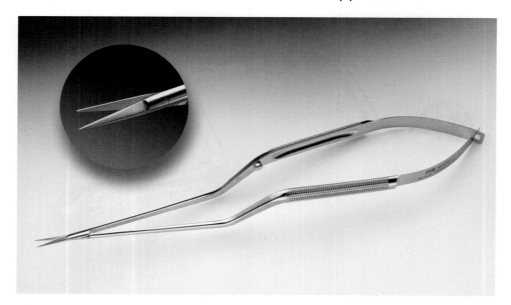

Instrument: RHOTON MICRO BAYONET SCISSORS

Use(s): Used for micro dissection of delicate tissues.

Description: Bayonet-style spring-action scissors that can have curved or straight blades.

Instrument Insight: Bayonet-shaped instruments are designed so that the user may see beyond his/her fingers.

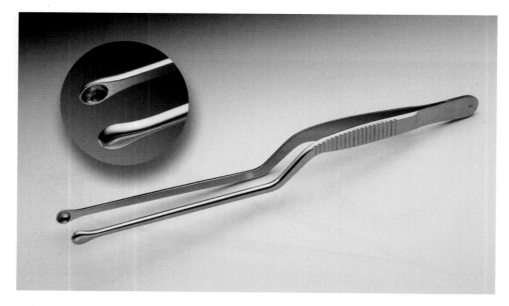

Instrument: ADSON HYPOPHYSEAL CUP TISSUE FORCEPS

Other Names: Baskin Robin, cup forceps, scoop forceps

Use(s): Used for grasping and removing tumors.

Description: Bayonet-shaped grasping forceps with a smooth cup tip.

Instrument Insight: Bayonet-shaped instruments are designed so that the user may see beyond his/her fingers. Tissue is removed from the cups with a moistened sponge.

GRASPING AND HOLDING INSTRUMENTS

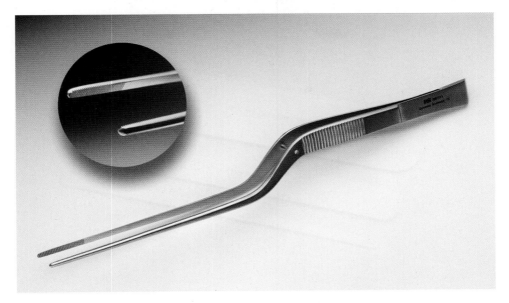

Instrument: CUSHING BAYONET TISSUE FORCEPS
Use(s): Used for grasping delicate tissues.
Description: Bayonet-shaped grasping forceps with serrated blunt tips.

Instrument Insight: Bayonet-shaped instruments are designed so that the user may see beyond his/her fingers.

PROBING AND DILATING INSTRUMENTS

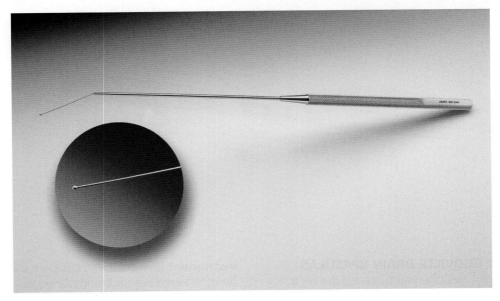

Instrument: BALL TIP PROBE
Use(s): Used for manipulating and probing blood vessels, nerves, and brain tissues.

Description: A round handle with a straight probe that leads to an angled wire with a solid ball tip.

RETRACTING AND EXPOSING INSTRUMENTS

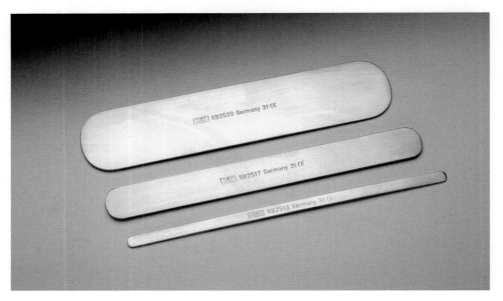

Instrument: DAVIS BRAIN SPATULAS
Other Names: Baby ribbons
Use(s): Retract the brain and tissues during a craniotomy.
Description: These are small, hand-held, malleable, smooth, flat, metal ribbons with rounded ends. The widths vary from ¼ inch to 1 ½ inches.

Instrument Insight: An assortment of sizes should be included in the set. Brain spatulas should always be moistened before being placed on the brain.

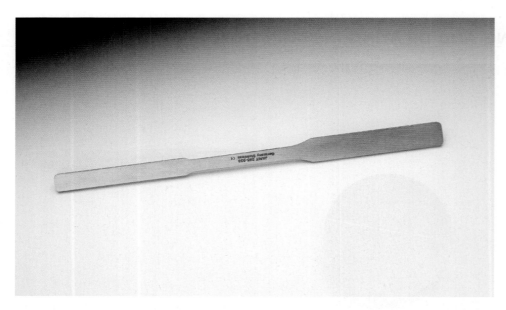

Instrument: SCOVILLE BRAIN SPATULAS
Use(s): Retract the brain and tissues during a craniotomy.
Description: These are small, handheld, double-ended, malleable, flat retractors with squared, blunt ends. One end is larger than the other end.

Instrument Insight: Brain spatulas should always be moistened before being placed on the brain.

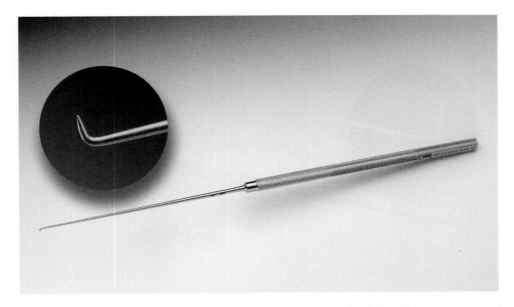

Instrument: DURA HOOK
Use(s): Used for elevating the dura.
Description: A sharp, right-angle hook with a round handle.

Instrument Insight: Exercise care when handling this sharp hook because it can easily compromise the integrity of your gloves or those of the surgeon.

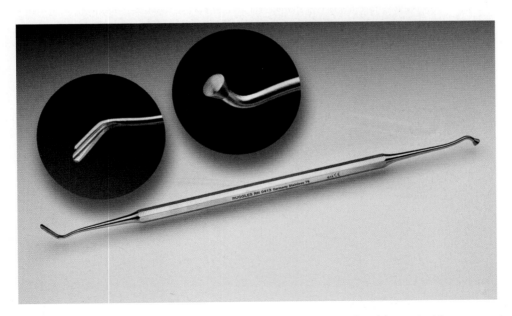

Instrument: WOODSON DURA SEPARATOR
Use(s): Separates the dura from the cranium when creating a burr hole or turning a bone flap.

Description: Double-ended instrument with a slightly angled, rounded spatula on one end and a blunt probe on the other end.

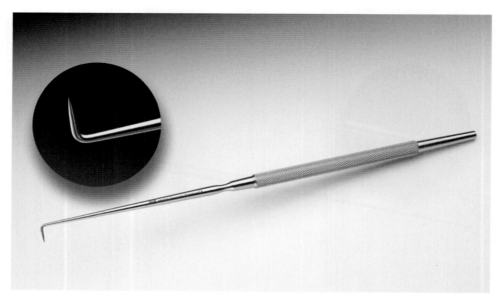

Instrument: ADSON HOOK, SHARP
Use(s): Used for elevating the dura.
Description: A sharp, right-angle, elongated hook with a round handle.

Instrument Insight: Exercise care when handling this sharp hook because it can easily compromise the integrity of your gloves or those of the surgeon.

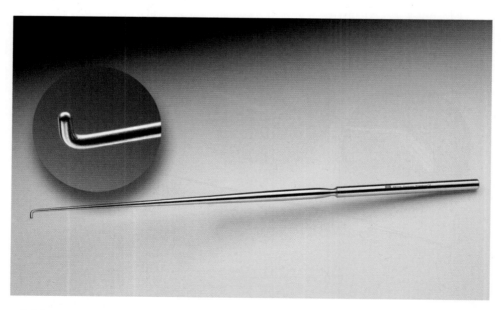

Instrument: DANDY NERVE HOOK
Use(s): Used for manipulation, probing, and dissection of very fine nerves, tissues, and vessels.

Description: A blunt, right-angle hook with a round handle.

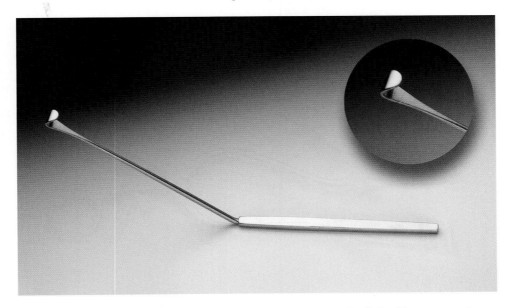

Instrument: LOVE NERVE ROOT RETRACTOR (ANGLED)

Use(s): Used for retracting the dura and the nerve root.

Description: A flattened handle that extends to a long, round shaft with a smooth, cup-shaped, curved blade with a crescent-shaped lip. The shaft of the retractor can be straight or angled.

Instrument Insight: To prevent damage to the nerve root, the retractor should not be moved after it has been placed by the surgeon. Because of the delicate nature of the tissue, care should be taken to not pull on the retractor but simply hold it in place.

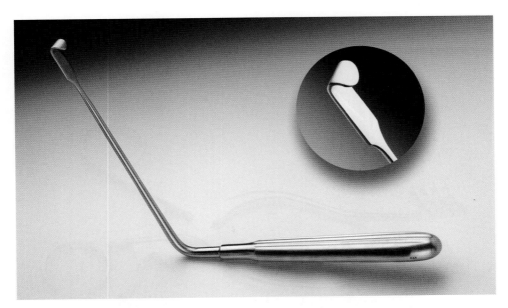

Instrument: SCOVILLE NERVE ROOT RETRACTOR (ANGLED)

Use(s): Used for retracting the dura and the nerve root.

Description: A round, tapered handle that extends to a long, round shaft with a smooth, flattened, elongated blade with a crescent-shaped lip. The shaft of the retractor can be straight or angled.

Instrument Insight: To prevent damage to the nerve root, the retractor should not be moved after it has been placed by the surgeon. Because of the delicate nature of the tissues, care should be taken to not pull on the retractor but simply hold it in place.

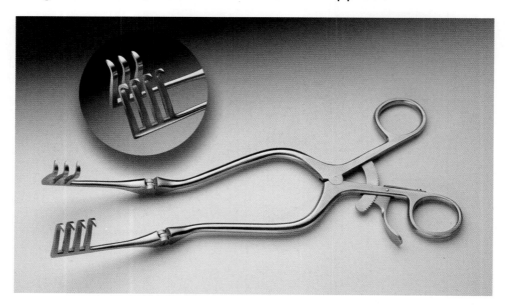

Instrument: BECKMAN RETRACTOR

Use(s): Used for retracting the wound edges during spinal surgery.

Description: Self-retaining, finger-ringed instrument with a ratcheted/release device on the shanks. Two hinged arms extend from the shank to three outward-curved prongs on one side and four on the other. These prongs can be sharp or dull.

Instrument Insight: Always hand this retractor to the surgeon with the prongs pointing down.

⚠ **CAUTION:** The prongs may be very sharp. Exercise care when handling sharp instruments to avoid puncture to gloves and/or skin.

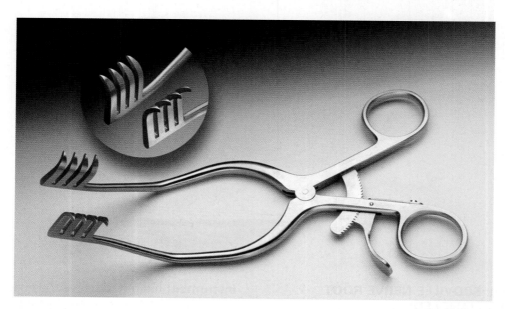

Instrument: CEREBELLAR RETRACTOR

Use(s): Used for retracting the scalp flap.

Description: Self-retaining, finger-ringed instrument with a ratcheted/release device on the shanks. Two arms extend from the shank to four outward-curved prongs on each. These prongs can be sharp or dull.

Instrument Insight: Always hand this retractor to the surgeon with the prongs pointing down.

⚠ **CAUTION:** The prongs may be very sharp. Exercise care when handling sharp instruments to avoid puncture to gloves and/or skin.

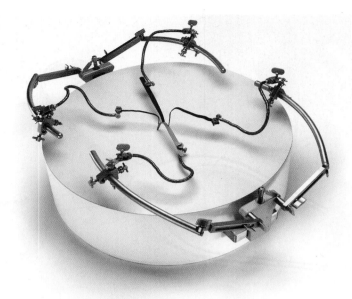

Instrument: LEYLA RETRACTOR

Other Names: Fukushima, Leyla-Yasargil

Use(s): Used to sustain gentle retraction of brain and neural tissues.

Description: Self-retaining table mounted retractor. This retractor has table clamps, U-bars, C-clamps, and snake arms. The flexible snake arms consist of a series of small metal tubes joined by a ball and socket. They are held together by a tension cable running through the middle of them, which is tightened by turning the knob on the distal end. When the cable is tightened the numerous metal components become rigid, thus maintaining the position in which they were placed. The brain spatulas are attached to the distal end of these flexible arms. At the proximal end the arms are fixed to a C-clamp, which allows the arms to be slid onto the U-bar.

⚠ **CAUTION:** Care should be taken not to inadvertently bump the retractor after it is placed.

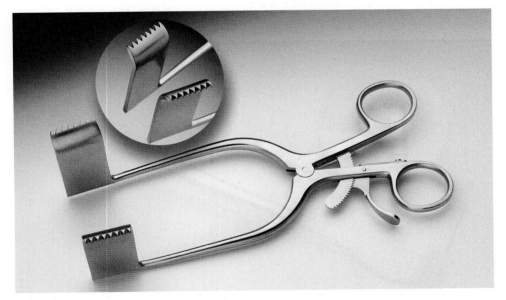

Instrument: MEYERDING LAMINECTOMY RETRACTOR

Use(s): Used for deep retraction during spinal surgery.

Description: Self-retaining, finger-ringed instrument with a ratcheted/release device on the shanks. Two arms extend from the shank to two outward-curved blades with multiple V-shaped teeth on each.

Instrument Insight: Always hand this retractor to the surgeon with the teeth pointing down.

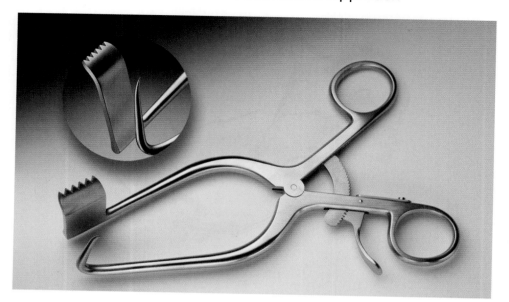

Instrument: WILLIAMS HEMILAMINECTOMY RETRACTORS

Other Names: Meyerding hemilaminectomy retractor

Use(s): Used for deep retraction during spinal surgery. Used when the lamina is being removed on one side of the spine only.

Description: Self-retaining, finger ringed instrument with a ratcheted/release device on the shanks. Two arms extend from the shank to an outward-curved blade with multiple V-shaped teeth on one side; the other arm has a sharp, angled prong. The blade will be on the right or the left side.

Instrument Insight: The surgeon will ask for a right or a left Williams retractor. Right or left is determined by which side contains the blade.

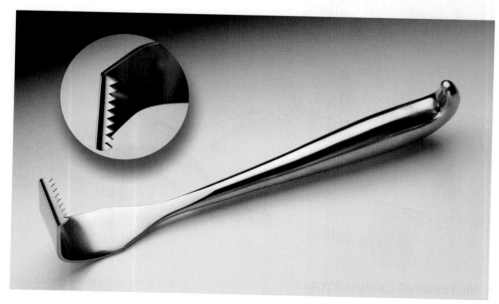

Instrument: MEYERDING HANDHELD RETRACTOR

Use(s): Retracts wound edges.

Description: Smooth-grip handle with a lateral-curved blade with multiple V-shaped teeth on the lip.

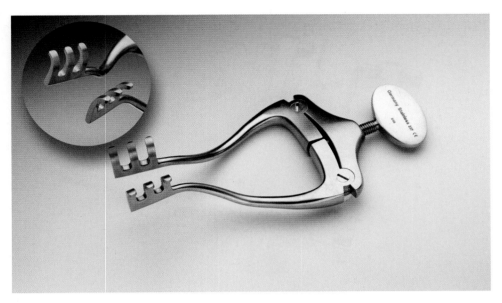

Instrument: DAVIS SCALP RETRACTOR

Use(s): Used for retracting the scalp when creating burr holes.

Description: A small self-retaining retractor with a screw-locking mechanism that has two elongated downward-curving arms with three outward (dull) curved prongs at each tip.

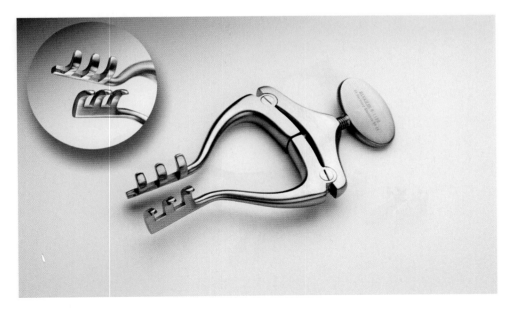

Instrument: JANSEN SCALP RETRACTOR

Use(s): Used for retracting the scalp when creating burr holes.

Description: A small self-retaining retractor with a screw-locking mechanism that has two arms with three outward-curved (dull) prongs at each tip.

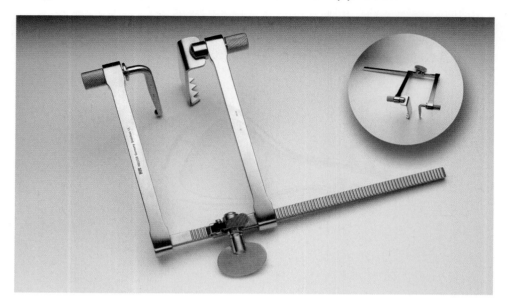

Instrument: SCOVILLE RETRACTOR
Other Names: Scofield/Meyerding self-retaining retractor
Use(s): Used for retracting wound edges during lumbar procedures.

Description: This is a key-ratcheted self-retaining frame with an interchangeable blade mechanism at the end of each arm. The interchangeable blades come in various sizes and styles.

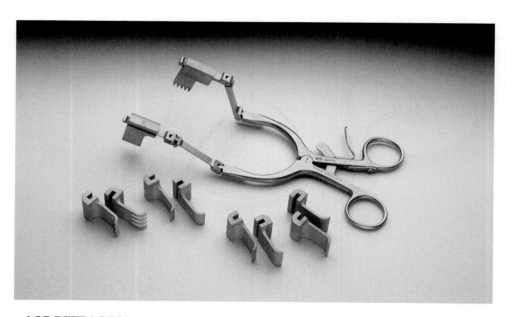

Instrument: ACF RETRACTOR
Use(s): Retracts wound edges during an anterior cervical diskectomy and fusion.

Description: A self-retaining retractor with two different style frames and a variety of interchangeable blades.

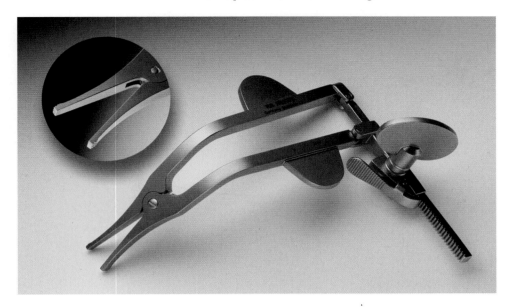

Instrument: CLOWARD VERTEBRA SPREADER
Use(s): Used for opening the vertebral space.
Description: This is a key-ratcheted device that has downward angle shanks with smooth, slightly outward bending jaws. The inner jaws are smooth, and they square off at the tips. On the outer edge is a small, crisscrossed grip patch.

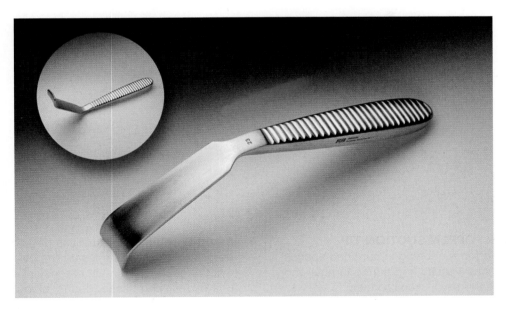

Instrument: CLOWARD CERVICAL RETRACTOR
Use(s): Used for retracting the wound during a cervical diskectomy and fusion.
Description: A solid grip handle with a smooth, elongated 45°-angle blade that has a crescent-shaped lip.

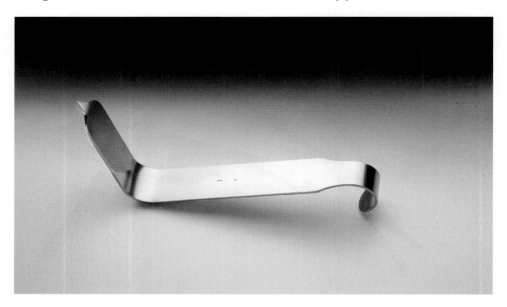

Instrument: TAYLOR SPINAL RETRACTOR

Use(s): Used for wound retraction during lumbar spinal procedures.

Description: This is a flat, stainless steel strip with a lateral-curved blade and a sharp V-shaped tip on the end. The width and length vary according to need.

SUCTIONING AND ASPIRATING INSTRUMENTS

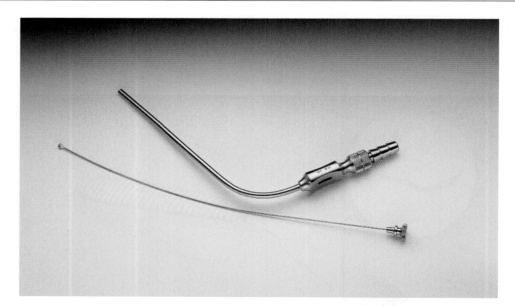

Instrument: POPPEN SUCTION TIP

Use(s): Used for suctioning in confined spaces such as the nasal cavity and during lumbar and cervical procedures or craniotomies.

Description: An angled, malleable, cylindrical tube with a relief opening/hole on the handgrip. The diameter of the suction tube is measured on the French (Fr) scale and ranges from 6Fr to 12Fr.

Instrument Insight: Usually is packaged with a metal stylet, which fits inside the cylinder. The stylet is used to maintain patency of the suction tube by relieving tissue, debris, blood, and other materials that may be caught inside the tube during suctioning. The suction is increased by covering the relief opening/hole.

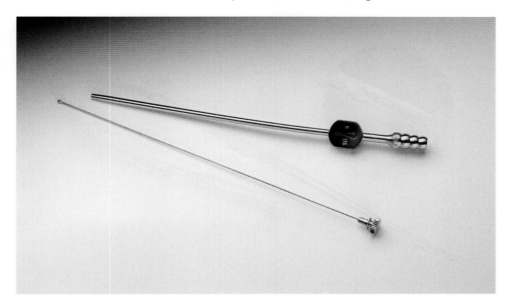

Instrument: TEARDROP SUCTION TIP
Other Names: Fukushima
Use(s): Used for suctioning of tissue, especially in hard-to-reach areas.
Description: This is a malleable, cylindrical tube with a teardrop-shaped control relief opening/hole on the handgrip. The diameter of the suction tube is measured on the French scale and ranges from 3Fr to 12Fr.

Instrument Insight: The malleable shaft gives the surgeon additional flexibility to adjust the configuration of the suction tube as necessary, allowing access in cases where difficult patient anatomy or tumor location may prevent the use of standard suction tubes. The suction is increased by covering the relief opening/hole.

SUTURING AND STAPLING INSTRUMENTS

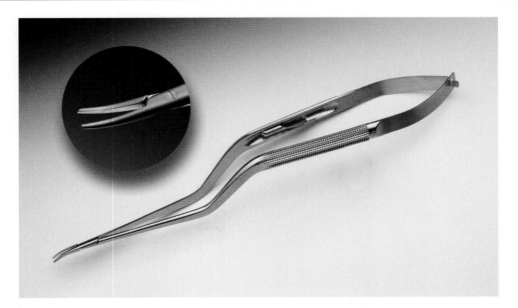

Instrument: RHOTON MICRO NEEDLE HOLDERS
Use(s): Used for holding very fine suture needles during microsurgical procedures.
Description: Bayonet-style spring-locking needle holder with curved or straight fine jaws.

Instrument Insight: Bayonet-shaped instruments are designed so that the user may see beyond his/her fingers.

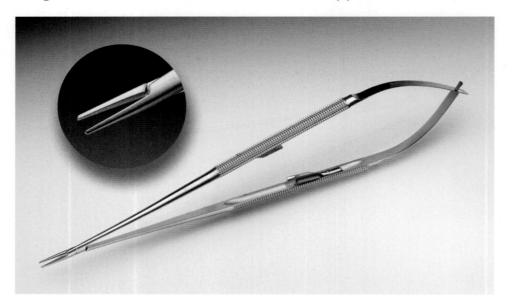

Instrument: JACOBSEN NEEDLES HOLDER
Use(s): Used for holding very fine suture needles during microsurgical procedures.

Description: Spring-locking needle holder with curved or straight fine jaws.

14

Cardiovascular Thoracic Instruments

ACCESSORY INSTRUMENTS

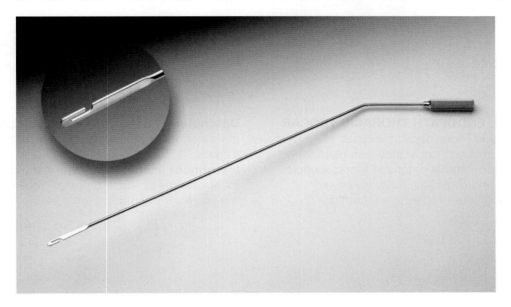

Instrument: RUMEL TOURNIQUET HOOK (STYLET)

Use(s): The surgeon encircles a vessel with umbilical tape or a vessel loop, and the loose ends are caught with the hook, pulled through a red rubber catheter shod or a plastic factory-made tubing tourniquet, and held taut with a hemostat to control flow in the vessel. Purse strings are also "snagged" this way when placing a cannula.

Description: Instrument has a hook or eyelet at the distal end.

Instrument Insight: Caution should be used when pulling the strings through the tourniquet because some tissues, such as an atrial appendage, are very fragile.

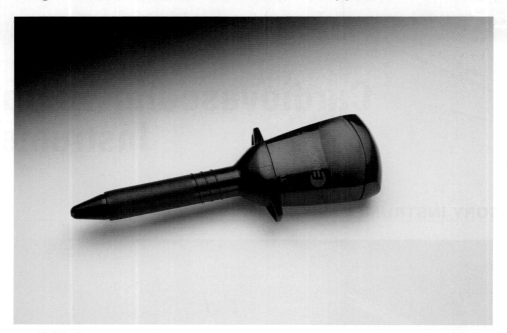

Instrument: ENDOPATH THORACIC TROCAR
Other Names: Thoracoport, Flexipath
Use(s): The thoracic trocar sleeve is used for an access port to internal organs in thoracoscopic procedures and other minimally invasive procedures that do not require insufflation.

Description: This trocar has a round tipped obturator and a thoracic sleeve with stability threads.
Instrument Insight: There are many different manufactures of these types of trocars, so there may be a variety of different styles.

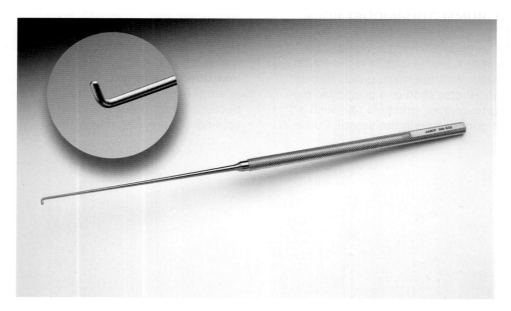

Instrument: BLUNT HOOK
Other Names: Nerve hook
Use(s): Used for "snagging" tangled or knotted fine suture. Also used for manipulating the leaflets in valve surgeries.

Description: This instrument has a right-angled hook.
Instrument Insight: This instrument can also be used to retract strings during placement of sutures during anastomosis.

CLAMPING AND OCCLUDING INSTRUMENTS

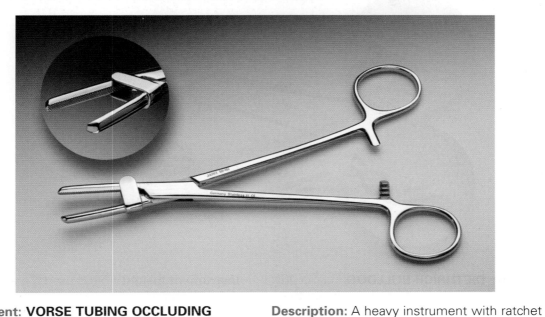

Instrument: VORSE TUBING OCCLUDING CLAMP
Other Names: Tube clamp
Use(s): This clamp is used to clamp off tubing and cannulas.

Description: A heavy instrument with ratchet handles and nonslip jaws.
Instrument Insight: Perfusionists use these on the heart-lung machine during bypass surgery; tube clamps are also used on the sterile field.

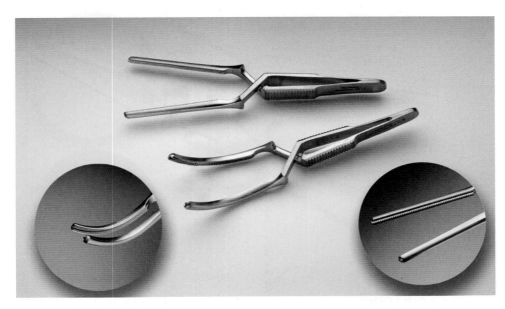

Instrument: DEBAKEY BULLDOG
Other Names: Bulldog
Use(s): Used for clamping off the flow in a vessel.
Description: This is a cross-action clamp. The jaws vary in length and can be straight or curved. The jaws are serrated with the DeBakey design.
Instrument Insight: This is often used to mark the end of a vein graft to specify flow direction.

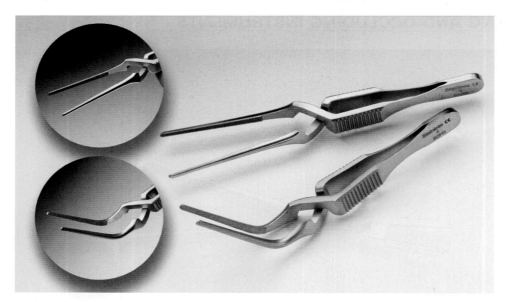

Instrument: DIETHRICH BULLDOG

Use(s): This small clamp is used to impede the flow in a vessel.

Description: This is a fine cross-action clamp. It can be straight or angled.

Instrument Insight: This is used more often than the heavier bulldog because there is less trauma to the vessel.

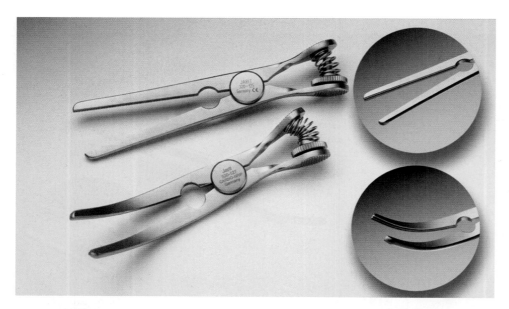

Instrument: GLOVER BULLDOG

Use(s): This is used to stop flow in a vessel and to clamp vessel loops encircling a vessel.

Description: This clamp is available in a variety of lengths. Serrations in the jaws are of the Cooley design.

Instrument Insight: This is seldom used because the Cooley jaws are more crushing.

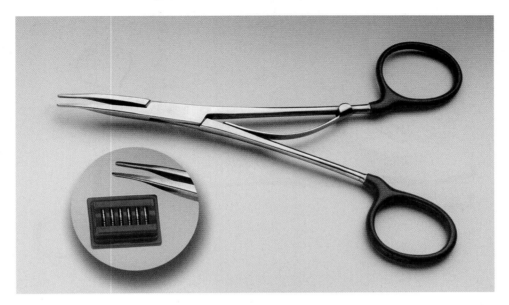

Instrument: HEMOCLIP APPLIERS
Other Names: Ligaclip applier
Use(s): This instrument is used to clip side branches on vessels instead of tying with suture material.
Description: These appliers are available in small, medium, medium/large, and large sizes.

They can also have an angled end. The clip bars that hold the actual clips come in the colors red, blue, green, and orange, and the applier handles have the same color.
Instrument Insight: "Load" by pushing instrument jaws onto clip and lifting. The surgeon "fires" the clip by squeezing the handles.

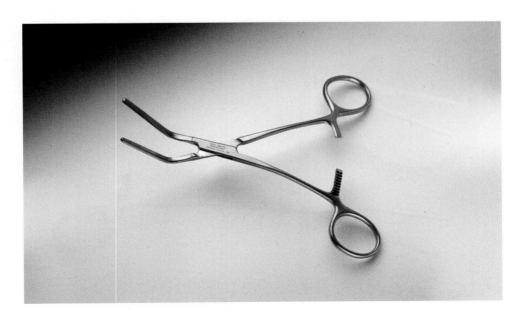

Instrument: COOLEY CLAMP
Other Names: Angled clamp
Use(s): Used for total occlusion of a vessel.
Description: This instrument has ratcheted handles and jaws. The angle is 45° or 55°. Serrations are of the Cooley design.

Instrument Insight: The ratchets allow the surgeon to adjust the clamp according to the blood pressure inside the vessel. They also allow gradual increase or decrease of blood flow.

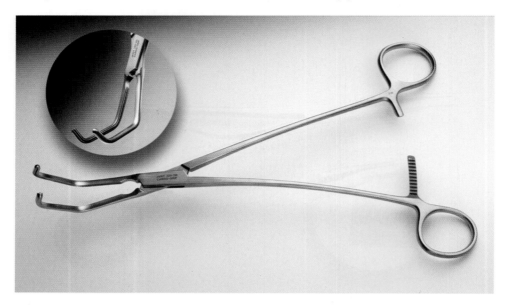

Instrument: SATINSKY VENA CAVA CLAMP

Other Names: Satinsky partial occlusion clamp

Use(s): Used for partially occluding vessels.

Description: This is a partial occlusion clamp. The clamp comes in a variety of lengths, with noncrushing jaws of the DeBakey design and ratchet handles.

Instrument Insight: This clamp is sometimes used to encircle the superior or inferior vena cava before placement of umbilical tape around the vessel. It is also sometimes used to clamp the atrial appendage.

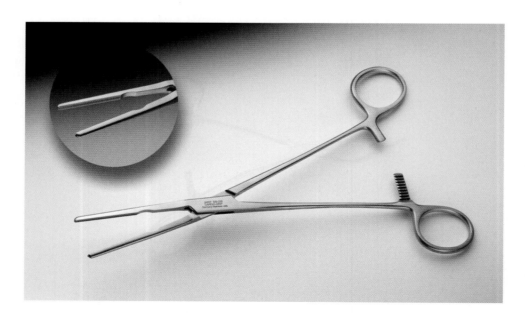

Instrument: GLOVER PATENT DUCTUS CLAMP

Use(s): This clamp can have a variety of uses and is a total occlusion clamp.

Description: This clamp is straight or angled slightly. They have ratcheted handles and DeBakey design serrated jaws.

Instrument Insight: Ratchets allow the doctor to adjust the clamp according to the blood pressure inside the vessel. They also allow gradual increase or decrease of blood flow.

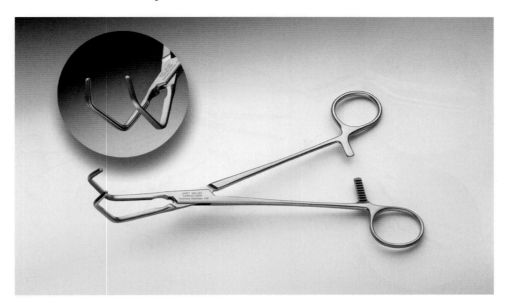

Instrument: BECK AORTIC CLAMP
Other Names: Pedicle clamp
Use(s): This is a partial occlusion clamp used in deep areas; it can also be used as a total occlusion clamp on larger vessels.

Description: This clamp comes in varying sizes, as do the jaws. They have the DeBakey design jaw serrations.

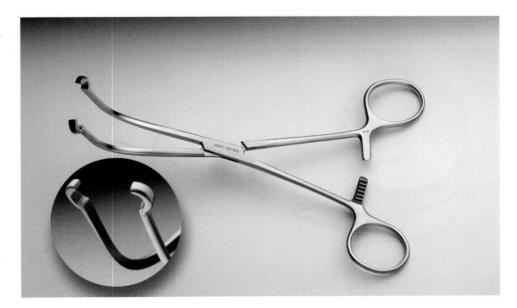

Instrument: JAVID CAROTID ARTERY CLAMP
Other Names: Javid carotid shunt clamp
Use(s): Used during a carotid endarterectomy procedure to secure the Javid shunt in the carotid artery when diverting the blood flow away from the operative site.

Description: A ratcheted, angled clamp in which the tip of each jaw is a half-circle that clamps around the artery and the shunt to hold it in place
Instrument Insight: This can be used with other shunts as well as for holding introducers in place during endovascular procedures.

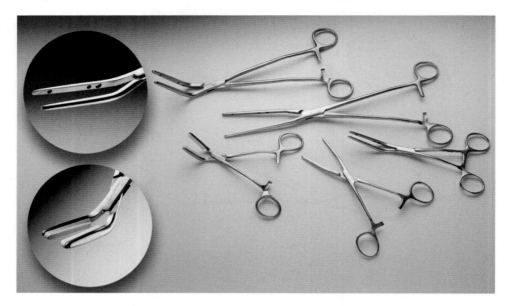

Instrument: FOGARTY CLAMP WITH JAW INSERTS
Other Names: Hydragrip
Use(s): This is a vascular clamp with soft jaws for vessels as well as graft material.

Description: These clamps can be angled and straight. The inserts come in a pair with one as a hydrajaw and one as a traction jaw.
Instrument Insight: These clamps are used in vascular, pulmonary, cardiac, and gastrointestinal procedures.

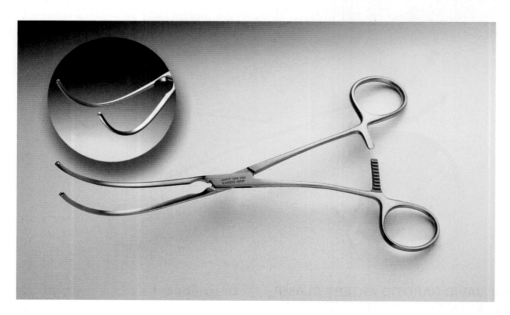

Instrument: DEBAKEY AORTIC CLAMP
Use(s): This is a multiple-use clamp. It can be used for partial occlusion or total occlusion. It is also used to tunnel under the tissues to pull a graft through to its distal anastomosis.
Description: This clamp has curved shanks with DeBakey design serrations in the jaws.

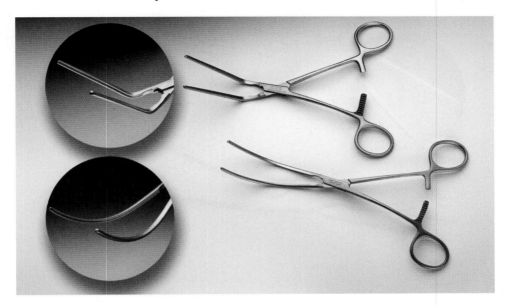

Instrument: DEBAKEY PERIPHERAL VASCULAR CLAMP

Other Names: Angled or sometimes referred to by degree such as a 35 or a 45.

Use(s): This is a total occlusion clamp.

Description: A ratcheted clamp with straight, curved, or various angled jaws that have DeBakey style serrations.

Instrument Insight: Ratchet handles allow the surgeon to adjust the clamp according to the blood pressure inside the vessel. They also allow gradual increase or decrease of blood flow.

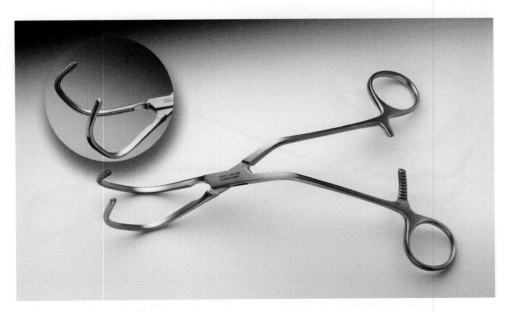

Instrument: LAMBERT-KAY AORTA CLAMP

Other Names: Side biter

Use(s): This is a partial occlusion clamp.

Description: This clamp has DeBakey design serrations in the jaws.

Instrument Insight: This is often used to partially occlude the aorta for proximal end anastomosis of saphenous vein grafts in coronary artery bypasses.

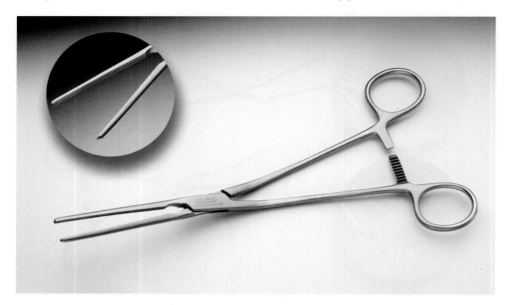

Instrument: DEBAKEY COARCTATION CLAMP
Other Names: Patent ductus
Use(s): This clamp is used on the iliac and femoral arteries during abdominal aortic aneurysm (AAA) repair.

Description: This clamp is slightly angled. The jaw has DeBakey design serrations.
Instrument Insight: This clamp is often used to occlude more than one vessel at a time such as the femoral and profunda femoris arteries.

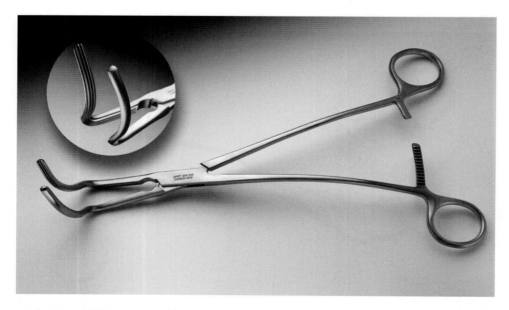

Instrument: DEBAKEY SIDEWINDER AORTA CLAMP
Other Names: Subramanian
Use(s): This is an aortic occlusion clamp.
Description: The clamp is angled and the jaws are curved.

Instrument Insight: This clamp is often used on the aorta during AAA repair when there is limited room for a cross-clamp.

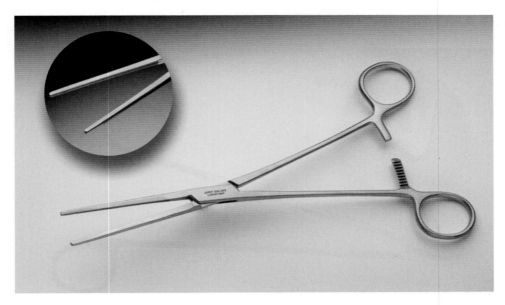

Instrument: COOLEY COARCTATION CLAMP
Other Names: Straight clamp
Use(s): This is often used when clamping deep anatomical vessels.

Description: A total occlusion clamp that has straight, cardio-grip jaws.

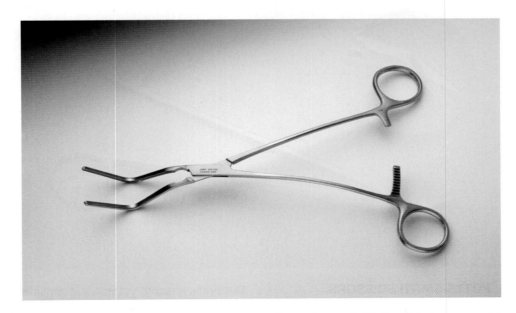

Instrument: LEE BRONCHUS CLAMP
Use(s): This is a clamp used for total occlusion of the bronchus during lung procedures.
Description: This clamp has 90°-angle tips.

Instrument Insight: This instrument is often used for occlusion of structures during lung procedures.

CUTTING AND DISSECTING INSTRUMENTS

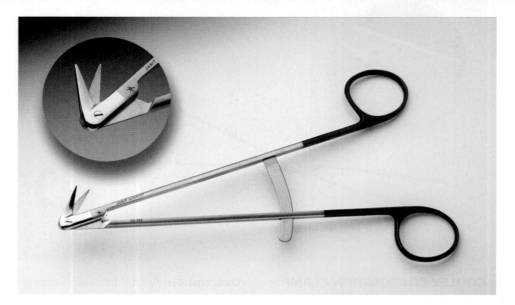

Instrument: DIETHRICH SCISSORS
Other Names: Ducks scissors
Use(s): These scissors are used to extend an opening in an artery or vein.
Description: These scissors vary in degrees of angles; they have a stabilizing bar on the handles, and the blades have a sharp point.

Instrument Insight: These are considered a delicate instrument and should never be used for anything except opening of a vessel. Wipe clean after each use with a damp sponge.

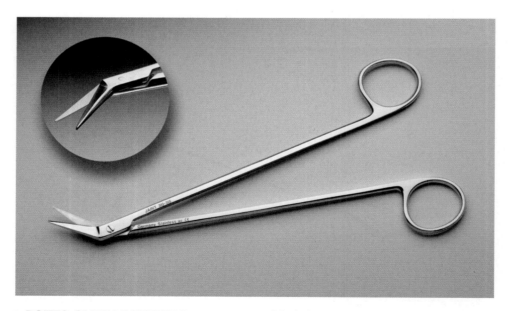

Instrument: POTTS-SMITH SCISSORS
Other Names: Potts
Use(s): These scissors are used to extend an opening in an artery or vein.
Description: These scissors come in a variety of degrees of angles. They are heavier than

Diethrich scissors yet are still considered a delicate instrument.
Instrument Insight: These scissors are to be used on vessels only. They are heavier and can cut through calcified plaque.

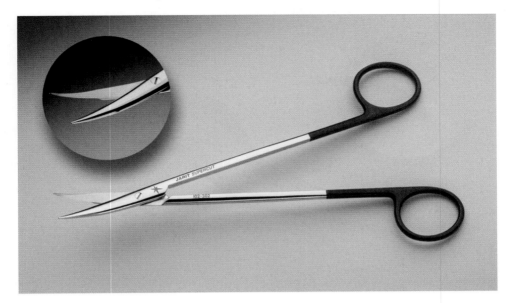

Instrument: JAMISON SCISSORS
Other Names: Tenotomy
Use(s): These scissors are used to dissect plaque out of an artery and to cut arterial branches when taking the mammary down. They are fine dissection scissors.

Description: These are fine scissors with sharp points and curved blades. They are available in a variety of lengths.
Instrument Insight: These delicate scissors should not be used to cut suture. The tips should be protected while sterilizing and packaging.

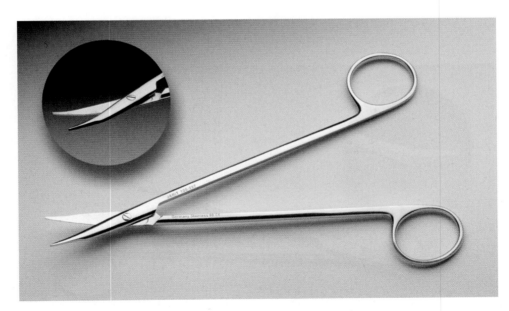

Instrument: REYNOLDS SCISSORS
Other Names: Jameson
Use(s): These are fine dissection scissors and are often used to bevel the vein when making an anastomosis.
Description: These scissors are available in a variety of lengths.

Instrument Insight: Jameson, Reynolds, and tenotomy scissors are often indiscernible. Reynolds scissors are delicate scissors and should be wiped clean after each use with a damp sponge. The tips should also be protected during sterilization and packaging.

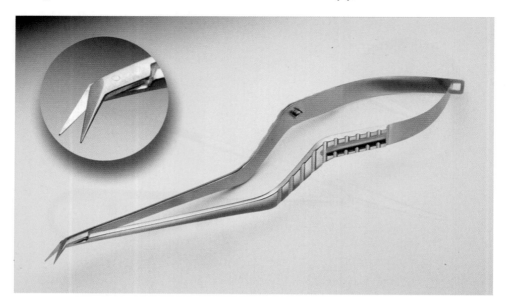

Instrument: YASARGIL SCISSORS
Other Names: Yasar scissors
Use(s): These scissors are used to extend an arteriotomy, usually in deep or hard to reach vessels such as a circumflex coronary artery.

Description: These are delicate, bayonet, spring-handled scissors.
Instrument Insight: These delicate scissors should be cleaned after each use with a damp sponge, and the tips should be protected during sterilization and packaging.

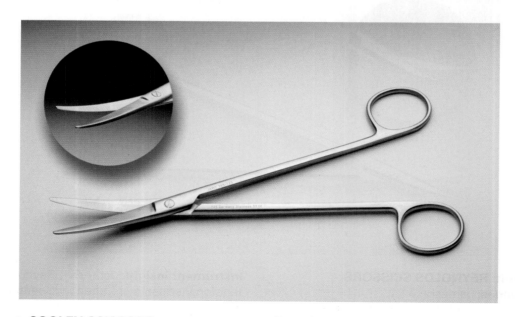

Instrument: COOLEY SCISSORS
Use(s): These are versatile scissors with many uses. They dissect tissue, cut suture, and can be used to cut grafts.

Description: These scissors have curved Mayo-type blades.

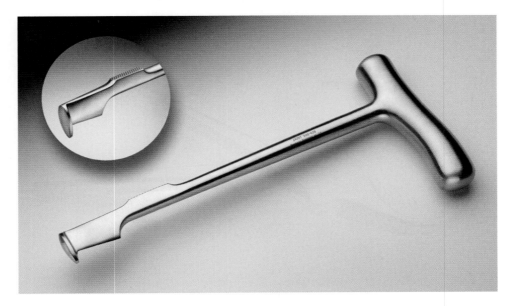

Instrument: LEBSCHE KNIFE
Other Names: Sternal knife
Use(s): Used for opening the sternum lengthwise.
Description: This is a heavy instrument with a flat, smooth distal end to protect the pericardium. The blade sits just above the flat end.
Instrument Insight: This is only used when a power saw is unavailable or during a power outage. Use it with a mallet.

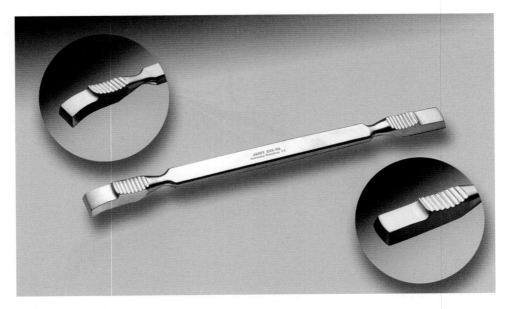

Instrument: FARABEUF RASP
Other Names: Alexander
Use(s): Used for scraping periosteum from rib bone.
Description: This is a heavy double-ended instrument with a blade. One end is curved and the other is straight.
Instrument Insight: Care should be taken to protect the edges of the blades against chipping or gouging.

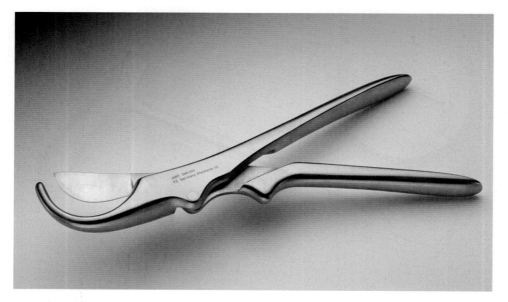

Instrument: GLUCK RIB SHEAR
Other Names: Rib cutter
Use(s): Used for resecting ribs.
Description: This is a heavy shear. The outside blade encircles the rib and the inside blade cuts down.

Instrument Insight: Patient anatomy as well as what rib is being excised dictates which rib cutter is preferred.

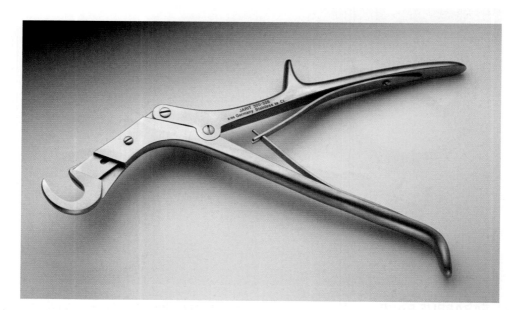

Instrument: STILLE-GIERTZ RIB SHEAR
Other Names: Shoemaker
Use(s): Used for resecting ribs.
Description: This shear is heavy. The distal end encircles the rib, and squeezing the handle brings the blade down, much like a guillotine, to cut the rib. The double-action handle allows for a more powerful cutting action.
Instrument Insight: Patient anatomy as well as what rib is being excised dictates which rib shear is preferred. Inspect the blade for nicks or gouges before use.

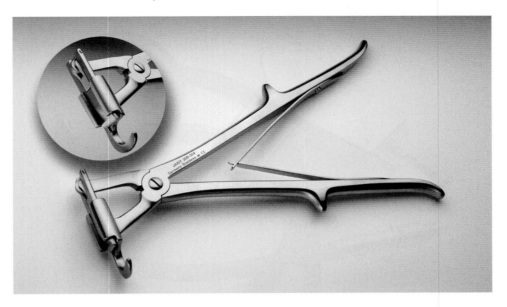

Instrument: SAUERBRUCH RIB RONGEUR
Other Names: Rib cutter
Use(s): Used for resecting a ribs.
Description: This rib shear is heavy. The working element encircles the rib, and squeezing the handles slides a blade out to cut the rib.

Instrument Insight: Patient anatomy, rib location, and doctor's preference dictate what rib shear is used. Inspect the blade for nicks or gouges before use.

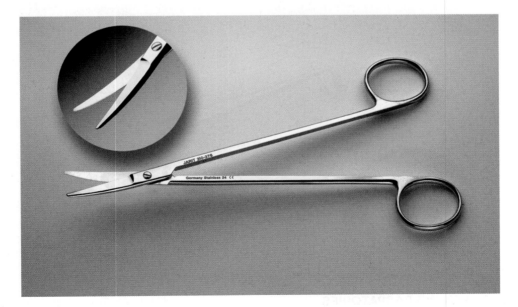

Instrument: LILLY SCISSORS
Use(s): These scissors are used for dissection of soft tissues.
Description: These scissors have blunt, pointed, slightly curved blades.

Instrument Insight: These scissors are similar to Metzenbaum scissors.

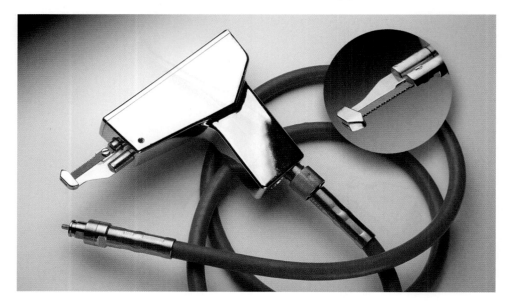

Instrument: STERNAL SAW
Other Names: Sarns sternal saw
Use(s): This is used to open the sternum by sawing lengthwise.
Description: This is a reciprocating-action saw with a disposable blade.

Instrument Insight: This saw needs a nitrogen tank and a foot pedal. Depending on the doctor's preference, the blade is loaded with the teeth up when sawing from xiphoid to sternal notch and the teeth down when sawing from the sternal notch to the xiphoid.

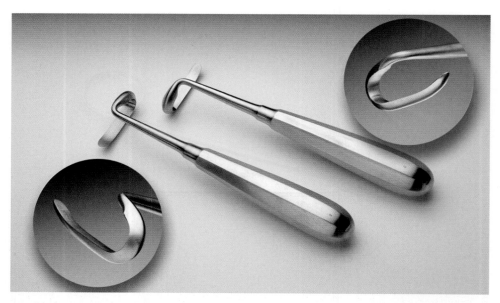

Instrument: DOYEN RIB RASPATORIES
Other Names: Doyen elevator and stripper
Use(s): This pair of instruments is used to scrape periosteum from rib bones before cutting.
Description: A solid, tapering handle attached to a straight shaft that leads to an outward C-shaped

curve at the distal end. The inside of the C-shape is flattened and has sharp edges.
Instrument Insight: The distal end encircles the rib and slides the length of rib to be excised, stripping the periosteum from the bone. Both right and left raspatories are available.

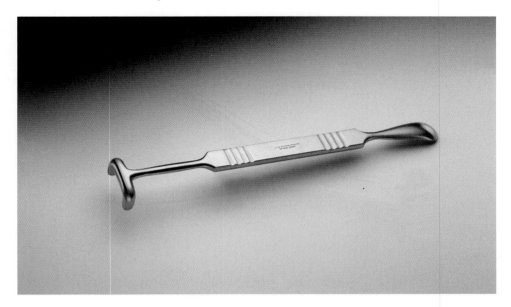

Instrument: MATSON RIB STRIPPER AND ELEVATOR
Other Names: Stripper
Use(s): Used for scraping periosteum from rib bone before cutting with a shear.

Description: This is a double-ended instrument with a flattened, tear-shaped elevator on one end and a U-shaped, sharp rib stripper on the other.
Instrument Insight: Before use, inspect the ends for gouges or nicks.

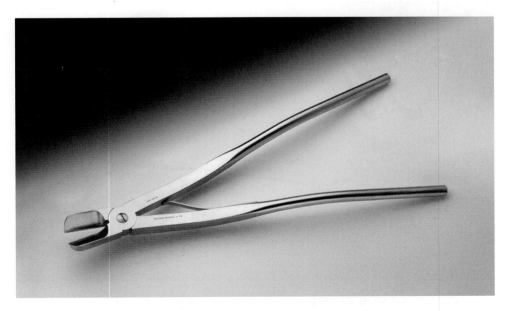

Instrument: BETHUNE RIB SHEARS
Use(s): Used for resecting ribs.
Description: This heavy shear has straight cutting blades.

Instrument Insight: The long handles provide greater force when cutting bone.

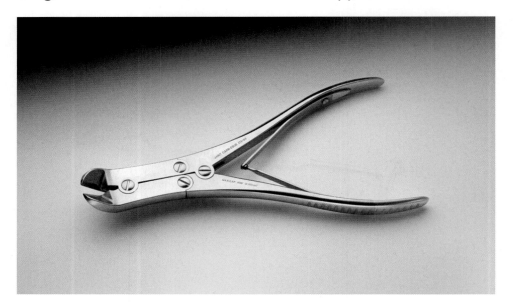

Instrument: HEAVY WIRE CUTTER
Other Names: Pin cutter
Use(s): This wire cutter is used to cut sternal wires.

Description: This wire cutter has double-action, angled blade tips.
Instrument Insight: Double action provides extra strength.

GRASPING AND HOLDING INSTRUMENTS

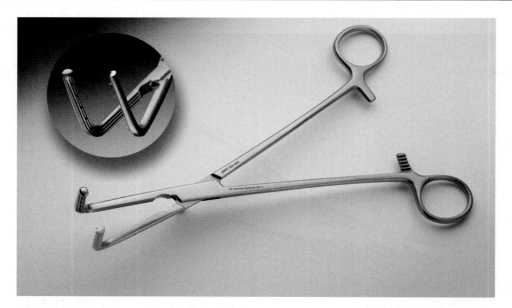

Instrument: SAROT BRONCHUS CLAMP
Use(s): During lung procedures, this clamp is used to hold and occlude the bronchus while stapling.
Description: These clamps come in a set of two: right and left, curved or angled. These have longitudinal serrations with holes on one side of jaws and pegs on the opposite jaw to match up and hold the tissue stable.
Instrument Insight: Take care to not snag gloves on pegs.

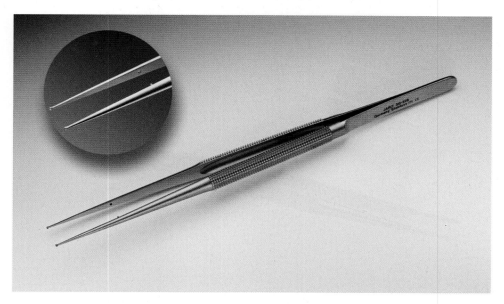

Instrument: MILLS/DENNIS MICRO RING TISSUE FORCEPS

Use(s): These forceps are used to take down the mammary from the chest wall and also to hold the mammary during anastomosis in bypass surgery.

Description: Very fine forceps with Barraquer-style handle and tiny ring tips with serrations.

Instrument Insight: These forceps are very fine with tiny serrations. The tips of these forceps should be protected during packaging and sterilization.

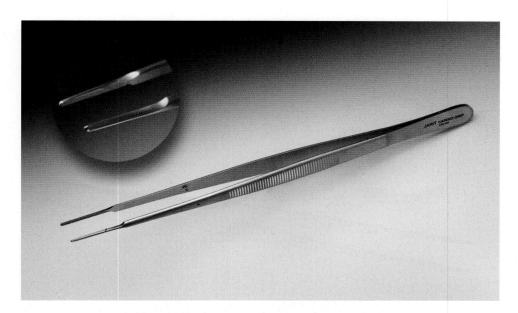

Instrument: GERALD TISSUE FORCEPS

Other Names: Mammary forceps

Use(s): Often used during a coronary artery bypass procedure to manipulate the vessel and tissues while taking down the mammary artery from the chest wall and to grasp the coronary artery and graft during the anastomosis.

Description: These forceps have very fine, narrowed tips with horizontal serrations.

Instrument Insight: These forceps are delicate and should be protected during sterilization and packaging. They are also used for opening the lumen of a vein and holding it open for suture placement.

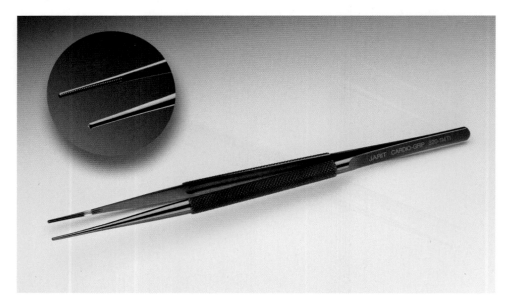

Instrument: DEBAKEY-DIETHRICH TISSUE FORCEPS
Other Names: Titaniums
Use(s): Used for holding the vein during bypass surgery.
Description: These fine forceps have Barraquer-style handles and noncrushing jaws of the DeBakey design.

Instrument Insight: These forceps are delicate, and tips should be protected during sterilization and packaging.

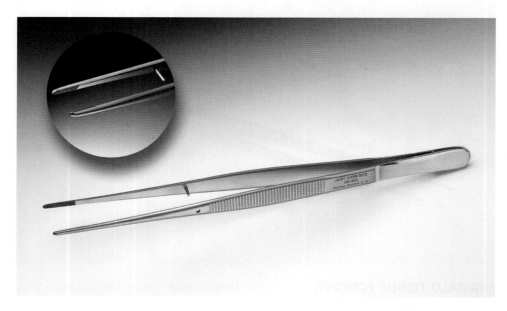

Instrument: POTTS-SMITH TISSUE FORCEPS
Other Names: Walters or goldies
Use(s): Used to hold and grasp tissue and vessels.
Description: These forceps have fine, serrated, carbide tips.

Instrument Insight: These are very sturdy forceps that are often used when the surgeon is suturing because the jaws do not bend or damage the needle.

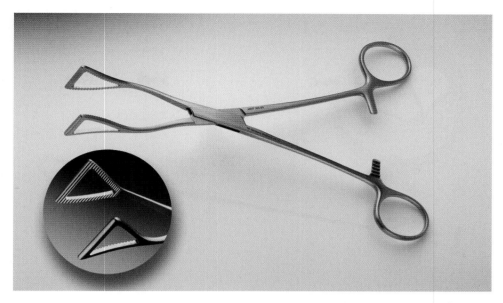

Instrument: DUVAL LUNG FORCEPS
Other Names: Lung clamp
Use(s): Used to grasp and hold lung tissue.
Description: This is an angled or straight forceps with triangular, fenestrated tips that have horizontal serrations.

Instrument Insight: These clamps are used for lung tissue but can be used on other friable tissue as well.

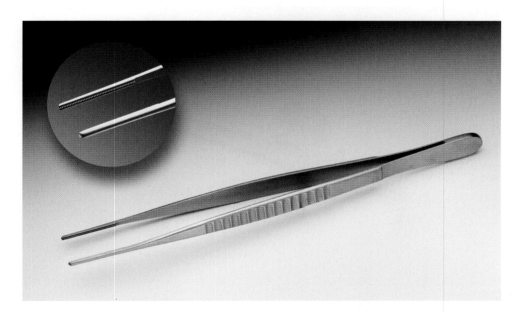

Instrument: DEBAKEY VASCULAR TISSUE FORCEPS
Use(s): These forceps are used for holding and grasping tissue.
Description: They come in a variety of lengths, and the jaws are of the DeBakey design.

Instrument Insight: The 7-inch and 8-inch DeBakey forceps are the most commonly used tissue forceps and are often used in other specialties.

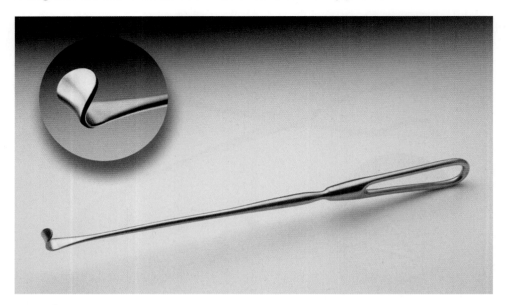

Instrument: CUSHING VEIN RETRACTOR

Use(s): Used for retracting vessels and tissues for exposure.

Description: This retractor has a plain, smooth, upward-curved end, and should be categorized as a retracting and exposing instrument.

Instrument Insight: Vein retractors should always be in your set.

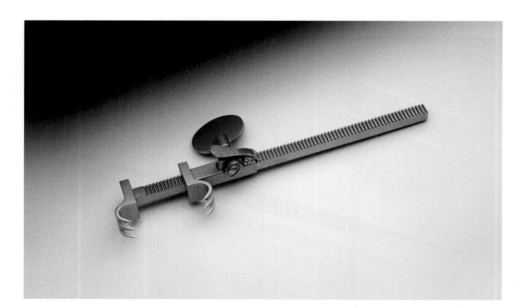

Instrument: BAILEY RIB CONTRACTOR

Other Names: Rib approximator

Use(s): This instrument is used to approximate the ribs and hold them until sutures can be placed and secured after a thoracotomy.

Description: This instrument has claws facing each other on a serrated post and a "paw" mechanism to tighten the claws, approximating the ribs.

Instrument Insight: When handling the Bailey, care must be taken; the jaws are sharp and may snag gloves, and it should be handed to the surgeon with the jaws closed.

PROBING AND DILATING INSTRUMENTS

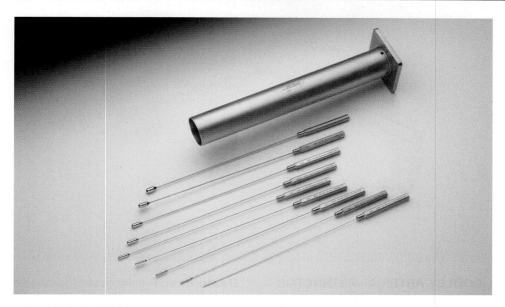

Instrument: GARRETT VASCULAR DILATORS
Use(s): These are used to dilate vessels gradually.
Description: They come in a set of nine and have tips of varying sizes. This instrument has an oval, solid, stainless-steel tip that attaches to a narrowed malleable stem, which extends to a solid, smooth handle.
Instrument Insight: The set comes in its own container or box to hold them in order of size. They are malleable but after a lot of use can actually break, so let the surgeon do the bending.

RETRACTING AND EXPOSING INSTRUMENTS

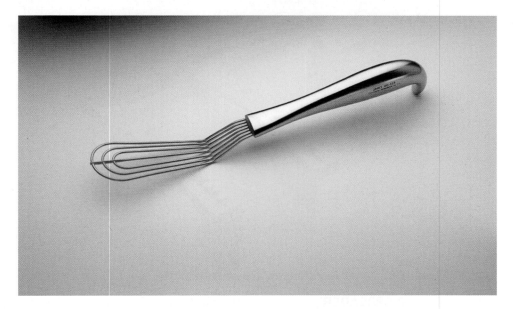

Instrument: ALLISON LUNG RETRACTOR
Other Names: Whisk
Use(s): This is used to retract lung tissue.
Description: A solid grip-handle that leads to multiple heavy wires that form a rounded spatula shape.
Instrument Insight: This retractor is not "pulled" but simply "held" in place.

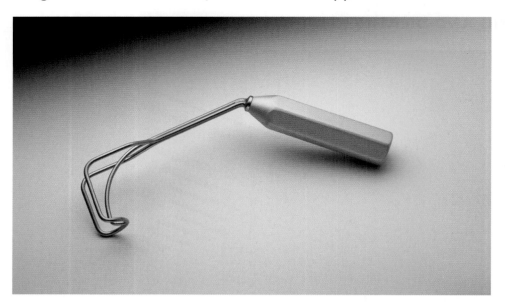

Instrument: COOLEY ARTERIAL RETRACTOR
Other Names: Mitral valve retractor
Use(s): Used to retract the atrium during mitral valve procedures.

Description: A solid octagonal handle that leads to a rod-like shaft that trifurcates to create a curved, open blade.
Instrument Insight: This retractor is seldom "pulled" but is placed and "held" in position.

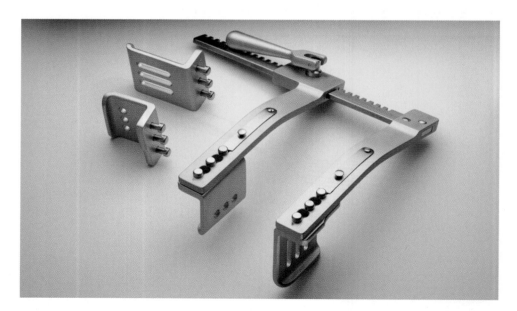

Instrument: BURFORD RIB SPREADER
Other Names: Chest spreader, Buford-Finochietto
Use(s): This instrument is used to retract ribs for lung procedures and to spread the sternum in cardiac procedures.

Description: A crank-ratcheted, self-retaining frame with interchangeable blades that attach to the end of each arm.
Instrument Insight: This chest spreader is lightweight. Both the blades and the arms are marked "R" and "L" to aid in assembly.

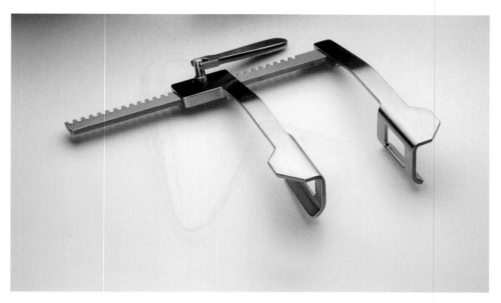

Instrument: FINOCHIETTO RIB SPREADER
Other Names: Chest or rib spreader
Use(s): Used for spreading ribs for exposure of the chest cavity.

Description: This self-retaining retractor has curved and straight blade arms, and the blades do not detach.

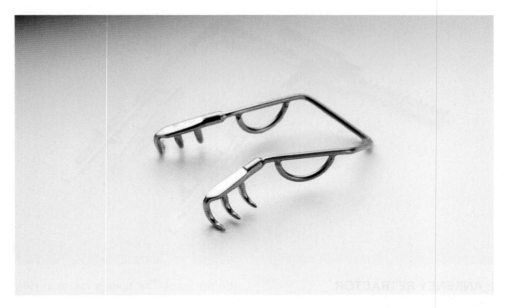

Instrument: PARSONNET EPICARDIAL RETRACTOR
Use(s): This is used to expose coronary arteries in adipose tissue during bypass surgery.

Description: This is a tiny, very light, self-retaining retractor that fits between the finger tips to place.
Instrument Insight: This is a delicate instrument and should be sterilized and packaged with care and protection.

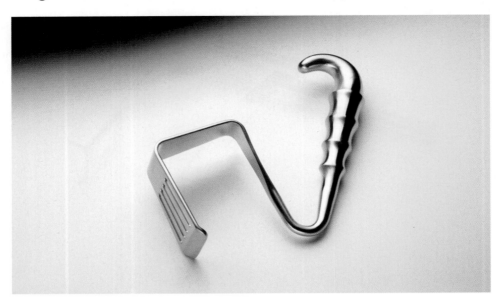

Instrument: DAVIDSON SCAPULA RETRACTOR
Use(s): Used for retracting the scapula to expose the ribs during thoracic entry and closure.
Description: A heavy retractor that resembles a spatula that is bent in the shape of an S.

Instrument Insight: This retractor is used for a short time during entry into the chest and sometimes during closure. It does not require pulling.

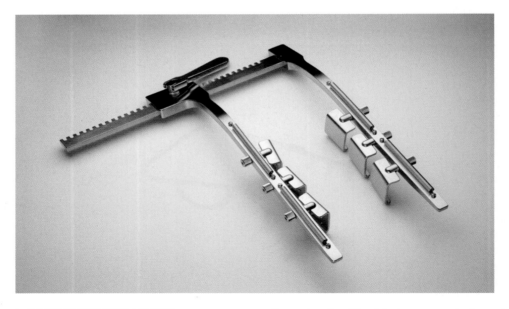

Instrument: ANKENEY RETRACTOR
Other Names: Chest spreader
Use(s): Used to spread the sternum open following a sternotomy during cardiac procedures.
Description: This is a self-retaining retractor with six blades that each screw onto the arms of

the retractor. The blades come in two depth lengths.
Instrument Insight: Retractor should be closed completely when handing it to the surgeon.

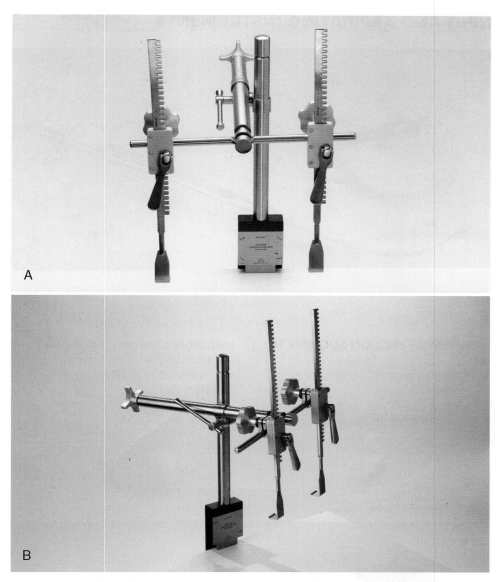

Instrument: INTERNAL MAMMARY RETRACTOR

Other Names: Mammary retractor, Favaloro

Use(s): Used for lifting up one side of the chest wall after a sternotomy to facilitate internal mammary dissection.

Description: The support bar clamps to the side rail of the operating table. Rake retractors are positioned on the sternum, and the ratchet assembly lifts the arms of rakes to the desired position or height the surgeon needs to take down the mammary.

Instrument Insight: An unsterile person clamps the support bar to the bed and unclamps it after mammary dissection.

SUCTIONING AND ASPIRATING INSTRUMENTS

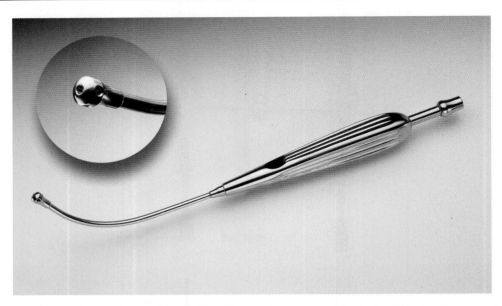

Instrument: ANDREWS-PYNCHON SUCTION TIP
Other Names: CV suction tip, baby Yankauer
Use(s): Used for suctioning of fluids to aid in exposure.
Description: This is a suction tip with four tiny holes on the sides of the tip and one larger hole at the end.

Instrument Insight: This is often used as a retractor at the same time as suctioning. The tip is somewhat malleable.

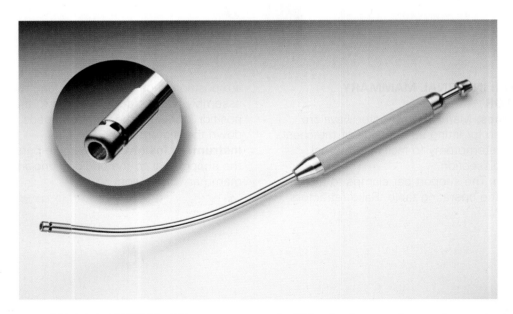

Instrument: VASCULAR SUCTION TIP
Other Names: Cardiac suction
Use(s): This instrument is used to suction fluids to aid in exposure.
Description: This suction has a large hole at the distal end and smaller holes on the sides of the

tip. This also is manufactured as a single use disposable tip.
Instrument Insight: This suction may be a retractor at the same time it is being used for suctioning.

SUTURING AND STAPLING INSTRUMENTS

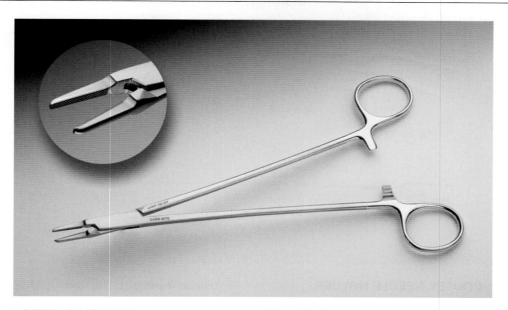

Instrument: NEEDLE HOLDER
Other Names: Fine Ryder needle holder
Use(s): Used for suturing of purse strings and valve sutures during heart surgery.

Description: Has finely tapered jaws with carbide inserts.
Instrument Insight: This is a fine but sturdy instrument. Wipe it clean every time when loading valve suture.

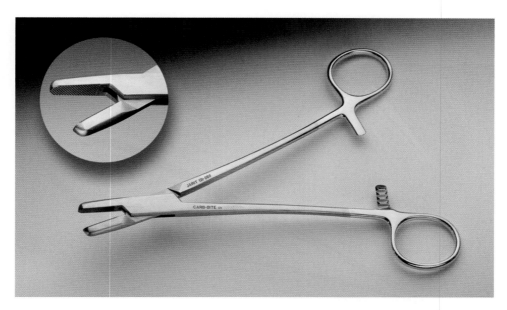

Instrument: STERNAL NEEDLE HOLDER AND WIRE TWISTER
Other Names: Big ugly
Use(s): Used for placement of sternal wires and as a wire twister.
Description: This needle holder type instrument has rounded, heavy jaws with carbide inserts to hold the needle.

Instrument Insight: Load heavy sternal wires at the center of the needle so the needle does not bend from the pressure of pushing it through hard bone.

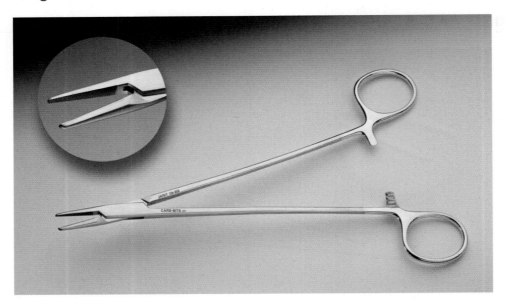

Instrument: COOLEY NEEDLE HOLDER

Use(s): Used for placement of purse strings and valve sutures.

Description: This is a needle holder with carbide jaws and fine tips.

Instrument Insight: The carbide jaws hold the needles so there is no slippage while placing the sutures.

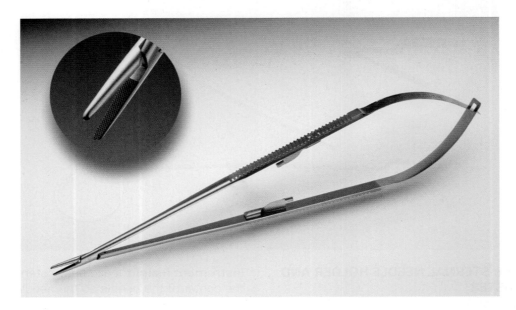

Instrument: CASTROVIEJO NEEDLE HOLDER

Other Names: Castro

Use(s): Used for anastomosis suturing.

Description: This needle holder comes in a variety of lengths. It has a flat, catch-spring handle.

Instrument Insight: This is a very delicate instrument and should be protected during sterilization and packaging. Use only 4-0 or smaller sutures with these needle holders.

Index

A

Abdominal sucker. *See* Poole suction tip
Abdominal wall retractor. *See* Mayo abdominal retractor
ACF retractor, 286–287, 286f
  description of, 286
  uses of, 286
Adson cranial rongeur, 263–264, 263f
  description of, 263
  insight on, 263
  uses of, 263
Adson dressing forceps. *See* Adson tissue forceps, plain
Adson forceps, 10, 10f. *See* Adson tonsil/Schnidt forceps
  description of, 10
  other names for, 10
  uses of, 10
Adson hook, sharp, 280, 280f
  description of, 280
  insight on, 280
  uses of, 280
Adson hypophyseal cup tissue forceps, 276, 276f
  description of, 276
  insight on, 276
  other names for, 276
  uses of, 276
Adson periosteal elevator, 272, 272f
  description of, 272
  other names for, 272
  uses of, 272
Adson tissue forceps, plain, 18–19, 18f
  description of, 18
  insight on, 18
  other names for, 18
  uses of, 18
Adson tissue forceps, toothed, 19, 19f
  description of, 19
  insight on, 19
  other names for, 19
  uses of, 19
Adson tonsil/Schnidt forceps, 143, 143f
  description of, 143
  other names for, 143
  uses of, 143
Adson with teeth forceps. *See* Adson tissue forceps, toothed
Alexander rasp. *See* Farabeuf rasp
Alligator forceps. *See* Wullstein ear forceps
Allis, big. *See* Allis-Adair

Allis-Adair, 90–91, 90f
  description of, 90
  insight on, 90
  other names for, 90
  uses of, 90
Allis forceps, 24, 24f
  description of, 24
  uses of, 24
Allis forceps, curved, 173–174, 173f
  description of, 173
  insight on, 173
  other names for, 173
  uses of, 173
Allis forceps, endoscopic, 62, 62f
  description of, 62
  uses of, 62
Allison lung retractor, 315–316, 315f
  description of, 315
  insight on, 315
  other names for, 315
  uses of, 315
Alm retractor, 244, 244f
  description of, 244
  uses of, 244
Andrews-Pynchon suction tip, 320, 320f
  description of, 320
  insight on, 320
  other names for, 320
  uses of, 320
Andrew's tongue depressor, 196, 196f
  categories of, 196
  description of, 196
  other names for, 196
  uses of, 196
Aneurysm clip applier and clips, 259, 259f
  cautions when using, 259–260
  description of, 259
  insight on, 259
  uses of, 259
Angle pick. *See* Root tip pick
Ankeney retractor, 318–319, 318f
  description of, 318
  insight on, 318
  other names for, 318
  uses of, 318
Anti-fog solution, 48–49, 48f
  description of, 48
  insight on, 48
  other names for, 48
  uses of, 48
Antrum rasp. *See* Wiener antrum rasp

Apical elevator, 188, 188f
  description of, 188
  insight on, 188
  other names for, 188
  uses of, 188
Apple needle holder, 69, 69f
  description of, 69
  insight on, 69
  uses of, 69
Arch bars, 186, 186f
  description of, 186
  insight on, 186
  uses of, 186
Areola marker, 197–198, 197f
  description of, 197
  insight on, 197
  other names for, 197
  uses of, 197
Army-Navy retractor, 25–26, 25f
  description of, 25
  insight on, 25
  other names for, 25
  uses of, 25
Army's retractor. *See* Army-Navy retractor
Arterial retractor, 79, 79f
  description of, 79
  insight on, 79
  other names for, 79
  uses of, 79
Arthroscope. *See* 25° 4-MM lens
Atraumatric towel clamp. *See* Towel clip (nonpenetrating)
Aufricht nasal rasps, 157, 157f
  description of, 157
  insight on, 157
  uses of, 157
Aufricht nasal retractor, 178–179, 178f
  description of, 178
  uses of, 178
Auvard weighted vaginal speculum, 95–96, 95f
  description of, 95
  insight on, 95
  other names for, 95
  uses of, 95

B

B. B. forceps. *See* Cushing bipolar forceps
Babcock forceps, 24–25, 24f
  description of, 24
  uses of, 24

Babcock forceps, endoscopic, 62–63, 62f
  description of, 62
  uses of, 62
Baby ribbons. *See* Davis brain spatulas
Baby sucker. *See* Bulb syringe
Backhaus towel clip. *See* Towel clip
  (penetrating)
Bacon cranial rongeur, 262–263, 262f
  description of, 262
  insight on, 262
  uses of, 262
Bailey rib contractor, 314, 314f
  description of, 314
  insight on, 314
  other names for, 314
  uses of, 314
Bakes common duct dilators, 40, 40f
  description of, 40
  insight on, 40
  other names for, 40
  uses of, 40
Balfour retractor, 43–44, 43f
  description of, 43
  insight on, 43
  other names for, 43
  uses of, 43
Ballenger swivel knife, 159–160, 159f
  description of, 159
  other names for, 159
  uses of, 159
Ballenger v-shaped osteotome,
  164–165, 164f
  description of, 164
  insight on, 164
  uses of, 164
Ball loop electrode, 105, 105f
  description of, 105
  insight on, 105
  uses of, 105
Balloon dilator, 112, 112f
  description of, 112
  insight on, 112
  uses for, 112
Ball tip probe, 277, 277f
  description of, 277
  uses of, 277
Bandage scissors. *See* Lister bandage
  scissors; Utility scissors
Barbara needle. *See* House-Barbara
  shattering needle
Barnhill adenoid curettes, 169, 169f
  description of, 169
  insight on, 169
  uses of, 169
Baron suction tips, 182–183, 182f
  description of, 182
  insight on, 182
  other names for, 182
  uses of, 182
Barraquer eye speculum, 134, 134f
  description of, 134
  other names for, 134
  uses of, 134
Barraquer iris scissors, 125, 125f
  description of, 125
  insight on, 125
  uses of, 125
Barraquer iris spatula, 122, 122f
  description of, 122

Barraquer iris spatula (*Continued*)
  other names for, 122
  uses of, 122
Barraquer needle holder, 138, 138f
  description of, 138
  uses of, 138
Baskin Robin. *See* Adson hypophyseal
  cup tissue forceps
Bayonet. *See* Jansen tissue forceps
Bean rongeur. *See* Cushing pituitary
  rongeur
Beaver handle, 18, 18f
  description of, 18
  insight on, 18
  other names for, 18
  uses of, 18
Beck aortic clamp, 297, 297f
  description of, 297
  other names for, 297
  uses of, 297
Becker septum scissors, 155–156, 155f
  description of, 155
  uses of, 155
Beckman retractor, 238, 238f, 282, 282f
  cautions when using, 238, 282
  description of, 238, 282
  insight on, 238, 282
  uses of, 238, 282
Bellucci scissors, 146–147, 146f
  description of, 146
  insight on, 146
  other names for, 146
  uses of, 146
Bennett retractor, 237, 237f
  description of, 237
  insight on, 237
  uses of, 237
Bethune rib shears, 309–310, 309f
  description of, 309
  insight on, 309
  uses of, 309
Beyer rongeur, 263, 263f
  description of, 263
  insight on, 263
  uses of, 263
Bifurcated prostate retractor. *See*
  Young bifurcated retractor
Big ugly. *See* Sternal needle holder and
  wire twister
Big Ugly's forceps. *See* Ferris-Smith
  tissue forceps
Billeau ear loop, 143, 144f
  description of, 143
  insight on, 143
  other names for, 143
  uses of, 143
Biopsy forceps, 109, 109f. *See also*
  Hysteroscope biopsy forceps
  description of, 109
  insight on, 109
  uses of, 109
Bipolar bayonet forceps. *See* Cushing
  bipolar forceps
Bipolar forceps. *See* Maryland bipolar
  forceps
Bishop-Harmon iris tissue forceps,
  132, 132f
  description of, 132
  uses of, 132

Bit block. *See* Mouth prop
Biter. *See* Cobra grasper
Bit wedge. *See* Mouth prop
Bivalve speculum. *See* Graves vaginal
  speculum
Blount knee retractor, 243, 243f
  description of, 243
  insight on, 243
  uses of, 243
Blunt curette. *See* Thomas uterine curette
Blunt dissector, 55, 55f
  description of, 55
  insight on, 55
  uses of, 55
Blunt grasper, 63, 63f
  description of, 63
  uses of, 63
Blunt hook, 292, 292f
  description of, 292
  insight on, 292
  other names for, 292
  uses of, 292
Blunt tip trocar. *See* Blunt trocar
Blunt trocar, 65, 65f
  description of, 65
  insight on, 65
  other names for, 65
  uses of, 65
Boettcher tonsil scissors, 168, 168f
  description of, 168
  insight on, 168
  other names for, 168
  uses of, 168
Bolt cutter. *See* Large pin cutter
Bone cement gun, 213, 213f
  description of, 213
  insight on, 213
  other names for, 213
  uses of, 213
Bone cement system, 213, 213f
  cautions when using, 213–214
  insight on, 213
  uses of, 213
Bone file, 223, 223f
  description of, 223
  insight on, 223
  other names for, 223
  uses of, 223
Bone hook, 239, 239f
  cautions when using, 239
  description of, 239
  insight on, 239
  uses of, 239
Bone skid. *See* Lever skid humeral
  head retractor
Bone tamp, 198, 199f
  description of, 212
  insight on, 212
  other names for, 212
  uses of, 212
Bookwalter, 44, 44f
  description of, 44
  insight on, 44
  other names for, 44
  uses of, 44
Boucheron ear speculum, 183–184, 183f
  description of, 183
  insight on, 183
  uses of, 183

Bovie pencil. *See* Electrosurgical pencil
Bovie spatula. *See* Permanent cautery
    spatula
Bowman lacrimal probe, 133, 133f
    description of, 133
    insight on, 133
    other names for, 133
    uses of, 133
Box curette. *See* Kevorkian endocervical
    curette
Bozeman uterine dressing forceps,
    91–92, 91f
    description of, 91
    other names for, 91
    uses of, 91
Braun tenaculum. *See* Schroeder
    tenaculum
Breast hook. *See* Mammoplasty hook
Bridge. *See* Telescope bridge
Briggs mammoplasty retractor, 208, 208f
    description of, 208
    uses of, 208
Brown-Adson tissue forceps, 19, 19f
    description of, 19
    other names for, 19
    uses of, 19
Browne deltoid retractor, 246–247, 246f
    description of, 246
    uses of, 246
Brown forceps. *See* Brown-Adson
    tissue forceps
Bruening septum forceps, 172, 172f
    description of, 172
    uses of, 172
Brun curettes. *See* Spinal curettes
Bruns oval bone curettes, 230, 230f
    description of, 230
    other names for, 230
    uses of, 230
Buck ear curette, 151–152, 151f
    description of, 151
    other names for, 151
    uses of, 151
Buford-Finochietto. *See* Burford rib
    spreader
Bugbee electrode, 105–106, 105f
    description of, 105
    insight on, 105
    uses of, 105
Bulb retractor. *See* Young bulb retractor
Bulb syringe, 98–99, 98f
    description of, 98
    insight on, 98
    other names for, 98
    uses of, 98
Bulldog. *See* DeBakey bulldog
Bullet nose dissector. *See* Cone tip
    dissector
Burford rib spreader, 316–317, 316f
    description of, 316
    insight on, 316
    other names for, 316
    uses of, 316

C

Caliper. *See* Townley caliper
Canal elevator. *See* House elevator
Canal knife. *See* House joint knife;
    House-sheehy knife curette

Cannulated pin cutter, 228–229, 228f
    description of, 228
    insight on, 228
    other names for, 228
    uses of, 228
Caplan scissors, 154–155, 154f
    description of, 154
    uses of, 154
Capsule retractor, 246, 246f
    description of, 246
    other names for, 246
    uses of, 246
Cardiac suction. *See* Vascular
    suction tip
Carmalt forceps, 9–10, 9f
    big curved (*See* Carmalt forceps)
    description of, 9
    other names for, 9
    uses of, 9
Carter-Glassman intestinal clamp, 36, 36f
    description of, 36
    other names for, 36
    uses of, 36
Castro. *See* Castroviejo corneal
    scissors; Castroviejo needle holder
Castroviejo caliper, 121, 121f
    description of, 121
    uses of, 121
Castroviejo corneal scissors, 125,
    125–126
    description of, 125
    other names for, 125
    uses of, 125
Castroviejo eye speculum, 134–135, 134f
    description of, 134
    uses of, 134
Castroviejo needle holder, 137, 137f,
    322, 322f
    description of, 137, 322
    insight on, 322
    other names for, 322
    uses of, 137, 322
Castroviejo suturing tissue forceps
    0.12 MM, 0.5 MM, 131, 131f
    description of, 131
    insight on, 131
    uses of, 131
Cath element. *See* Catheter deflecting
    element
Catheter deflecting element, 103–104,
    103f
    description of, 103
    insight on, 103
    other names for, 103
    uses of, 103
Cat paw. *See* Mathieu retractor
Cat paw retractor. *See* Senn retractor
Cautery pencil. *See* Electrosurgical pencil
Cautery spatula. *See* Permanent
    cautery spatula
Cawood retractor. *See* Minnesota
    cheek retractor
CEEA stapler. *See* Intraluminal stapler
Cement gun. *See* Bone cement gun
Cerebellar retractor, 282, 282f
    cautions when using, 282–283
    description of, 282
    insight on, 282
    uses of, 282

Cervical dilators. *See* Hank dilators;
    Hegar dilators; Pratt uterine dilators
Chandler elevator. *See* Chandler retractor
Chandler retractor, 239–240, 239f
    description of, 239
    insight on, 239
    other names for, 239
    uses of, 239
Channel locks. *See* Pliers
Cheek retractor. *See* Minnesota cheek
    retractor
Chest spreader. *See* Ankeney retractor;
    Burford rib spreader; Finochietto rib
    spreader
Chuck and key, 217–218, 217f
    description of, 217
    other names for, 217
    uses of, 217
Cicherelli mastoid rongeur, 149–150,
    149f
    description of, 149
    insight on, 149
    other names for, 149
    uses of, 149
Cinelli guarded osteotome, 167–168,
    167f
    description of, 167
    insight on, 167
    uses of, 167
Circular stapler. *See* Intraluminal stapler
Clamp. *See* Crile forceps; Kelly forceps
    angled (*See* Cooley clamp; DeBakey
    peripheral vascular clamp)
Claw grasper, 63, 63f
    cautions when using, 63–64
    description of, 63
    insight on, 63
    other names for, 63
    uses of, 63
Clayman lens forceps. *See* Lens
    insertion forceps
Clip applier. *See* Endo clip applier;
    Hemoclip applier
Cloweard cervical retractor, 287–288,
    287f
    description of, 287
    uses of, 287
Cloweard vertebra spreader, 287, 287f
    description of, 287
    uses of, 287
Coag scissors. *See* Endoscopic scissors
Coakley antrum curettes, 163–164, 163f
    description of, 163
    other names for, 163
    uses of, 163
Cobb curettes, 271, 271f
    description of, 271
    uses of, 271
Cobb elevators, 270–271, 270f
    description of, 270
    insight on, 270
    uses of, 270
Cobb ring curettes, 271–272, 271f
    description of, 271
    uses of, 271
Coblation wand, 142, 142f
    description of, 142
    insight on, 142
    uses of, 142

Cobra. *See* Cobra grasper
Cobra grasper, 77–78, 77f
　description of, 77
　other names for, 77
　uses of, 77
Cobra retractor, 242–243, 242f
　description of, 242
　insight on, 242
　uses of, 242
Cold cone knife. *See* Long angled #3
　knife handle
Colibri tissue forceps, 130–131, 130f
　description of, 130
　insight on, 130
　uses of, 130
Columella retractor. *See* Cottle
　columella forceps
Common duct dilators. *See* Bakes
　common duct dilators
Cone tip dissector, 56, 56f
　description of, 56
　insight on, 56
　other names for, 56
　uses of, 56
Cookie cutter. *See* Areola marker
Cooley arterial retractor, 316, 316f
　description of, 316
　insight on, 316
　other names for, 316
　uses of, 316
Cooley clamp, 295–296, 295f
　description of, 295
　insight on, 295
　other names for, 295
　uses of, 295
Cooley coarctation clamp, 301, 301f
　description of, 301
　other names for, 301
　uses of, 301
Cooley needle holder, 322, 322f
　description of, 322
　insight on, 322
　uses of, 322
Cooley scissors, 304–305, 304f
　description of, 304
　uses of, 304
Cord clamp, 83, 83f
　description of, 83
　insight on, 83
　uses of, 83
Cottle angular scissors, 155, 155f
　description of, 155
　insight on, 155
　other names for, 155
　uses of, 155
Cottle bone crusher, 140–141, 140f
　description of, 140
　insight on, 140
　uses of, 140
Cottle chisels, 167, 167f
　description of, 167
　insight on, 167
　other names for, 167
　uses of, 167
Cottle columella forceps, 175, 175f
　description of, 175
　insight on, 175
　other names for, 175
　uses of, 175

Cottle double hook retractor, 177–178,
　177f
　description of, 177
　insight on, 177
　uses of, 177
Cottle knife guide and retractor, 177, 177f
　description of, 177
　uses of, 177
Cottle mallet, 141, 141f
　description of, 141
　insight on, 141
　other names for, 141
　uses of, 141
Cottle nasal knife, 162, 162f
　description of, 162
　insight on, 162
　uses of, 162
Cottle nasal speculum, 175–176, 175f
　description of, 175
　uses of, 175
Cottle osteotomes, 166–167, 166f
　description of, 166
　insight on, 166
　uses of, 166
Cottle septal elevator, 162–163, 162f
　description of, 162
　insight on, 162
　uses of, 162
Cottle tenaculum, double, 205, 205f
　cautions when using, 205–206
　description of, 205
　insight on, 205
　other names for, 205
　uses of, 205
Cottle tenaculum, single, 205, 205f
　cautions when using, 205
　description of, 205
　insight on, 205
　uses of, 205
Crabtree dissector, 153–154, 153f
　description of, 153
　insight on, 153
　other names for, 153
　uses of, 153
Crane elevator, 187, 187f
　description of, 187
　other names for, 187
　uses of, 187
Crego elevator, 225, 225f
　description of, 225
　insight on, 225
　uses of, 225
Cricket retractor. *See* Jarit cross action
　retractor
Crile forceps, 7–8, 7f. *See also* Kelly
　forceps
　description of, 7
　insight on, 7
　other names for, 7
　uses of, 7
Crile-Wood needle holder, 32, 32f
　description of, 32
　other names for, 32
　uses of, 32
Crimper. *See* McGee wire crimping
　forceps
Cryer elevator, 187–188, 187f
　description of, 187
　insight on, 187

Cryer elevator *(Continued)*
　other names for, 187
　uses of, 187
Cryer forceps. *See* Lower anterior
　extraction forceps (151); Upper
　anterior extraction forceps (150)
Cup forceps. *See* Adson hypophyseal
　cup tissue forceps
Curettes. *See* Bruns oval bone curettes
　angled (*See* Lucas bone curette)
Curved needle holder. *See* Heaney
　needle holder
Curved scissors, 76, 76f
　description of, 76
　other names for, 76
　uses of, 76
Cushing bayonet tissue forceps, 277,
　277f
　description of, 277
　insight on, 277
　uses of, 277
Cushing bipolar forceps, 260, 260f
　description of, 260
　insight on, 260
　other names for, 260
　uses of, 260
Cushing pituitary rongeur, 265, 265f
　description of, 265
　insight on, 265
　uses of, 265
Cushing rongeur, 231–232, 231f
　description of, 231
　insight on, 231
　uses of, 231
Cushing vein contractor, 314, 314f
　description of, 314
　insight on, 314
　uses of, 314
CV suction tip. *See* Andrews-Pynchon
　suction tip
Cystoscope sheath and obturator, 116,
　116f
　description of, 116
　insight on, 116
　uses of, 116

D

Dandy clamp. *See* Dandy hemostatic
　forceps
Dandy hemostatic forceps, 261, 261f
　description of, 261
　other names for, 261
　uses of, 261
Dandy nerve hook, 280–281, 280f
　description of, 280
　uses of, 280
Davidson scapula retractor, 318, 318f
　description of, 318
　insight on, 318
　uses of, 318
Davis brain spatulas, 278, 278f
　description of, 278
　insight on, 278
　other names for, 278
　uses of, 278
Davis scalp retractor, 285, 285f
　description of, 285
　uses of, 285

Dean rongeur, 144, 144f
  description of, 144
  insight on, 144
  uses of, 144
Dean scissors, 191, 191f
  description of, 191
  insight on, 191
  other names for, 191
  uses of, 191
Deaver, small. *See* Deaver retractor, baby
Deaver retractor, 42, 42f
  description of, 42
  insight on, 42
  uses of, 42
Deaver retractor, baby, 98, 98f
  description of, 98
  other names for, 98
  uses of, 98
DeBakes forceps. *See* Debakey tissue
  forceps
DeBakey aortic clamp, 298–299, 298f
  description of, 298
  uses of, 298
DeBakey bulldog, 293–294, 293f
  description of, 293
  insight on, 293
  other names for, 293
  uses of, 293
DeBakey coarctation clamp, 300, 300f
  description of, 300
  insight on, 300
  other names for, 300
  uses of, 300
DeBakey-Diethrich tissue forceps, 312,
  312f
  description of, 312
  insight on, 312
  other names for, 312
  uses of, 312
DeBakey forceps, 78, 78f. *See also*
  Debakey tissue forceps
  description of, 78
  insight on, 78
  uses of, 78
DeBakey forceps, endoscopic, 61–62, 61f
  description of, 61
  uses of, 61
DeBakey peripheral vascular clamp,
  299, 299f
  description of, 299
  insight on, 299
  other names for, 299
  uses of, 299
DeBakey sidewinder aorta clamp,
  300–301, 300f
  description of, 300
  insight on, 300
  other names for, 300
  uses of, 300
Debakey tissue forceps, 21, 21f
  description of, 21
  insight on, 21
  other names for, 21
  uses of, 21
DeBakey vascular tissue clamp,
  313–314, 313f
  description of, 313
  insight on, 313
  uses of, 313

Deflecting bridge. *See* Catheter
  deflecting element
Delee suction, 99, 99f
  cautions when using, 99
  description of, 99
  insight on, 99
  other names for, 99
  uses of, 99
Delicate grasper. *See* Prograsp
  forceps
Dental mirror. *See* Mouth mirror
Dental pick. *See* Root tip pick
Depth gauge, 210–211, 210f. *See also*
  Sims uterine sound
  description of, 210
  insight on, 210
  other names for, 210
  uses of, 210
Dermamesher, 198–199, 198f
  description of, 198
  insight on, 198
  other names for, 198
  uses of, 198
Dermatome, 199, 199f
  caution when using, 199
  description of, 199
  insight on, 199
  other names for, 199
  uses of, 199
Dermatome blade, 199, 199f
  cautions when using, 199–200
  description of, 199
  insight on, 199
  other names for, 199
  uses of, 199
Desjardin gallstone forceps, 39, 39f
  description of, 39
  other names for, 39
  uses of, 39
Desmarres chalazion clamp, 129, 129f
  description of, 129
  insight on, 129
  other names for, 129
  uses of, 129
Desmarres lid retractor, 135–136,
  135f
  description of, 135
  uses of, 135
Diamond-flex retractor. *See* Endoflex
  retractor
Diamond pin cutter, 229, 229f
  description of, 229
  insight on, 229
  other names for, 229
  uses of, 229
Diathermy pencil. *See* Electrosurgical
  pencil
Dietrich bulldog, 294, 294f
  description of, 294
  insight on, 294
  uses of, 294
Dietrich scissors, 302, 302f
  description of, 302
  insight on, 302
  other names for, 302
  uses of, 302
Dissector. *See* Endo kittner
Ditto. *See* House strut hook
Dr. Fog. *See* Anti-fog solution

Dolphin nose dissector, 55–56, 55f
  description of, 55
  insight on, 55
  uses of, 55
Doyen clamp. *See* Doyen intestinal
  clamp
Doyen elevator and stripper. *See* Doyen
  rib raspatories
Doyen intestinal clamp, 36–37, 36f
  description of, 36
  insight on, 36
  other names for, 36
  uses of, 36
Doyen rib raspatories, 308–309, 308f
  description of, 308
  insight on, 308
  other names for, 308
  uses of, 308
Dressing forceps. *See* Bozeman uterine
  dressing forceps
Drill bit set, 221f, 234
  description of, 221
  other names for, 221
  uses of, 221
Drill box. *See* Drill bit set
Drill chuck. *See* Chuck and key
Duckbill right and left biter, 232, 232f
  description of, 232
  insight on, 232
  uses of, 232
Duckbill speculum. *See* Graves vaginal
  speculum
Duckbill straight biter, 232–233, 232f
  description of, 232
  uses of, 232
Duck scissors. *See* Dietrich scissors
Duct probes. *See* Bowman lacrimal
  probe
Dura hook, 279, 279f
  description of, 279
  insight on, 279
  uses of, 279
Dura scissors, angled. *See* Taylor dural
  scissors
Duval forceps. *See* Pennington forceps
Duval lung forceps, 313, 313f
  description of, 313
  insight on, 313
  other names for, 313
  uses of, 313

E

Ear cup forceps. *See* Oval cup forceps,
  straight, right, left
Ear curette. *See* Billeau ear loop;
  House double-ended curettes; Spratt
  mastoid curettes
Ear knife. *See* House sickle knife;
  Myringotomy knife
Ear suction. *See* Baron suction tips
Ear syringe. *See* Bulb syringe
Eastman retractor, 97–98, 97f. *See also*
  Richardson-Eastman retractor
  description of, 97
  insight on, 97
  other names for, 97
  uses of, 97
EEA stapler. *See* Intraluminal stapler

Electrosurgical pencil, 6, 6f
    cautions when using, 6–7
    description of, 6
    insight on, 6
    other names for, 6
    uses of, 6
Elevator, angular. *See* Crane elevator
Ellik evacuator, 114–115, 114f
    description of, 114
    insight on, 114
    uses of, 114
Endo catch, 53, 53f
    description of, 53
    insight on, 53
    other names for, 53
    uses of, 53
Endocervical curette. *See* Kevorkian
    endocervical curette
Endo clip applier, 70, 70f
    description of, 70
    other names for, 70
    uses of, 70
Endo fan retractor, 66, 66f
    description of, 66
    insight on, 66
    other names for, 66
    uses of, 66
Endoflex retractor, 67, 67f
    description of, 67
    insight on, 67
    other names for, 67
    uses of, 67
Endo-fog. *See* Anti-fog solution
Endo GIA stapler, 70, 70f
    description of, 70
    insight on, 70
    uses of, 70
Endo harmonic scalpel, 53, 53f
    description of, 53
    insight on, 53
    other names for, 53
    uses of, 53
Endo KD. *See* Endo kittner
Endo kit. *See* Endo kittner
Endo kittner, 49–50, 49f
    description of, 49
    insight on, 49
    other names for, 49
    uses of, 49
Endo paddle retractor, 66–67, 66f
    description of, 66
    insight on, 66
    uses of, 66
Endopath thoracic trocar, 257, 258f
    description of, 292
    insight on, 292
    other names for, 292
    uses of, 292
Endo Peanut. *See* Endo kittner
Endo Pouch. *See* Endo catch
Endo right angle forceps, 54–55, 54f
    description of, 54
    insight on, 54
    other names for, 54
    uses of, 54
Endosac. *See* Endo catch
Endoscopic aspirating needle, 68, 68f
    cautions when using, 68
    description of, 68
    uses of, 68

Endoscopic biopsy forceps, 58, 58f
    description of, 58
    insight on, 58
    uses of, 58
Endoscopic biopsy punch, 58–59, 58f
    description of, 58
    insight on, 58
    uses of, 58
Endoscopic camera, 71, 71f, 117, 117f,
    248, 248f
    description of, 71, 117, 248
    insight on, 71, 117, 248
    uses of, 71, 117, 248
Endoscopic cholangiogram forceps, 61,
    61f
    description of, 61
    insight on, 61
    other names for, 61
    uses of, 61
Endoscopic hook scissors, 57–58, 57f
    description of, 57
    insight on, 57
    uses of, 57
Endoscopic scissors, 57, 57f
    description of, 57
    insight on, 57
    other names for, 57
    uses of, 57
Endo shears. *See* Endoscopic
    scissors
EndoWrist, 74, 74f
    description of, 74
    insight on, 74
    uses of, 74
Enucleation scissors, 127–128, 127f
    description of, 127
    uses of, 127
Evacuator, disposable. *See* Microvasive
    evacuator
Eye suture scissors, 127, 127f
    description of, 127
    insight on, 127
    uses of, 127

F

Fancy clamp. *See* Adson forceps;
    Adson tonsil/Schnidt forceps
Fan finger retractor. *See* Endo fan
    retractor
Fan retractor. *See* Arterial retractor
Farabeuf rasp, 305–306, 305f
    description of, 305
    insight on, 305
    other names for, 305
    uses of, 305
Farrior ear speculum, 184, 184f
    description of, 184
    insight on, 184
    uses of, 184
Favoloro. *See* Internal mammary
    retractor
Female dilators. *See* Walther female
    urethral sounds
Female sounds. *See* Walther female
    urethral sounds
Fenestrated grasper. *See* Prograsp
    forceps
Fenestrated rongeur. *See* Wilde
    rongeur

Ferguson gallstone scoop, 35, 35f
    description of, 35
    insight on, 35
    other names for, 35
    uses of, 35
Ferris-Smith tissue forceps, 21, 21f
    description of, 21
    insight on, 21
    other names for, 21
    uses of, 21
Fiberoptic light cord, 50, 50f, 101, 101f,
    214, 214f
    cautions when using, 50–51,
        101–102, 214
    description of, 50, 101, 214
    insight on, 50, 101, 214
    other names for, 50, 101, 214
    uses of, 50, 101, 214
Fine needle holder. *See* Crile-Wood
    needle holder
Finger-control suction. *See* Baron
    suction tips
Finger retractor. *See* Arterial retractor;
    Jarit cross action retractor
Finochietto rib spreader, 317, 317f
    description of, 317
    other names for, 317
    uses of, 317
5-mm 0° endscope, 73, 73f
    description of, 73
    insight on, 73
    other names for, 73
    uses of, 73
Flag elevators. *See* Cryer elevator
Flap knife. *See* House joint knife
Fletcher forceps. *See* Forester sponge
    forceps
Flexible ureteroscope, 118, 118f
    description of, 118
    insight on, 118
    uses of, 118
Flexipath. *See* Endopath thoracic trocar
Fogarty clamp with jaw inserts, 298, 298f
    description of, 298
    insight on, 298
    other names for, 298
    uses of, 298
Forceps. *See* Simpson obstetrical forceps
Forester sponge forceps, 23–24, 23f
    description of, 23
    insight on, 23
    other names for, 23
    uses of, 23
Fork. *See* Capsule retractor
45 clamp. *See* DeBakey peripheral
    vascular clamp
4-MM sheath and sharp obturator,
    215–216, 215f
    description of, 215
    insight on, 215
    uses of, 215
4-MM sheath with blunt obturator,
    215, 215f
    description of, 215
    insight on, 215
    uses of, 215
Fox eye shield, 120, 120f
    description of, 120
    insight on, 120
    uses of, 120

Frazier suction tip, 30–31, 30f
  description of, 30
  insight on, 30
  uses of, 30
Freer elevator, 225–226, 225f. *See*
  Freer septum elevator
  description of, 225
  insight on, 225
  uses of, 225
Freer septum elevator, 161, 161f
  description of, 161
  other names for, 161
  uses of, 161
Freer septum knife, 160, 160f
  description of, 160
  insight on, 160
  other names for, 160
  uses of, 160
Fukuda. *See* Fukuda humeral head
  retractor
Fukuda humeral head retractor, 245,
  245f
  description of, 245
  other names for, 245
  uses of, 245
Fukushima. *See* Leyla retractor; Teardrop
  suction tip

G

Gallbladder trocar, 38, 38f
  description of, 38
  insight on, 38
  uses of, 38
Garrett vascular dilators, 315, 315f
  description of, 315
  insight on, 315
  uses of, 315
Gaylor punch. *See* Thomas-Gaylor
  uterine biopsy forceps
Gelfoam masher. *See* House gelfoam
  press
Gelpi retractor, 30, 30f
  cautions when using, 30
  description of, 30
  insight on, 30
  uses of, 30
Gemini clamp, 37, 37f
  description of, 37
  insight on, 37
  other names for, 37
  uses of, 37
Gemini forceps. *See* Lahey gall duct
  forceps; Mixter forceps
Gerald tissue forceps, 311–312,
  311f
  description of, 311
  insight on, 311
  other names for, 311
  uses of, 311
GIA stapler. *See* Linear cutter-stapler
Gigli saw, 219, 219f
  cautions when using, 219–220
  description of, 219
  uses of, 219
Gillies hook. *See* Skin hook
Gimmick. *See* House elevator
Glassman clamp. *See* Carter-Glassman
  intestinal clamp
Glidewire. *See* Guidewire

Glover bulldog, 294–295, 294f
  description of, 294
  insight on, 294
  uses of, 294
Glover patient ductus clamp, 296–297,
  296f
  description of, 296
  insight on, 296
  uses of, 296
Gluck rib shear, 306, 306f
  description of, 306
  insight on, 306
  other names for, 306
  uses of, 306
Goelet retractor, 26, 26f
  description of, 26
  insight on, 26
  uses of, 26
Goldies. *See* Potts-Smith tissue forceps
Graspers. *See* Hysteroscope grasping
  forceps
Graves vaginal speculum, 96, 96f
  description of, 96
  insight on, 96
  other names for, 96
  uses of, 96
Green retractor, 181–182, 181f
  description of, 181
  other names for, 181
  uses of, 181
Guidewire, 106, 106f
  description of, 106
  insight on, 106
  other names for, 106
  uses of, 106
Gynecare morcellex, 87, 87f
  cautions when using, 87
  description of, 87
  insight on, 87
  other names for, 87
  uses of, 87

H

Halsey needle holder, 209, 209f
  description of, 209
  uses of, 209
Halstead forceps, 8, 8f
  description of, 8
  other names for, 8
  uses of, 8
Hammer. *See* Mallet
Hank dilators, 93–94, 93f
  description of, 93
  insight on, 93
  other names for, 93
  uses of, 93
Harmonic scalpel, 7, 7f
  description of, 7
  insight on, 7
  other names for, 7
  uses of, 7
Harrington heart retractor. *See*
  Harrington retractor
Harrington retractor, 42–43, 42f
  description of, 42
  other names for, 42
  uses of, 42
Hartman forceps. *See* Halstead forceps
Hasson trocar. *See* Blunt trocar

Heaney-Ballentine hysterectomy
  forceps, 82–83, 82f
  description of, 82
  insight on, 82
  other names for, 82
  uses of, 82
Heaney clamp. *See* Heaney-Ballentine
  hysterectomy forceps
Heaney hysterectomy forceps, 82, 82f
  description of, 82
  insight on, 82
  other names for, 82
  uses of, 82
Heaney needle holder, 99, 99f
  description of, 99
  insight on, 99
  other names for, 99
  uses of, 99
Heaney retractor, 97, 97f
  description of, 97
  insight on, 97
  other names for, 97
  uses of, 97
Heaney uterine biopsy curette, 85, 85f
  description of, 85
  uses of, 85
Heavy tissue scissors. *See* Mayo
  scissors, curved
Heavy wire cutter, 310, 310f
  description of, 310
  insight on, 310
  other names for, 310
  uses of, 310
Hegar dilators, 94, 94f
  description of, 94
  insight on, 94
  other names for, 94
  uses of, 94
Heiss retractor. *See* Jarit cross action
  retractor
Hemoclip applier, 34, 34f, 295, 295f. *See*
  Endo clip applier; Surgiclip applier
  description of, 34
  description of, 295
  insight on, 34, 295
  other names for, 34, 295
  uses of, 34, 295
Hemostat forceps. *See* Crile forceps;
  Kelly forceps
Herd elevator. *See* Hurd dissector
Herrick kidney clamp, 107, 107f
  description of, 107
  other names for, 107
  uses of, 107
Heymann-Knight angular scissors. *See*
  Knight angular scissors
Hibbs retractor, 237–238, 237f
  description of, 237
  uses of, 237
Hoen periosteal elevator, 272–273,
  272f
  description of, 272
  uses of, 272
Hohmann retractor, blunt, 241, 241f
  description of, 241
  uses of, 241
Hohmann retractor, mini, 240, 240f
  description of, 240
  insight on, 240
  uses of, 240

Hohmann retractor, sharp, 240–241, 240f
  description of, 240
  insight on, 240
  uses of, 240
Holzheimer retractor. *See* Jarit cross
  action retractor
Hooks. *See* Cottle tenaculum, double
House-Barbara shattering needle, 153,
  153f
  description of, 153
  insight on, 153
  other names for, 153
  uses of, 153
House-dieter malleus nipper, 146, 146f
  description of, 146
  other names for, 146
  uses of, 146
House double-ended curettes, 151, 151f
  description of, 151
  insight on, 151
  other names for, 151
  uses of, 151
House elevator, 148–149, 148f
  description of, 148
  insight on, 148
  other names for, 148
  uses of, 148
House gelfoam press, 140, 140f
  description of, 140
  other names for, 140
  uses of, 140
House hough, 152–153, 152f
  description of, 152
  insight on, 152
  uses of, 152
House joint knife, 148, 148f
  description of, 148
  insight on, 148
  other names for, 148
  uses of, 148
House oval window pick, 150–151, 150f
  description of, 150
  insight on, 150
  other names for, 150
  uses of, 150
House picks, 150, 150f. *See also* House
  oval window pick
  description of, 150
  insight on, 150
  uses of, 150
House-sheehy knife curette, 147–148,
  147f
  description of, 147
  insight on, 147
  other names for, 147
  uses of, 147
House sickle knife, 147, 147f
  description of, 147
  insight on, 147
  other names for, 147
  uses of, 147
House strut caliper, 139–140, 139f
  description of, 139
  other names for, 139
  uses of, 139
House strut hook, 154, 154f
  description of, 154
  insight on, 154
  other names for, 154
  uses of, 154

Hudson brace. *See* Hudson
  handheld drill
Hudson handheld drill, 275, 275f
  description of, 275
  insight on, 275
  other names for, 275
  uses of, 275
Hulka tenaculum, 90, 90f
  description of, 90
  other names for, 90
  uses of, 90
Humby. *See* Watson skin graft knife
Humeral head. *See* Fukuda humeral
  head retractor
Humeral head retractor, 244–245,
  244f
  description of, 244
  uses of, 244
Hunt chalazion clamp, 129–130, 129f
  description of, 129
  insight on, 129
  other names for, 129
  uses of, 129
Hunter bowel grasper, 64, 64f
  description of, 64
  uses of, 64
Hupp tracheal hook, 174, 174f
  description of, 174
  insight on, 174
  other names for, 174
  uses of, 174
Hurd dissector, 181, 181f
  description of, 181
  other names for, 181
  uses of, 181
Hydragrip. *See* Fogarty clamp with jaw
  inserts
Hyster clamps. *See* Heaney hysterectomy forceps
Hysteroscope, 100, 100f
  description of, 100
  insight on, 100
  uses of, 100
Hysteroscope biopsy forceps, 88, 88f
  description of, 88
  insight on, 88
  other names for, 88
  uses of, 88
Hysteroscope grasping forceps, 93, 93f
  description of, 93
  insight on, 93
  other names for, 93
  uses of, 93
Hysteroscope scissors, 87–88, 87f
  description of, 87
  insight on, 87
  other names for, 87
  uses of, 87
Hysteroscopic scissors. *See*
  Hysteroscope scissors

I

Iglesias. *See* Working element
Insufflation needle. *See* Verres
  needle
Insufflation tubing, 50, 50f
  description of, 50
  insight on, 50
  uses of, 50

Internal mammary retractor, 319,
  319f
  description of, 319
  insight on, 319
  other names for, 319
  uses of, 319
Intraluminal stapler, 47, 47f
  description of, 47
  insight on, 47
  other names for, 47
  uses of, 47
Irish retractor. *See* O'Sullivan-O'Connor
  retractor
Iris scissors, 200, 200f
  cautions when using, 200–201
  description of, 200
  insight on, 200
  uses of, 200
Iris spatula. *See* Barraquer iris spatula
Irrigation tubing, 102, 102f
  description of, 102
  insight on, 102
  other names for, 102
  uses of, 102
Israeli retractor. *See* Volkman retractor
Israel rake retractor, 242, 242f
  description of, 242
  insight on, 242
  uses of, 242

J

Jacobsen needles holder, 290, 290f
  description of, 290
  uses of, 290
Jacobs tenaculum. *See* Jacobs
  vulsellum
Jacobs uterine forceps. *See* Jacobs
  vulsellum
Jacobs vulsellum, 88, 88f
  cautions when using, 88–89
  description of, 88
  insight on, 88
  other names for, 88
  uses of, 88
Jameson forceps, 132, 132f
  description of, 132
  other names for, 132
  uses of, 132
Jameson muscle hook, 136, 136f
  description of, 136
  uses of, 136
Jamison scissors, 202–203, 202f, 303,
  303f. *See also* Reynolds scissors
  description of, 202, 303
  insight on, 303
  other names for, 303
  uses of, 202, 303
Janesn mastoid retractor, 174–175,
  174f
  description of, 174
  uses of, 174
Jansen-Middleton septum forceps, 165,
  165f
  description of, 165
  insight on, 165
  uses of, 165
Jansen scalp retractor, 285–286, 285f
  description of, 285
  uses of, 285

Jansen tissue forceps, 172–173, 172f
  description of, 172
  insight on, 172
  other names for, 172
  uses of, 172
Jarit cross action retractor, 207–208, 207f
  description of, 207
  other names for, 207
  uses of, 207
Jaritrack retractor. *See* Bookwalter
Javid carotid artery clamp, 297–298, 297f
  description of, 297
  insight on, 297
  other names for, 297
  uses of, 297
Javid carotid shunt clamp. *See* Javid carotid artery clamp
Jennings mouth gag, 180–181, 180f
  description of, 180
  uses of, 180
Jeweler's bipolar forceps, 120–121, 120f
  description of, 120
  insight on, 120
  uses of, 120
Jeweler's forceps, 130, 130f
  description of, 130
  insight on, 130
  uses of, 130
J hook, 52, 52f
  description of, 52
  insight on, 52
  uses of, 52
Jimmy. *See* Crabtree dissector
Joker. *See* Adson periosteal elevator
Jones towel clip. *See* Towel clip (penetrating)
Joplin. *See* Lewin bone-holding forceps
Joseph button-end knife, 161–162, 161f
  description of, 161
  uses of, 161
Joseph double skin hook, 204, 204f
  cautions when using, 204–205
  description of, 204
  insight on, 204
  uses of, 204
Joseph hook. *See* Skin hook
Joseph scissors, 156–157, 156f
  description of, 156
  insight on, 156
  uses of, 156
Joseph single skin hook, 204, 204f
  cautions when using, 204
  description of, 204
  insight on, 204
  uses of, 204
Joseph skin hooks, 178, 178f
  description of, 178
  other names for, 178
  uses of, 178

K

Kaye facelift scissors, 201, 201f
  description of, 201
  other names for, 201
  uses of, 201

Kelly forceps, 8–9, 8f. *See also* Crile forceps
  description of, 8
  other names for, 8
  uses of, 8
Kelly retractor, 41–42, 41f
  description of, 41
  insight on, 41
  uses of, 41
Kelly scissors, 190–191, 190f
  description of, 190
  insight on, 190
  other names for, 190
  uses of, 190
Kelppinger bipolar forceps, 52–53, 52f
  description of, 52
  insight on, 52
  uses of, 52
Kern bone-holding forceps, 234–235, 234f
  description of, 234
  insight on, 234
  uses of, 234
Kerrison-Costen rongeur, 159, 159f
  description of, 159
  insight on, 159
  uses of, 159
Kerrison rongeur, 158–159, 158f, 264, 264f
  description of, 158, 264
  insight on, 158, 264
  other names for, 158, 264
  uses of, 158, 264
Kevorkian endocervical curette, 84–85, 84f
  description of, 84
  other names for, 84
  uses of, 84
Key elevator, 224–225, 224f
  description of, 224
  insight on, 224
  uses of, 224
Killian nasal speculum, 176–177, 176f
  description of, 176
  uses of, 176
Kirschner wires, 216, 216f
  description of, 216
  insight on, 216
  other names for, 216
  uses of, 216
Knapp iris scissors, 124–125, 124f
  description of, 124
  uses of, 124
Knee arthroplasty set. *See* Total knee instruments
Knight angular scissors, 156, 156f
  description of, 156
  other names for, 156
  uses of, 156
Knot pusher, 69–70, 69f
  description of, 69
  insight on, 69
  uses of, 69
Kocher forceps, 25, 25f
  curved (*See* Ochsner forceps, curved)
  description of, 25
  insight on, 25
  other names for, 25
  uses of, 25

Koch forceps. *See* Kocher forceps
Kolbel self-retaining Glenoid retractor, 247, 247f
  description of, 247
  uses of, 247
K wires. *See* Kirschner wires

L

Lacrimal dilators. *See* Bowman lacrimal probe
Lahey clamp. *See* Gemini clamp
Lahey forceps. *See* Mixter forceps
Lahey gall duct forceps, 37, 37f
  description of, 37
  insight on, 37
  other names for, 37
  uses of, 37
Lambert-Kay aorta clamp, 299–300, 299f
  description of, 299
  insight on, 299
  other names for, 299
  uses of, 299
Lambotte osteotome, 228, 228f
  description of, 228
  insight on, 228
  uses of, 228
Lampert elevator, 149, 149f
  description of, 149
  insight on, 149
  uses of, 149
Langenbeck periosteal elevator, 273, 273f
  description of, 273
  uses of, 273
Large bone cutters. *See* Liston bone cutting forceps
Large fragment set, 249–250, 249f
  description of, 249
  insight on, 249
  other names for, 249
  uses of, 249
Large frag set. *See* Large fragment set
Large mouth rongeur. *See* Stille-Luer rongeur
Large needle driver, 80, 80f
  description of, 80
  insight on, 80
  other names for, 80
  uses of, 80
Large needle holder. *See* Large needle driver
Large pin cutter, 229, 229f
  description of, 229
  insight on, 229
  other names for, 229
  uses of, 229
Laryngeal mirror, 141–142, 141f. *See also* Mouth mirror
  description of, 141
  insight on, 141
  uses of, 141
Lateral retractor. *See* Eastman retractor; Heaney retractor
LDS stapler. *See* Ligating and dividing stapler
Lead hand, 219, 219f
  description of, 219
  insight on, 219
  uses of, 219

Lebsche knife, 305, 305f
  description of, 305
  insight on, 305
  other names for, 305
  uses of, 305
Lee bronchus clamp, 301, 301f
  description of, 301
  insight on, 301
  uses of, 301
Leep loop electrode, 81, 81f
  description of, 81
  insight on, 81
  other names for, 81
  uses of, 81
Left upper molar extraction forceps
  (88L), 192, 192f
  description of, 192
  insight on, 192
  other names for, 192
  uses of, 192
Leksell rongeur, 264, 264f
  description of, 264
  insight on, 264
  uses of, 264
Lens endoscope. *See* 10-mm
  0° endoscope; 10-mm 30° endoscope
Lens inserter. *See* Lens insertion
  forceps
Lens insertion forceps, 128–129, 128f
  description of, 128
  other names for, 128
  uses of, 128
Lens rigid endoscope. *See* 5-mm
  0° endoscope
Lens warmer, 49, 49f
  description of, 49
  insight on, 49
  uses of, 49
Lever skid humeral head retractor,
  245–246, 245f
  description of, 245
  other names for, 245
  uses of, 245
Lewin bone-holding forceps, 235–236,
  235f
  description of, 235
  insight on, 235
  other names for, 235
  uses of, 235
Lewis rasp, 157–158, 157f
  description of, 157
  insight on, 157
  uses of, 157
Leyla retractor, 283, 283f
  cautions when using, 283
  description of, 283
  other names for, 283
  uses of, 283
Leyla-Yasargil. *See* Leyla retractor
L hook, 51–52, 51f
  description of, 51
  insight on, 51
  uses of, 51
Lift scissors. *See* Kaye facelift scissors
Ligaclip. *See* Surgiclip applier
Ligaclip applier. *See* Hemoclip applier
Ligasure, 51, 51f
  description of, 51
  insight on, 51
  uses of, 51

Ligating and dividing stapler, 46–47, 46f
  description of, 46
  insight on, 46
  other names for, 46
  uses of, 46
Light cord. *See* Fiberoptic light cord
Lilly scissors, 307–308, 307f
  description of, 307
  insight on, 307
  uses of, 307
Linear cutter-stapler, 45–46, 45f
  description of, 45
  insight on, 45
  other names for, 45
  uses of, 45
Linear stapler, 46, 46f
  description of, 46
  insight on, 46
  other names for, 46
  uses of, 46
Liposuction cannula, 208, 208f
  description of, 208
  insight on, 208
  uses of, 208
Lister bandage scissors, 12, 12f
  description of, 12
  insight on, 12
  other names for, 12
  uses of, 12
Liston bone cutting forceps, 226, 226f
  description of, 226
  insight on, 226
  other names for, 226
  uses of, 226
Litler's. *See* Littler plastic surgery
  scissors
Littler plastic surgery scissor
  description of, 201
  insight on, 201
  other names for, 201
  uses of, 201
Littler plastic surgery scissors, 201–202,
  201f
Littler scissors, 222, 222f
  description of, 222
  insight on, 222
  uses of, 222
Long angled #3 knife handle,
  86–87, 86f
  description of, 86
  insight on, 86
  other names for, 86
  uses of, 86
Long handle. *See* #3 long knife handle
Long knife. *See* #3 long knife handle
Loop. *See* Leep loop electrode; Loop
  electrode
Loop electrode, 104–105, 104f
  description of, 104
  insight on, 104
  other names for, 104
  uses of, 104
Lothrop uvula retractor, 179–180, 179f
  description of, 179
  uses of, 179
Love nerve root retractor (angled), 281,
  281f
  description of, 281
  insight on, 281
  uses of, 281

Lower anterior extraction forceps (151),
  194, 194f
  description of, 194
  insight on, 194
  other names for, 194
  uses of, 194
Lower molar extraction forceps (17),
  193, 193f
  description of, 193
  insight on, 193
  other names for, 193
  uses of, 193
Lowman bone clamp, 235, 235f
  description of, 235
  insight on, 235
  uses of, 235
Lowsley prostatic retractor, 110, 110f
  description of, 110
  insight on, 110
  uses of, 110
Lucas bone curette, 189–190, 189f
  description of, 189
  other names for, 189
  uses of, 189
Lung clamp. *See* Duval lung forceps;
  Pennington forceps
Luxating elevator. *See* Apical elevator

M

Male sounds. *See* Van Buren urethral
  sounds
Malleable retractor. *See* Ribbon
  retractor
Mallet, 211–212, 211f, 260, 260f. *See*
  Cottle mallet
  description of, 198, 260
  insight on, 198, 260
  other names for, 198
  uses of, 198, 260
Maltz-Lipsett. *See* Maltz rasp
Maltz rasp, 158, 158f
  description of, 158
  insight on, 158
  other names for, 158
  uses of, 158
Mammary forceps. *See* Gerald tissue
  forceps
Mammary retractor. *See* Internal
  mammary retractor
Mammoplasty hook, 203, 203f
  cautions when using, 203–204
  description of, 203
  insight on, 203
  other names for, 203
  uses of, 203
Mandibular forceps (17), #17. *See*
  Lower molar extraction forceps (17)
Mandibular universal forceps.
  See Lower anterior extraction
  forceps (151)
Martin cartilage clamp, 233–234, 233f
  description of, 233
  other names for, 233
  uses of, 233
Maryland bipolar forceps, 75, 75f
  description of, 75
  insight on, 75
  other names for, 75
  uses of, 75

Maryland dissector, 56–57, 56f
  description of, 56
  insight on, 56
  uses of, 56
Maryland forceps. *See* Maryland
  bipolar forceps
Masterson clamp. *See* Heaney-
  Ballentine hysterectomy forceps
Mastoid rongeur. *See* Cicherelli mastoid
  rongeur
Mathieu retractor, 206, 206f
  cautions when using, 206
  description of, 206
  insight on, 206
  other names for, 206
  uses of, 206
Matson rib stripper and elevator, 309,
  309f
  description of, 309
  insight on, 309
  other names for, 309
  uses of, 309
Maxillary left forceps, No. 88L, 88L.
  See Left upper molar extraction
  forceps (88L)
Maxillary right forceps, No. 88R, 88R.
  See Right upper molar extractio
  forceps (88R)
Maxillary universal forceps. *See* Upper
  anterior extraction forceps (150)
Mayo abdominal retractor, 43, 43f
  description of, 43
  other names for, 43
  uses of, 43
Mayo forceps. *See* Rochester-Péan
  forceps
Mayo-Guyon vessel clamp, 108, 108f
  description of, 108
  uses of, 108
Mayo-Hegar needle holder, 32–33, 32f
  description of, 32
  uses of, 32
Mayo scissors, curved, 11, 11f
  description of, 11
  insight on, 11
  other names for, 11
  uses of, 11
Mayo scissors, straight, 11, 11f
  description of, 11
  insight on, 11
  other names for, 11
  uses of, 11
Mayo uterine scissors, 85, 85f
  description of, 85
  other names for, 85
  uses of, 85
McGee wire crimping forceps, 170, 170f
  description of, 170
  insight on, 170
  other names for, 170
  uses of, 170
McIvor mouth gag, 180, 180f
  description of, 180
  insight on, 180
  uses of, 180
McKissock keyhole, 198, 198f
  description of, 198
  insight on, 198
  other names for, 198
  uses of, 198

McPherson needle holder, 137–138,
  137f
  description of, 137
  uses of, 137
McPherson tying forceps, 131–132,
  131f
  description of, 131
  insight on, 131
  uses of, 131
Measuring stick. *See* Ruler
Measuring tool. *See* House strut caliper
Meltzer adenoid punch, 168–169, 168f
  description of, 168
  insight on, 168
  other names for, 168
  uses of, 168
Meniscus clamp. *See* Martin cartilage
  clamp
Metacarpal pins. *See* Kirschner wires
Metzenbaum scissors, curved, 12, 12f
  description of, 12
  insight on, 12
  other names for, 12
  uses of, 12
Metz scissors. *See* Metzenbaum
  scissors, curved
Meyerding finger retractor, 206–207,
  206f
  description of, 206
  uses of, 206
Meyerding handheld retractor,
  284–285, 284f
  description of, 284
  uses of, 284
Meyerding hemilaminectomy retractor.
  See Williams hemilaminectomy
  retractors
Meyerding laminectomy retractor,
  283–284, 283f
  description of, 283
  insight on, 283
  uses of, 283
Meyhoeffer Chalazion curettes,
  123–124, 123f
  description of, 123
  insight on, 123
  uses of, 123
Micro cups. *See* Oval cup forceps,
  straight, right, left
Micro knife, 270, 270f
  description of, 270
  uses of, 270
Micro scissors. *See* Rhoton micro
  scissors
Microvasive evacuator, 115, 115f
  description of, 115
  insight on, 115
  other names for, 115
  uses of, 115
Midas rex drill, 274–275, 274f
  description of, 274
  insight on, 274
  uses of, 274
Middle ear scissors. *See* Bellucci
  scissors
Miller rasp, 223–224, 223f
  description of, 223
  insight on, 223
  other names for, 223
  uses of, 223

Mills/Dennis micro ring tissue forceps,
  311, 311f
  description of, 311
  insight on, 311
  uses of, 311
Minnesota cheek retractor, 194–195,
  194f
  description of, 194
  other names for, 194
  uses of, 194
Mitral valve retractor. *See* Cooley
  arterial retractor
Mixter clamp. *See* Gemini clamp
Mixter forceps, 10, 10f. *See* Endo
  right angle forceps; Lahey gall duct
  forceps
  description of, 10
  other names for, 10
  uses of, 10
Molt bone curette, 190, 190f
  description of, 190
  other names for, 190
  uses of, 190
Molt mouth gag, 195, 195f
  description of, 195
  other names for, 195
  uses of, 195
Monopolar pencil. *See* Electrosurgical
  pencil
Morcellator. *See* Gynecare morcellex
Mosquito forceps. *See* Halstead forceps
Mother-in-law grasper. *See* Claw grasper
Mouth gag. *See* Molt mouth gag
Mouth mirror, 185–186, 185f
  description of, 185
  insight on, 185
  other names for, 185
  uses of, 185
Mouth prop, 195–196, 195f
  description of, 195
  insight on, 195
  other names for, 195
  uses of, 195
Mucous trap. *See* Delee suction
Murphy-Lane bone skid, 238–239, 238f
  description of, 238
  insight on, 238
  uses of, 238
Murphy retractor, 27, 27f
  cautions when using, 27
  description of, 27
  insight on, 27
  other names for, 27
  uses of, 27
Muscle clamp. *See* Jameson forceps
Muscle hook. *See* Von Graefe strabismus hook
Myringotomy knife, 143f, 144–145
  description of, 144
  insight on, 144
  other names for, 144
  uses of, 144

N

Nasal chisels. *See* Cottle chisels
Nasal curettes. *See* Coakley antrum
  curettes
Navy's retractor. *See* Army-Navy
  retractor

Needle holder, 321, 321f
  description of, 321
  insight on, 321
  other names for, 321
  uses of, 321
Needlenose pliers, 236, 236f
  description of, 236
  uses of, 236
Neivert-Anderson guarded osteotome, 164, 164f
  description of, 164
  insight on, 164
  uses of, 164
Nerve hook. *See* Blunt hook
Nested right angle retractor. *See* Parker retractor
Neurocautery suction. *See* Suction coagulator tip
Nezhat-Dorsey suction tips, 68, 68f
  description of, 68
  uses of, 68
Nipper. *See* House-dieter malleus nipper
Nipple washer. *See* Areola marker
Notched retractor. *See* Young bulb retractor
#11 blade, 15, 15f
  description of, 15
  insight on, 15
  uses of, 15
#15 blade, 16, 16f
  description of, 16
  insight on, 16
  uses of, 16
#5 penfield dissector, 269, 269f
  description of, 269
  uses of, 269
#4 knife handle, 14f, 17
  description of, 17
  insight on, 17
  uses of, 17
#4 penfield dissector, 268–269, 268f
  description of, 268
  insight on, 268
  uses of, 268
#1 penfield dissector, 267, 267f
  desription of, 267
  uses of, 267
#7 knife handle, 14, 17f
  cautions when using, 14–15
  description of, 14
  uses of, 14
#10 blade, 15, 15f
  cautions when using, 15
  description of, 15
  insight on, 15
  uses of, 15
#3 handle. *See* #3 knife handle
#3 knife handle, 13, 13f
  cautions when using, 13–14
  description of, 13
  insight on, 13
  other names for, 13
  uses of, 13
#3 long knife handle, 14, 14f
  cautions when using, 14
  description of, 14
  other names for, 14
  uses of, 14

#3 penfield dissector, 268, 268f
  description of, 268
  uses of, 268
#12 blade, 16, 16f
  description of, 16
  insight on, 16
  other names for, 16
  uses of, 16
#20 blade, 17–18, 17f
  description of, 17
  insight on, 17
  uses of, 17
#2 penfield dissector, 267–268, 267f
  description of, 267
  uses of, 267

O

Obtuse clamp. *See* Mixter forceps
Ochsner forceps. *See also* Kocher forceps
  curved, 91, 91f
  description of, 91
  other names for, 91
  uses of, 91
O'Connor retractor. *See* O'Sullivan-O'Connor retractor
Olsen clamp. *See* Endoscopic cholangiogram forceps
150. *See* Upper anterior extraction forceps (150)
151. *See* Lower anterior extraction forceps (151)
Optical trocar. *See* Visiport
Oral suction. *See* Yankauer suction tip, nondisposable
Oral suction tip. *See* Yankauer suction tip
Oral tip. *See* Yankauer suction tip, nondisposable
O'Sullivan-O'Connor retractor, 96–97, 96f
  description of, 96
  insight on, 96
  other names for, 96
  uses of, 96
O'Sullivan retractor. *See* O'Sullivan-O'Connor retractor
Otis urethrotome, 109, 109f
  description of, 109
  insight on, 109
  uses of, 109
Oval chalazion clamp. *See* Desmarres Chalazion clamp
Oval cup forceps, straight, right, left, 145–146, 145f
  description of, 145
  insight on, 145
  other names for, 145
  uses of, 145
Overstreet endometrial polyp forceps, 92, 92f
  description of, 92
  other names for, 92
  uses of, 92

P

Packing forceps. *See* Bozeman uterine dressing forceps
Paget blade. *See* Dermatome blade

Paget dermatome. *See* Dermatome
Paper clip. *See* Barraquer eye speculum
Park bench retractor. *See* Parker retractor
Parker retractor, 28–29, 28f
  description of, 28
  insight on, 28
  other names for, 28
  uses of, 28
Parsonnet epicardial retractor, 317–318, 317f
  description of, 317
  insight on, 317
  uses of, 317
Patent ductus. *See* DeBakey coarctation clamp
Peacock retractor. *See* Endo fan retractor
Péan forceps. *See* Rochester-Péan forceps
Peapod rongeur, 266, 266f
  description of, 266
  insight on, 266
  uses of, 266
Pedicle clamp. *See* Beck aortic clamp; Herrick kidney clamp; Wertheim-Cullen pedicle clamp
Pennington forceps, 38–39, 38f
  description of, 38
  other names for, 38
  uses of, 38
Periosteal elevator. *See* West periosteal
Permanent cautery spatula, 75, 75f
  description of, 75
  insight on, 75
  other names for, 75
  uses of, 75
Pierce double ended elevator, 160–161, 160f
  description of, 160
  insight on, 160
  uses of, 160
Pillar retractor. *See* Hurd dissector
Pin cutter. *See* Cannulated pin cutter; Diamond pin cutter; Heavy wire cutter
Pituitary forceps. *See* Cushing pituitary rongeur
PK dissecting forceps, 77, 77f
  description of, 77
  insight on, 77
  other names for, 77
  uses of, 77
PK forceps. *See* PK dissecting forceps
Plain tissue forceps, 20, 20f
  description of, 20
  other names for, 20
  uses of, 20
Plate bender. *See* Plate bending pliers
Plate bending pliers, 218–219, 218f
  description of, 218
  insight on, 218
  other names for, 218
  uses of, 218
Plate clamp. *See* Plate forceps
Plate forceps, 221–222, 234f
  description of, 234
  other names for, 234
  uses of, 234
Plate holders. *See* Plate forceps

Plate holding foceps. *See* Plate forceps
Pliers, 236, 236f
    description of, 236
    other names for, 236
    uses of, 236
Polyp forceps. *See* Overstreet endome-
    trial polyp forceps
Poole suction tip, 31, 31f
    description of, 31
    insight on, 31
    other names for, 31
    uses of, 31
Poppen suction tip, 288–289, 288f
    description of, 288
    insight on, 288
    uses of, 288
Posterior scissors. *See* Cottle angular
    scissors
Potts. *See* Potts-Smith scissors
Potts elevator, 186–187, 186f
    description of, 186
    insight on, 186
    other names for, 186
    uses of, 186
Potts scissors, 76–77, 76f
    description of, 76
    uses of, 76
Potts-Smith scissors, 302–303, 302f
    description of, 302
    insight on, 302
    other names for, 302
    uses of, 302
Potts-Smith tissue forceps, 312–313,
    312f
    description of, 312
    insight on, 312
    other names for, 312
    uses of, 312
Pratt rectal speculum, 44–45, 44f
    description of, 44
    insight on, 44
    uses of, 44
Pratt uterine dilators, 94–95, 94f
    description of, 94
    insight on, 94
    other names for, 94
    uses of, 94
Probe and grooved director, 39–40, 39f
    description of, 39
    uses of, 39
Prograsp forceps, 79, 79f
    description of, 79
    other names for, 79
    uses of, 79
Prop. *See* Molt mouth gag
Prostate retractor, anterior. *See* Young
    anterior retractor
Pulsavac, 247, 247f
    description of, 247
    other names for, 247
    uses of, 247
Pulse lavage. *See* Pulsavac
Pump tubing, 214–215, 214f
    description of, 214
    uses of, 214
Punch. *See* Meltzer adenoid punch
Punctal lacrimal dilator. *See* Wilder
    lacrimal dilator
Pusher. *See* Endo kittner

Putti bone rasp, 224, 224f
    cautions when using, 224
    description of, 224
    insight on, 224
    other names for, 224
    uses of, 224
Putti Platte. *See* Putti bone rasp

R

Ragnell retractor, 207, 207f, 241–242,
    241f
    description of, 207, 241
    uses of, 207, 241
Rake retractor. *See* Murphy retractor;
    Volkman retractor
Randall stone forceps, 111, 111f. *See
    also* Desjardin gallstone forceps
    description of, 111
    uses of, 111
Raney clip appliers, 257–258, 257f
    description of, 257
    insight on, 257
    other names for, 257
    uses of, 257
Raney clips, 258, 258f
    description of, 258
    insight on, 258
    uses of, 258
Rasp. *See* Bone file
Rat tail. *See* Putti bone rasp
Rat tooth forceps. *See* Adson tissue
    forceps; Toothed tissue forceps,
    toothed
Reducer caps, 102–103, 102f
    description of, 102
    insight on, 102
    other names for, 102
    uses of, 102
Reduction marker. *See* McKissock
    keyhole
Resano forceps, 78–79, 78f
    description of, 78
    other names for, 78
    uses of, 78
Resectoscope sheath and obturator,
    116–117, 116f
    description of, 116
    insight on, 116
    uses of, 116
Reynolds scissors, 203, 203f, 303–304,
    303f
    description of, 203, 303
    insight on, 303
    other names for, 303
    uses of, 203, 303
Rhoton dissector extended set,
    269–270, 269f
    description of, 269
    insight on, 269
    uses of, 269
Rhoton micro bayonet scissors, 276, 276f
    description of, 276
    insight on, 276
    uses of, 276
Rhoton micro needle holders, 289–290,
    289f
    description of, 289
    insight on, 289
    uses of, 289

Rhoton micro scissors, 275–276, 275f
    description of, 275
    other names for, 275
    uses of, 275
Rib approximator. *See* Bailey rib
    contractor
Ribbon retractor, 28, 28f
    description of, 28
    insight on, 28
    other names for, 28
    uses of, 28
Rib cutter. *See* Gluck rib shear;
    Sauerbruch rib rongeur
Rib spreader. *See* Finochietto rib
    spreader
Richardson-Eastman retractor, 40–41, 40f
    description of, 40
    insight on, 40
    other names for, 40
    uses of, 40
Richardson retractor, 41, 41f
    description of, 41
    insight on, 41
    other names for, 41
    uses of, 41
Rich retractor. *See also* Richardson
    retractor
    big (*See* Richardson-Eastman
        retractor)
    double-ended (*See* Richardson-
        Eastman retractor)
Right angle clamp. *See* Gemini clamp
Right angle forceps. *See* Lahey gall
    duct forceps; Mixter forceps
Right angle retractor. *See* Heaney
    retractor
Right-angle scissors. *See* Dean scissors
Right upper molar extractio forceps
    (88R), 192–193, 192f
    description of, 192
    insight on, 192
    other names for, 192
    uses of, 192
Rigid endoscope. *See* 10-mm
    0° endscope; 10-mm 30° endscope
Ring curette. *See* Buck ear curette
Ring forceps. *See* Forester sponge
    forceps
Rochester-Péan forceps, 9, 9f
    description of, 9
    other names for, 9
    uses of, 9
Rod cutter. *See* Large pin cutter
Roeder towel clip. *See* Towel clip
    (penetrating)
Root elevators. *See* Cryer elevator
Root tip pick, 188–189, 188f. *See* Crane
    elevator
    description of, 188
    other names for, 188
    uses of, 188
Rosen knife. *See* House-sheehy knife
    curette
Rosen needle, 152, 152f
    description of, 152
    insight on, 152
    uses of, 152
Round chalazion clamp. *See* Hunt
    chalazion clamp

Round handle. *See* Beaver handle
Rubin morselizer, 171–172, 171f
  description of, 171
  uses of, 171
Ruler, 211, 211f
  description of, 211
  insight on, 211
  other names for, 211
  uses of, 211
Rumel tourniquet hook (stylet),
  291–292, 291f
  description of, 291
  insight on, 291
  uses of, 291
Russians forceps. *See* Russian tissue
  forceps
Russian star forceps. *See* Russian
  tissue forceps
Russian tissue forceps, 22, 22f
  description of, 22
  other names for, 22
  uses of, 22
Ryder needle holder, 33, 33f
  fine (*See* Needle holder)
  insight on, 33
  uses of, 33

S

Sarns sternal saw. *See* Sternal saw
Sarot bronchus clamp, 310–311, 310f
  description of, 310
  insight on, 310
  uses of, 310
Satinsky partial occlusion clamp. *See*
  Satinsky vena cava clamp
Satinsky vena cava clamp, 296, 296f
  description of, 296
  insight on, 296
  other names for, 296
  uses of, 296
Sauerbruch rib rongeur, 307, 307f
  description of, 307
  insight on, 307
  other names for, 307
  uses of, 307
Sawyer rectal retractor, 45, 45f
  description of, 45
  insight on, 45
  uses of, 45
Scalp clip applier. *See* Raney clip
  appliers
Scalp clip gun, 258–259, 258f
  description of, 258
  insight on, 258
  uses of, 258
Scalpel handle. *See* #3 knife handle
Schiotz tonometer. *See* Tonometer
Schnidt forceps. *See* Adson tonsil/
  Schnidt forceps
Schroeder tenaculum, 89, 89f
  cautions when using, 89
  description of, 89
  insight on, 89
  other names for, 89
  uses of, 89
Schroeder uterine vulsellum, 89, 89f
  cautions when using, 89–90
  description of, 89
  insight on, 89

Schroeder uterine vulsellum (*Continued*)
  other names for, 89
  uses of, 89
Scoffield/Meyerding self-retaining
  retractor. *See* Scoville retractor
Scoop. *See* Ferguson gallstone scoop
Scoop forceps. *See* Adson hypophyseal
  cup tissue forceps
Scoville brain spatulas, 278–279, 278f
  description of, 278
  insight on, 278
  uses of, 278
Scoville nerve root retractor (angled),
  281–282, 281f
  description of, 281
  insight on, 281
  uses of, 281
Scoville retractor, 286, 286f
  description of, 286
  other names for, 286
  uses of, 286
Screw depth gauge. *See* Depth gauge
Screwdriver kit. *See* Universal screwdriver set
Seals. *See* Reducer caps
Self-retaining retractor. *See* Balfour
  retractor
Semken dressing forceps. *See* Plain
  tissue forceps
Semken tissue forceps. *See* Toothed
  tissue forceps
Senn retractor, 26, 26f
  cautions when using, 26–27
  description of, 26
  insight on, 26
  other names for, 26
  uses of, 26
Septal knife. *See* Freer septum knife
Serrefine clamps, 123, 123f
  description of, 123
  insight on, 123
  uses of, 123
70° endoscope. *See* 70° telescope
70° lens. *See* 70° telescope
70° telescope, 118, 118f
  cautions when using, 118
  description of, 118
  insight on, 118
  other names for, 118
  uses of, 118
Shark forceps. *See* Resano forceps
Sharp curettes. *See* Sims uterine curette
Shattering needle. *See* House-Barbara
  shattering needle
Shaver, 233, 233f
  description of, 233
  insight on, 233
  uses of, 233
Shears. *See* Curved scissors
Shoemaker rib shear. *See* Stille-Giertz
  rib shear
Shoulder skid. *See* Lever skid humeral
  head retractor
Sickle knife. *See* #12 blade
Side biter. *See* Lambert-Kay aorta clamp
Simpson obstetrical forceps, 92–93, 92f
  description of, 92
  other names for, 92
  uses of, 92

Sims uterine curette, 84, 84f
  description of, 84
  insight on, 84
  other names for, 84
  uses of, 84
Sims uterine sound, 95, 95f
  description of, 95
  other names for, 95
  uses of, 95
Single-tooth tenaculum. *See* Schroeder
  tenaculum
Sinskey hook, 122, 122f
  description of, 122
  uses of, 122
Skin hook, 29, 29f
  cautions when using, 29
  description of, 29
  other names for, 29
  single (*See* Joseph skin hooks)
  uses of, 29
Skin mesher. *See* Dermamesher
Skin stapler, 33–34, 33f
  description of, 33
  insight on, 33
  uses of, 33
Small bone curettes. *See* House
  double-ended curettes
Small frag. *See* Small fragment set
Small fragment set, 250–253, 250f
  description of, 250
  insight on, 250
  other names for, 250
  uses of, 250
Small-mouthed rongeur. *See*
  Zaufel-Jansen rongeur
Small rasp. *See* Miller rasp
Smooth forceps. *See* Plain tissue
  forceps
Smooth pins. *See* Steinman pins,
  smooth
Snake retractor. *See* Endoflex retractor
Snap forceps. *See* Crile forceps
Sound. *See* Sims uterine sound
Spencer suture scissors, 191, 191f
  description of, 191
  insight on, 191
  other names for, 191
  uses of, 191
Spinal curettes, 274, 274f
  description of, 274
  other names for, 274
  uses of, 274
Sponge stick forceps. *See* Forester
  sponge forceps
Spoon. *See* Ferguson gallstone scoop
Spratt mastoid curettes, 145, 145f
  description of, 145
  other names for, 145
  uses of, 145
Spurling rongeur (straight), 265, 265f
  description of, 265
  insight on, 265
  uses of, 265
Star forceps. *See* Russian tissue
  forceps
Stat forceps. *See* Crile forceps
Steinman pins, smooth, 216–217, 216f
  description of, 216
  insight on, 216

Steinman pins, smooth (Continued)
   other names for, 216
   uses of, 216
Steinman pins, threaded, 217, 217f
   description of, 217
   insight on, 217
   other names for, 217
   uses of, 217
Sternal knife. See Lebsche knife
Sternal needle holder and wire twister,
   321–322, 321f
   description of, 321
   insight on, 321
   other names for, 321
   uses of, 321
Sternal saw, 308, 308f
   description of, 308
   insight on, 308
   other names for, 308
   uses of, 308
Stevens scissors. See Stevens
   tenotomy scissors
Stevens tenotomy scissors, 126–127,
   126f, 202, 202f
   description of, 126, 202
   other names for, 126
   uses of, 126, 202
Stille bone chisel, 227, 227f
   description of, 227
   insight on, 227
   uses of, 227
Stille bone gouge, 225–226, 226f
   description of, 226
   insight on, 226
   uses of, 226
Stille bone osteotome, 227–228, 227f
   description of, 227
   insight on, 227
   uses of, 227
Stille-Giertz rib shear, 306–307, 306f
   description of, 306
   insight on, 306
   other names for, 306
   uses of, 306
Stille-Luer rongeur, 230, 230f
   description of, 230
   insight on, 230
   other names for, 230
   uses of, 230
Stone basket, 110–111, 110f
   description of, 110
   insight on, 110
   uses of, 110
Strabismus scissors, 124, 124f
   description of, 124
   uses of, 124
Straight clamp. See Cooley coarctation
   clamp
Straight curette. See Molt bone curette
Straight elevator. See Apical elevator
Straight rongeur. See Stille-Luer
   rongeur
Stripper. See Matson rib stripper and
   elevator
Strully scissors, 261, 261f
   description of, 261
   insight on, 261
   uses of, 261
Strut. See House strut caliper

Stryker core system, 221, 221f
   description of, 221
   insight on, 221
   other names for, 221
   uses of, 221
Stryker system 6 power, 220–221, 220f
   description of, 220
   insight on, 220
   uses of, 220
Subramanian. See DeBakey sidewinder
   aorta clamp
Suction coagulator tip, 142, 142f
   description of, 142
   insight on, 142
   other names for, 142
   uses of, 142
Suctioning irrigator, 67–68, 67f
   description of, 67
   insight on, 67
   uses of, 67
Surgical curette. See Molt bone curette
Surgiclip applier, 34, 34f
   description of, 34
   other names for, 34
   uses of, 34
Suturecut needle driver, 80, 80f
   description of, 80
   insight on, 80
   uses of, 80
Suture scissors. See Mayo scissors,
   straight; Spencer suture scissors
Sweetheart retractor. See Harrington
   retractor
Swivel knife. See Ballenger swivel knife

T

Takahashi nasal forceps, 165–166, 165f
   description of, 165
   insight on, 165
   uses of, 165
Tamp. See Bone tamp
TA stapler. See Linear stapler
Taylor dural scissors, 262, 262f
   description of, 262
   other names for, 262
   uses of, 262
Taylor hip retractor, 243–244, 243f
   description of, 243
   insight on, 243
   uses of, 243
Taylor spinal retractor, 288, 288f
   description of, 288
   uses of, 288
T-bar Potts elevators. See Potts elevator
Teardrop suction tip, 289, 289f
   description of, 289
   insight on, 289
   other names for, 289
   uses of, 289
Telescope bridge, 103, 103f
   description of, 103
   insight on, 103
   other names for, 103
   uses of, 103
Tenaculums, double-tooth. See
   Schroeder uterine vulsellum
10-mm 30° endscope, 72, 72f
   description of, 72
   insight on, 72

10-mm 30° endscope (Continued)
   other names for, 72
   uses of, 72
10-mm 0° endscope, 71–72, 71f
   description of, 71
   insight on, 71
   other names for, 71
   uses of, 71
Tentomy. See Jamison scissors
30° endoscope. See 30° telescope
35 clamp. See DeBakey peripheral
   vascular clamp
30° lens. See 30° telescope
30° telescope, 117, 117f
   cautions when using, 117–118
   description of, 117
   insight on, 117
   other names for, 117
   uses of, 117
Thomas-Gaylor uterine biopsy forceps,
   86, 86f
   description of, 86
   other names for, 86
   uses of, 86
Thomas uterine curette, 83–84, 83f
   description of, 83
   other names for, 83
   uses of, 83
Thoracoport. See Endopath thoracic
   trocar
Threaded pins. See Steinman pins,
   threaded
Thyroid retractor. See Green retractor
Tissue forceps
   with teeth (See Toothed tissue
     forceps)
   without teeth (See Plain tissue
     forceps)
Tissue scissors. See Kelly scissors;
   Metzenbaum scissors, curved
Titaniums. See DeBakey-Diethrich
   tissue forceps
Tongs. See Simpson obstetrical forceps
Tongue blade. See Andrew's tongue
   depressor
Tongue depressor. See Wieder tongue
   blade
Tonometer, 119–120, 119f
   description of, 119
   other names for, 119
   uses of, 119
Tonsil forceps. See Allis forceps,
   curved
Tonsil grasper. See Allis forceps, curved
Tonsil Schnidt forceps. See Adson
   forceps
Tonsil scissors. See Boettcher tonsil
   scissors
Tonsil snare, 169, 169f
   description of, 169
   insight on, 169
   uses of, 169
Tonsil suction tip. See Yankauer
   suction tip
Toomey syringe, 115, 115f
   description of, 115
   insight on, 115
   uses of, 115
Toothed grasper. See Cobra grasper

Toothed tissue forceps, 20, 20f
  description of, 20
  insight on, 20
  other names for, 20
  uses of, 20
Total hip instruments, 256, 256f
  description of, 256
  insight on, 256
  other names for, 256
  uses of, 256
Total knee instruments, 253–256, 253f
  description of, 253
  insight on, 253
  other names for, 253
  uses of, 253
Towel clip (nonpenetrating), 23, 23f
  caution when using, 23
  description of, 23
  other names for, 23
  uses of, 23
Towel clip (penetrating), 22, 22f
  cautions when using, 22–23
  description of, 22
  insight on, 22
  other names for, 22
  uses of, 22
Townley caliper, 212–213, 212f
  description of, 212
  other names for, 212
  uses of, 212
TPS system. *See* Stryker core system
Tracheal spreader. *See* Trousseau
  tracheal dilator
Trach hook. *See* Hupp tracheal hook
Triangle forceps. *See* Pennington forceps
Trousseau tracheal dilator, 182, 182f
  description of, 182
  other names for, 182
  uses of, 182
Tube clamp. *See* Vorse tubing occluding
  clamp
Turbinate scissors. *See* Cottle angular
  scissors
25° 4-MM lens, 248, 248f
  description of, 248
  insight on, 248
  other names for, 248
  uses of, 248
Tympanostomy knife. *See* Myringotomy
  knife

U

Ultrasonic scalpel. *See* Endo harmonic
  scalpel; Harmonic scalpel
U.S. retractor. *See* Army-Navy retractor
Universal screwdriver set, 218, 218f
  description of, 218
  insight on, 218
  other names for, 218
  uses of, 218
University of Minnesota retractor. *See*
  Minnesota cheek retractor
Up-biter. *See* Kerrison rongeur
Upper anterior extraction forceps (150),
  193–194, 193f
  description of, 193
  insight on, 193
  other names for, 193
  uses of, 193

Ureter clamp. *See* Mixter forceps
Urethral dilators. *See* Van Buren
  urethral sounds; Walther female
  urethral sounds
Uterine dilators. *See* Hank dilators;
  Hegar dilators; Pratt uterine
  dilators
Uterine manipulator. *See* Hulka
  tenaculum
Uterine scissors. *See* Mayo uterine
  scissors
Utility scissors, 222–223, 222f
  description of, 222
  insight on, 222
  other names for, 222
  uses of, 222

V

Van Buren. *See* Van Buren urethral
  sounds
Van Buren urethral sounds, 112, 112
  description of, 112
  insight on, 112
  other names for, 112
  uses of, 112
Vannas. *See* Vannas capsulotomy
  scissors
Vannas capsulotomy scissors, 128,
  128f
  description of, 128
  other names for, 128
  uses of, 128
Vascular suction tip, 320, 320f
  description of, 320
  insight on, 320
  other names for, 320
  uses of, 320
Verres needle, 54, 54f
  description of, 54
  insight on, 54
  other names for, 54
  uses of, 54
Versa port trocars, 59–60, 59f
  description of, 59
  insight on, 59
  uses of, 59
Versa step trocars, 65, 65f
  description of, 65
  insight on, 65
  uses of, 65
Vienna nasal speculum, 176, 176f
  description of, 176
  uses of, 176
Visiport, 60, 60f
  description of, 60
  insight on, 60
  other names for, 60
  uses of, 60
Volkman retractor, 27, 27f
  cautions when using, 27–28
  description of, 27
  insight on, 27
  other names for, 27
  uses of, 27
Von Graefe strabismus hook, 136,
  136f
  description of, 136
  other names for, 136
  uses of, 136

Vorse tubing occluding clamp, 293, 293f
  description of, 293
  insight on, 293
  other names for, 293
  uses of, 293
Vulsellum. *See* Jacobs vulsellum

W

Walsham septum straightener, 171, 171f
  description of, 171
  insight on, 171
  uses of, 171
Walters forceps. *See* Potts-Smith tissue
  forceps
Walther female urethral sounds,
  111–112, 111f
  description of, 111
  insight on, 111
  other names for, 111
  uses of, 111
Water tubing. *See* Irrigation tubing
Watson skin graft knife, 200, 200f
  description of, 200
  insight on, 200
  other names for, 200
  uses of, 200
Webster needle holder, 209, 209f
  description of, 209
  uses of, 209
Weighted speculum. *See* Auvard
  weighted vaginal speculum
Weitlaner retractor, 29, 29f
  cautions when using, 29–30
  description of, 29
  insight on, 29
  uses of, 29
Wells enucleation spoon, 121–122, 121f
  description of, 121
  uses of, 121
Wertheim clamp, 108, 108f
  description of, 108
  uses of, 108
Wertheim-Cullen pedicle clamp,
  107–108, 107f
  description of, 107
  other names for, 107
  uses of, 107
Westcott tenotomy scissors, 126, 126f
  description of, 126
  uses of, 126
West periosteal, 189, 189f
  description of, 189
  other names for, 189
  uses of, 189
Whisk. *See* Allison lung retractor
Wieder tongue blade, 179, 179f
  description of, 179
  other names for, 179
  uses of, 179
Wiener antrum rasp, 163, 163f
  description of, 163
  other names for, 163
  uses of, 163
Wilde dressing forceps. *See* Wilde tissue forceps
Wilde Ehtmoid forceps, 166, 166f
  description of, 166
  insight on, 166
  uses of, 166

Wilder lacrimal dilator, 133, 133f
  description of, 133
  other names for, 133
  uses of, 133
Wilde rongeur, 266, 266f
  description of, 266
  insight on, 266
  other names for, 266
  uses of, 266
Wilde tissue forceps, 173, 173f
  description of, 173
  other names for, 173
  uses of, 173
Williams eye speculum, 135, 135f
  description of, 135
  uses of, 135
Williams hemilaminectomy retractors, 284, 284f
  description of, 284
  insight on, 284
  other names for, 284
  uses of, 284
Wire cutters. *See* Wire scissors
Wire scissors, 13, 13f
  description of, 13
  insight on, 13
  other names for, 13
  uses of, 13
Wire speculum. *See* Barraquer eye speculum
Woodson dura separator, 279–280, 279f
  description of, 279
  uses of, 279

Woodson elevator, 273–274, 273f
  description of, 273
  uses of, 273
Working element, 104, 104f
  description of, 104
  insight on, 104
  other names for, 104
Wullstein ear forceps, 170–171, 170f
  description of, 170
  other names for, 170
  uses of, 170

X
Xcel blunt port. *See* Blunt trocar
Xcel trocars, 64–65, 64f
  description of, 64
  insight on, 64
  uses of, 64

Y
Yankauer, baby. *See* Andrews-Pynchon suction tip
Yankauer suction tip, 31, 31f
  description of, 31
  insight on, 31
  other names for, 31
  uses of, 31
Yankauer suction tip, nondisposable, 183, 183f
  description of, 183
  insight on, 183
  other names for, 183
  uses of, 183

Yasargil scissors, 304, 304f
  description of, 304
  insight on, 304
  other names for, 304
  uses of, 304
Yasar scissors. *See* Yasargil scissors
Young anterior retractor, 113, 113f
  description of, 113
  other names for, 113
  uses of, 113
Young bifurcated retractor, 114, 114f
  description of, 114
  insight on, 114
  other names for, 114
  uses of, 114
Young bulb retractor, 113–114, 113f
  description of, 113
  insight on, 113
  other names for, 113
  uses of, 113
Young renal clamps, 106–107, 106f
  description of, 106
  uses of, 106

Z
Zaufel-Jansen rongeur, 231, 231f
  description of, 231
  insight on, 231
  other names for, 231
  uses of, 231